PALLIATIVE CARE:
THE NURSING ROLE

SECOND EDITION

EDITED BY

Jean Lugton
MA MSc PhD RGN RNT HV
Health Visitor, Lothian NHS Trust,

Rosemary McIntyre
PhD MN DipN (Lond) RGN NDN RNT
Head of Studies (Scotland and Northern Ireland),
Marie Curie Cancer Care (Education), Edinburgh, UK

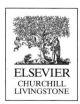

ELSEVIER
CHURCHILL
LIVINGSTONE

Edinburgh London New York Oxford Philadelphia St Louis Sydney Toronto 2005

ELSEVIER
CHURCHILL LIVINGSTONE

© Elsevier Limited 1999, 2005. All rights reserved.

The right of Jean Lugton and Rosemary McIntyre to be identified as editors of this work has been asserted by them in accordance with the Copyright, Designs and Patents Act 1988

First edition 1999
Reprinted 2000, 2002
Second edition 2005
  Reprinted 2008

ISBN 978 0 44307458 5

British Library Cataloguing in Publication Data
A catalogue record for this book is available from the British Library

Library of Congress Cataloging in Publication Data
A catalog record for this book is available from the Library of Congress

Note
Medical knowledge is constantly changing. Standard safety precautions must be followed, but as new research and clinical experience broaden our knowledge, changes in treatment and drug therapy may become necessary or appropriate. Readers are advised to check the most current product information provided by the manufacturer of each drug to be administered to verify the recommended dose, the method and duration of administration, and contraindications. It is the responsibility of the practitioner, relying on experience and knowledge of the patient, to determine dosages and the best treatment for each individual patient. Neither the Publisher nor the editors assume any liability for any injury and/or damage to persons or property arising from this publication.

The Publisher

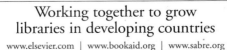
Printed in China

PALLIATIVE
THE NURSIN

For Elsevier:
Senior Commissioning Editor: Ninette Premdas
Development Editor: Katrina Mather
Project Manager: Andrew Palfreyman
Design: Stewart Larkin

CONTENTS

CONTRIBUTORS

Brenda Bottrill DipDY MISPA MLD MSR

Relaxation Therapist/Aromatherapist,
Oncology Department and Maggie's Centre,
Western General Hospital, Edinburgh, UK and
MacMillan Centre, St John's Hospital,
Livingston, UK

Jacquelyn Chaplin
MN (Cancer Care) BA RGN RCNT RNT

Advisor to Clinical Services
Marie Curie (Scotland),
Glasgow, UK

Anthony Duffy
MSc BSc (Hons) PG Dip (HE) RN RNT

Lecturer in Cancer and Palliative Care, Marie
Curie Hospice, Penarth, UK

Fran Duncan

Senior Social Worker, Marie Curie Centre,
Newcastle upon Tyne, UK

Doreen Frost
RGN DipDW BA SPS RGW BA Diploma District
Nursing BA

Specialist Practice Supervisor, Whitburn
Health Centre, Whitburn, UK

Richard Gamlin MPhil RN DipNurs CertEd

Senior Lecturer, St Benedicts Hospice,
Sunderland, UK

Jacqueline Husband
RGN Post Graduate Diploma in Palliative Care
RNT

Lecturer, Marie Curie Cancer Care, Fairmile,
Edinburgh, UK

Bridget M Johnston
PhD BN (Hons) RN PGCE (FE)

Lecturer in Palliative Care, Strathcarron
Hospice, Denny, Stirlingshire, UK

Kate Jones RGN NDN Cert HV Cert
Diploma in Nurse Education Post Grad Dip
Health Care Ethics

Lecturer, Marie Curie Cancer Care, Fairmile
Education Dept, Edinburgh, UK

Catriona M Kennedy
PLD BA (Hons) DipNurs RN Dn
PWT RNT DNT

Senior Lecturer, School of Acute and
Continuing Care Nursing, Napier University,
Edinburgh, UK

Shaun Kinghorn
MSc BA (Hons) RN RNT CertEd RCNT ITOL
LETTOL

Senior Lecturer, (Learning Development)
Marie Curie Cancer Care, Marie Curie
Hospice, Newcastle Upon Tyne, UK

Ishbel Kirkwood RGN SCM LLSA

Staff Nurse, Recovery, Western General
Hospital, Edinburgh, UK

Karen Lockhart
MSc BSc PGCert RGN RNT

Lecturer, School of Acute and Continuing
Care Nursing, Napier University,
Edinburgh, UK

Jean Lugton
MA MSc PhD RGN RNT HV

Health Visitor, Lothian NHS Trust

Paula McCormack
MSc BA (Hons) DipN (Con) RGN
SCM DN RNT

Director of Clinical and Education
Services,
Highland Hospice, Ness House,
Inverness, UK

Rosemary McIntyre
PhD MN DipN (Lond) RGN NDN RNT

Head of Studies (Scotland and Northern Ireland), Marie Curie Cancer Care (Education), Edinburgh, UK

David Mitchell BD DipPTheo MSC

Lecturer, Marie Curie Centre, Glasgow, UK

Jacqueline S Nicol
PGCert (HE) BSc RGN RNT

Lecturer, Education Department, Marie Curie Hospice, Edinburgh, UK

Christine M Pearce RGN RNT

Senior Lecturer in Palliative Care, Marie Curie Cancer Care, Ipswich, UK

Noreen Reid
MPH MN (Hons) Grad Dip Palliative Care PGCert (HE) BHLthSc RGN RNT

Lecturer Practitioner, Highland Hospice, Ness House, Inverness, UK

Susan Scavizzi
RGN DipDW BA SPS RGW BA
Diploma District Nursing BA

Specialist Practice Supervisor, Whitburn Health Centre, Whitburn, UK

PREFACE

This second edition of Palliative Care; The Nursing Role builds on the very successful first edition which was published in 1999 edited by Jean Lugton and Margaret Kindlen.

In this second edition a number of changes have been made. Firstly, Rosemary McIntyre joined Jean Lugton as a new co-editor. They have each undertaken doctoral research within the field of palliative care. Jean's clinical experience lieswithin primary care and Rosemary has experience as Head of Education with Marie Curie Cancer Care.

Since the first edition was published in 1999, the pace of change within palliative care has been such that the book has required a substantial re-write and update. As a result this second edition reflects new research evidence and recent developments within palliative care policy and practice.

Whilst some of the original chapter titles and authors remain unchanged, apart from updating the literature, other chapters were substantially rewritten. In addition, a significant number of new authors joined the team and they have written new chapters for this edition. Many of the new authors were drawn from the Marie Curie Education Service and brought their experience in palliative care to their writing.

Every effort has been made to ensure that this new edition remains very accessible and clinically relevant. It provides a comprehensive introduction to palliative care for pre-registration and post-registration nurses who are studying palliative care or delivering care in hospital, community or specialist palliative care settings.

The multidisciplinary, holistic nature of palliative care, the wider diagnostic focus and the need to include the family and carers, are acknowledged throughout this new edition. This ensures that it is also useful to Allied Health Professionals seeking to update their knowledge within the field of palliative care.

The range of chapters included, and the strong clinical focus of the chapters, should ensure that the key principles of palliative care are comprehensively covered. For example, physical, psychosocial, spiritual and ethical aspects of care are included as are contextual and policy influences on palliative care practice. Developments in palliative care education and palliative care research and audit are also included.

Case studies and reflection points are used liberally in order to encourage readers to consider the issues being presented in terms of their implications for palliative care practice. Further study is also encouraged by provision of comprehensive reference lists, and in some cases other resources are suggested at the end of the chapter.

Jean Lugton
Rosemary McIntyre
2005

CHAPTER ONE

Introduction to palliative care:
Overview of nursing developments

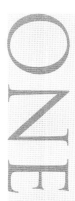

Bridget M Johnston

The word 'palliative' is derived from the Latin word *pallium*, meaning a cloak or cover. The Oxford English dictionary defines palliative as 'to relieve without curing'.

In its most literal use it refers to the provision of active care for a person whose condition is not responsive to curative treatment. The development of modern-day palliative care in the UK is closely bound to the development of the hospice movement.

CHAPTER AIMS

This chapter will introduce the reader to the concept of palliative nursing by: outlining what palliative care is, discussing the development of contemporary palliative care services and outlining the role of the nurse in palliative care.

By the end of the chapter the reader will be able to:

- Identify the key features of palliative care services in hospital, in hospices and in the community

- Understand the key research studies related to the role and function of the nurse in palliative care
- Distinguish the characteristics of the role of the nurse in palliative care.

INTRODUCTION

The World Health Organization (2005, p. 1) recently redefined palliative care as: 'an approach that improves the quality of life of patients and their families facing the problem associated with life-threatening illness, through the prevention and relief of suffering by means of early identification and impeccable assessment and treatment of pain and other problems, physical, psychosocial and spiritual'.

According to this definition, palliative care:

- Provides relief from pain and other distressing symptoms
- Affirms life and regards dying as a normal process
- Intends neither to hasten nor to postpone death
- Integrates the psychological and spiritual aspects of patient care
- Offers a support system to help patients live as actively as possible until death
- Offers a support system to help the family cope during the patient's illness and in their own bereavement
- Uses a team approach to address the needs of patients and their families, including bereavement counselling, if indicated
- Will enhance quality of life and may also positively influence the course of illness
- Is applicable early in the course of illness in conjunction with other therapies that are intended to prolong life, such as chemotherapy or radiation therapy, and includes those investigations needed to better understand and manage distressing clinical complications.

This is the first time that the definition does not overtly refer to cancer, reflecting the 21st century view that palliative care is applicable whatever the life-threatening illness. Indeed, more and more hospices and specialist palliative care units accept referrals of patients with diseases other than cancer.

The objectives of palliative care are, therefore, to palliate physical symptoms, alleviate disease and maintain independence for as long and as comfortably as possible; alleviate isolation, anxiety and fear associated with advancing disease; provide as dignified a death as possible; and support those who are bereaved.

The palliative care movement was born out of the hospice movement and the term was first coined by Professor Mount, a Canadian who worked with Cicely Saunders at St Christopher's Hospice in London. Since 1987, palliative medicine has been recognised as a distinct medical specialty (HMSO 1992).

Palliative nursing, as a term, was introduced by a specialist nursing group of the RCN – the Palliative Nursing Group – in 1989. It is now a widely used term in the UK and is recognised as a distinct nursing specialty with diploma, undergraduate and postgraduate degree programmes.

The premise put forward in this chapter is that all life-threatening illnesses – be they cancer, neurological, cardiac or respiratory disease – have implications for physical, social, psychological and spiritual health, for both the individual and their family. The role of palliative nursing is therefore to assess needs in each of these areas and to plan, implement and evaluate appropriate interventions. It aims to improve the quality of life and to enable a dignified death.

With the growth of palliative care as a specialty, there can be some confusion as to what specialist palliative care is and where and how this should be practised. The National Council for Hospice and Specialist Palliative Care Services (NCHSPCS 1995) advocates the palliative care approach as a vital and integral part of all clinical practice, whatever the illness or its stage. A knowledge and practice of palliative care principles inform such an approach.

Palliative intervention, on the other hand, concerns intervention when the disease is not curable. Both of these are sometimes known as generic palliative care.

Specialist palliative care requires a high level of professional skills from trained staff, as well as a high staff:patient ratio. It refers to a service provided by a multiprofessional team led by clinicians with recognised specialist palliative care training. The aim is also to support patients and their families, wherever they may be – hospital, home or hospice. In Scotland these services are now assessed and monitored using nationally recognised standards (NHS Quality Improvement Scotland (QIS) 2004)

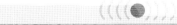

REFLECTION POINT 1.1
Palliative care services

- In your experience, what aspects of palliative care are difficult to integrate into the general care setting? Why do you think this is so?

- What palliative care services are available in your area? In your judgement, how appropriate/adequate are these?

HISTORY AND DEVELOPMENT OF PALLIATIVE CARE

PALLIATIVE CARE IN HOSPICES

Although Mme Jeanne Garnier opened the first hospice, specifically for the dying, in France during the middle of the 19th century, the founding of the modern hospice movement is attributed to Dame Cicely Saunders. Her vision arose from discussions with a Jewish patient, David Tasma, who had been in the Warsaw ghetto. Cicely Saunders, a former nurse, was at the time working as a social worker in London. When he died, David Tasma left a legacy to Cicely Saunders to be 'a window in your home'. This home, St Christopher's Hospice, opened for inpatient care in 1967. It was the first hospice with an academic model of integrated care that combined clinical care, research and teaching and provided a joint emphasis on medical and psychosocial enquiry. Cicely Saunders's ultimate vision for hospices was 'moving out of the NHS so that attitudes and knowledge could move back in' (Saunders 1991/2, 1993).

The modern hospice movement has proliferated since 1967. It has a worldwide philosophy, which has adapted to the needs of different cultures and settings, and is established in six continents. Hospices now often provide home care services, inpatient facilities and day care centres and are staffed by a multidisciplinary team including nurses, doctors, physiotherapists, occupational therapists, social workers, chaplains and volunteers. Currently, there are now 237 hospice inpatient units in the UK and Ireland (Directory of Hospice Services 2003; Tables 1.1, 1.2).

TABLE 1.1

UK hospice and palliative care services, January 2003: inpatient units

	Units			Beds			Children	
	Total	NHS	Vol.	Total	NHS	Vol.	Units	Beds
London	16	6	10	370	86	284	0	0
Midlands and east of England	54	12	42	744	171	573	10	82
North	61	9	52	752	46	706	7	45
South	57	13	44	816	183	633	5	41
Total England	**188**	**40**	**148**	**2682**	**486**	**2196**	**22**	**168**
Scotland	25	10	15	358	101	257	1	8
Wales	18	11	7	162	76	86	1	10
N. Ireland	6	1	5	79	4	75	1	10
Total	**237**	**62**	**175**	**3281**	**667**	**2614**	**25**	**196**

The voluntary services (vol.) include 11 Marie Curie Centres with 250 beds and six Sue Ryder units with 110 beds. The remainder are independent local charities, including three services exclusively for HIV/AIDS, with 64 beds.
Source: Directory of Hospice Services 2003

TABLE 1.2

UK hospice and palliative care services, January 2003: community and hospital support services

	Home care	Extended nursing care: 'Hospice at Home'	Day care	Hospital support nurses	Hospital support teams
London	26	7	17	12	34
Midlands and east of England	85	32	61	43	48
North	71	25	66	39	59
South	63	23	63	32	48
Total England	**245**	**87**	**207**	**126**	**189**
Scotland	48	10	22	24	22
Wales	30	7	21	9	20
N Ireland	10	4	4	8	11
Total	**333**	**108**	**254**	**167**	**242**

Source: Directory of Hospice Services 2003

In the early years of the modern hospice movement there was little evaluative research on its role. Much of the existing research is American, although a number of studies have now been completed in the UK. There is little research that compares how hospices differ from each other and whether the quality of care differs from other institutions. The role of the hospice movement in revolutionising the concept of pain control and symptom management in the care of the dying is unchallenged and widely acknowledged. The hospice movement has also paved the way in the disclosure of diagnosis, demonstrating that this can be done for the benefit of all parties concerned, although hospital doctors and general practitioners (GPs) are now the main source of such information (Seale 1991). Despite the absence of clear research evidence, it is thought that the management of physical symptoms, in combination with attention to the person's psychosocial needs, is rarely implemented as well in other settings (Field & James 1993).

The hospice movement is not without its critics. Douglas (1992) argues the following:

- Why should care at the end of an illness be separate from all that has gone before and why should collective dying be a good thing?
- Why should only a minority of a minority (i.e. only those who die from malignancies) be singled out for special treatment?

- Why should a large and general need be left to the 'scanty and scandalously choosy efforts of a patchwork of local charities'?

These issues are starting to be addressed, although specialist palliative care services are still largely cancer-dominated. There is now a UK-wide government initiative to look at the needs of people dying from non-malignant disease and to explore the appropriate palliative care provision. For instance, the Scottish Partnership Agency has recently been commissioned to explore these issues for Scotland.

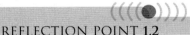

REFLECTION POINT 1.2

Care in hospices

What do you understand by the term 'disadvantaged dying'? Find an interested friend/colleague and discuss the subject. A useful article to read is Harris (1990), 'The disadvantaged dying'.

Nursing and medical research and audit need to evaluate the effectiveness of care and show what it is that is special about hospice care and hospice nursing, particularly from a psychosocial perspective. Furthermore, there is a need for education and exchange of ideas to ensure that the concept of palliative care is integrated into the mainstream of the NHS, community and private sectors.

PALLIATIVE CARE IN HOSPITALS

The most common place for people to die of a terminal illness is in a variety of settings within an NHS hospital (Cartwright 1991, Field & James 1993). Moreover, while dying is unique and highly personal to the person experiencing it and those close to them, it is part of the routine and ritual of the hospital staff caring for them (Field & James 1993, Walsh & Ford 1989). The ways in which staff define and perform their role of caring for dying patients has an important effect on patients and their relatives. According to Field (1989), care of the dying is, to a certain extent, determined by the organisational demands and routines of hospital life.

Inadequate and ineffective communication is another factor that may limit the effectiveness of caring for dying people in acute settings (Faulkner & Maguire 1994, Field 1989). Stedeford (1994) asserted that poor communication can cause more suffering than many of the symptoms of terminal disease. Another factor is the conflict between acute and palliative care (Dunn 1992, Williams 1982). It can be difficult for staff to decide when curative care ends and palliative care begins. A number of researchers have identified caring for dying patients in acute hospitals as a major source of stress for nurses and other health-care professionals (Reisetter & Thomas 1986, Vachon 1987).

There is, in addition, a tendency for hospital staff to pay lip service to the multidisciplinary team rather than working within it. Often in hospital there are inadequate facilities for relatives to stay overnight and for staff to interview them and provide support (Griffin 1991, Irvine 1993). Finally, nurses often receive inadequate preparation and support for their role in caring for dying patients in the acute setting (Hockley 1989, B M Irvine, unpublished work 1990, Reisetter & Thomas 1986).

Specialist palliative care in hospitals commenced as a concept in 1976, with the first support team being established at St Thomas' Hospital in London. The idea was based on a model that originated in 1975, at St Luke's Hospital in New York (Bates et al 1981). The team initially included a chaplain, a social worker, a nurse and two part-time voluntary doctors. It operated as an advisory service and was able to facilitate a level of symptom control that enabled many patients to be discharged home earlier than anticipated. There are now 409 hospitals in the UK with support teams, or support nurses. Many of these have been pump-primed by Macmillan Cancer Relief (Directory of Hospice Services 2003). Support teams (or palliative care teams, as they are sometimes known) advise and support the primary care team, usually hospital doctors and nurses, by providing support and advice on pain and symptom control, management of pain, psychosocial and spiritual needs, bereavement support and support for staff (Anstey 1993, Dunlop & Hockley 1990, Hockley et al 1988).

PALLIATIVE CARE IN THE COMMUNITY

At the beginning of the 20th century, the majority of people died at home. The number of people who now die at home has fallen to 19% with 23% dying from cancer, concurrent with the number of deaths in institutions rising to 66.5% (55.5% with cancer) (Ellershaw and Word 2003). These figures relate to urban populations, as opposed to populations in rural areas, 80% of whom die in hospital. In Herd's study (1990) it was noted that the further people live from hospital the greater their chance of dying at home.

The first home-care team was established in 1969 as an extension to inpatient care at St Christopher's Hospice in London. This pattern continues. However, much specialist palliative care in the community is carried out by Macmillan nurses, who may or may not be attached to an inpatient hospice unit. Macmillan nurses operate specialist palliative care services. The first community Macmillan nurse post was established in 1975. The success of this venture prompted the then Cancer Relief Macmillan Fund (now Macmillan Cancer Relief) to initiate a programme whereby health authorities could apply for a 3-year grant to create pump-priming Macmillan nurse posts with the proviso that the health authority became responsible for continuing the service beyond the grant period. In 2005 there are over 2000 Macmillan nurses working in hospitals and the community throughout the UK (Macmillan Cancer Relief 2004). These nurses are often viewed as a model for clinical nurse specialists. The role has evolved over the years in response to a growing body of knowledge in palliative care, political changes in the health service and developments in nursing. Today, Macmillan nurses act in an advisory and supportive role towards patients, professionals and the primary carer.

The debate about home death versus hospital or hospice for those dying from life-threatening illnesses has continued since the early work of Hinton (1979), Lamerton (1980) and Parkes (1985). These studies contended that patients tended to choose home as their preferred place of death. More recent studies have reinforced that patients, when asked and given a choice, would prefer to die at home (Hockley et al 1988, Townsend et al 1990, Higginson et al 2000). Despite government policy about care in the community, the majority of people still die of terminal illness in hospital (Addington-Hall & McCarthy 1995). Studies carried out in the 1990s, however, revealed that there was a discrepancy between how patients and their carers perceived care at home (Higginson et al 1990, Norum 1995, Spiller & Alexander 1993). The deciding factors for the families appeared to be support, coordination of care and respite care. Seale (1992) further identified that, in order to care effectively for dying patients, home community nurses themselves need support.

Field & James (1993) indicated that the experience of patients dying in their own homes appeared to vary widely, partly because homes and families differ in terms of social, psychological and spiritual make up and partly because of the nature, conduct and availability of support given to unpaid carers. Moreover, according to Cartwright (1991), Field & James (1993) and Thorpe (1993), symptom control is often less effective at home than in hospital or a hospice. In his study, Parkes (1985) proposed that people might be prepared to relinquish ideal physical symptom control for the social and psychological benefits of remaining in their own home.

Field & James (1993) noted that, should a person choose to die at home and receive adequate support, they might have up to 25 different paid carers visiting their home during the course of their terminal illness. Not surprisingly, communication and coordination of their care becomes inadequate, leading to fragmentation of care between health carers such as doctors, nurses and home helps. These circumstances may also result in marginalisation or exclusion of the dying person and their family from decision-making. Field & James (1993) go on to assert that the paradox for terminal care in the community is that, at a time when professions in palliative care are being encouraged to deliver 'holistic' care, current trends in the NHS may limit the opportunity to do just that. They conclude that: 'the care of dying people is of such central importance to all members of our society that the manifold inadequacies are something which must be readdressed, rediscussed and improved' (Field & James 1993, p. 27).

$((((\bullet))))$

REFLECTION POINT 1.3
Care in the community

People being cared for at home very often have a multiplicity of health-care personnel involved in their care. Drawing on your experience, consider in what ways patients' autonomy may be supported or denied when many agencies are involved. Who, in your view, might most effectively act as advocate for patients and families?

Day care

Day hospices are relatively new in the UK. These are units, normally based in hospices, where patients with advancing disease can attend on a day basis. Staff usually comprise nurses and paramedics, such as occupational therapists and physiotherapists, assisted by volunteers.

The purpose of a day hospice is to provide respite care for relatives as well as social and therapeutic benefits for the patient. These can range from craft activities through aromatherapy to direct care such as a wound dressing or a bath. Without a doubt, the provision of day care has enhanced the care that can be offered to patients and their relatives in the community. The day centre established in 1990 at St Christopher's Hospice in London stated that its primary aim was to improve the quality of life for patients by adding a new dimension to the total package of care already in place for the patient and their family. They viewed their aims as fivefold, to provide:

- Stimulation and enjoyment through activities, focusing on the individual's needs and choices and encouraging self-esteem
- Social support and help to alleviate feelings of isolation and depression
- Respite for carers
- Basic nursing, where appropriate, to aid and improve physical wellbeing
- Rehabilitation by adapting the patient's physical and social environment so that independence can be maintained for as long as possible.

((((●))))
REFLECTION POINT 1.4
Day care and day therapy

How would you differentiate between day care and day therapy? From a service provider's perspective, what advantages/disadvantages might each model of care have?

Care homes

Care homes are another area where palliative care is practised. Katz et al (1999) carried out an exploratory study to determine if the principles of palliative care had permeated the ethos of care homes and whether it was appropriate to apply aspects of palliative care to people in these care settings. They found that there was a great need for support and training in this area. Although staff demonstrated a willingness to care, they did not have the expertise or training to do it. However, there are several new initiatives to increase education and practice in this area. For instance, there are clinical nurse specialists working with and developing practice in nursing homes (Avis et al 1999, Froggatt & Hoult 2002), as well as educational programmes and initiatives specifically designed for teaching palliative care to nursing home staff (Froggatt 2000, Hill 2003).

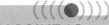

REFLECTION POINT 1.5
Palliative care in nursing homes

If you work in a care home:

- Think about your work over the last 6 months. How often have you been involved in providing palliative care? What challenges did that present?

- Consider a difficult palliative care situation that you have managed. Who did you turn to for specialist advice and support?

TEAMWORK

Teamwork is central to effective palliative care (Hull et al 1989, Maynard 2003). The question arises of who the key members of the team are. Many different health-care professionals can make up a palliative care team (Box 1.1).

Box 1.1
An example of a typical hospice team with integrated education and research

Hospice – 24 beds
- Director

- Administrator

- Matron

Nurses
- Deputy (Matron)

- Staff nurses (19.3 full-time equivalents (FTE))

- Nursing assistants (15 FTE)

- Home care staff (Macmillan nurses, 8.7 FTE)

- Ward sister

- Lymphoedema nurse specialist

- Day care sister

- Day care nurses – Registered nurses (1.81 FTE), nursing assistants (1.67 FTE)

Doctors
- Two consultants
- Hospice physicians (total, including consultants, 4.5 FTE)

Professions allied to medicine
- Social worker
- Physiotherapist
- Occupational therapist
- Pharmacist

Other professionals
- Clinical effectiveness coordinator
- Research nurse practitioner

Clergy
- Chaplain

Education department
- Three FTE lecturers
- Education secretary

Support staff
- Secretaries
- Switchboard operator
- Appeals and finance staff

Kitchen and domestic staff
- Cook
- Catering staff
- Housekeeping staff
- Domestic staff

Maintenance
- Caretaker/handyman
- Groundsman

Voluntary staff
- Volunteer coordinator
- Volunteers (210).

The key person in the team is the patient (and also their family). To exclude the patients from the team is to render them passive recipients of their care rather than partners in decision-making. Health care in modern society is often based on paternalism – 'the professional knows best' – rather than being about partnership and patient autonomy. Palliative care seeks to redress this balance.

What, then, is the function of the team? It could be argued that the primary goal of teamwork is to offer the best possible quality of life for the patient. Effective teamwork depends on good communication, effective leadership and coordination. Individual team members require to know their own limitations and to share in decision-making and formal review (Hull et al 1989). Several factors, therefore, contribute to successful team management. In addition to an individual's role within the team, there is shared decision-making, effective communication and common goals. Certain role functions and dysfunction also need to be taken into account. These include role expectations, ambiguity, conflict and overload.

Without a doubt the members of the team in palliative care face particular stresses and strains as a result of working with dying patients and their families. It is therefore of paramount importance to pay attention to staff support and continuing education.

$((((\bullet))))$

REFLECTION POINT 1.6
Teamwork

Mary is a 45-year-old lady with advanced breast cancer with a prognosis of 6–8 weeks. She is divorced, unemployed and has four school-age children. Mary is an inpatient at a hospice but wishes her remaining care to take place at home. Reflect on Mary's situation and consider the following questions:

- Which professionals might be involved in her care?

- How would they ensure that Mary's care is not duplicated and that her needs and wishes are met?

- Who do you think should coordinate this care?

You may wish to discuss this scenario with a district nursing sister or Macmillan nurse.

COMMUNICATION

Many authors have asserted that communication is a key aspect of the role of the nurse (Gooch 1988, Macleod Clark 1983, Wilkinson 1991). Indeed, Buckman (1993) proposed that effective symptom control is impossible without effective communication. Patients also state that communication is key to their care being effective (Johnston 2002). Moreover, Johnston (2002) found that expert nurses in palliative care should have effective communication skills and that these skills should be a prerequisite for working in specialist palliative care. Yet, despite the efforts of expert trainers, such as Faulkner & Maguire (1994), to improve communication skills, there remains evidence that these remain largely ineffective throughout the profession (Heaven & Maguire 1996, Wilkinson 1991).

A number of studies have identified the problems that professionals have with communication. These include distancing or blocking tactics, ignoring cues, false reassurance and avoidance tactics (Faulkner & Maguire 1994, Heaven & Maguire 1996, Macleod Clark 1983, Wilkinson 1991).

In order to communicate effectively with patients and their families, nurses must be supported in the workplace. This can be achieved through clinical supervision (Heaven 2001). If nurses' morale is low or if they feel under-valued by colleagues and managers, they may not have the courage or will to communicate effectively.

So what are effective communication skills and strategies? Most authors would agree that effective communication in palliative care incorporates effective listening skills and appropriate non-verbal communication; coun-selling skills, such as reflection, clarification and empathy; supportiveness; and, above all, self-awareness.

Faulkner & Maguire (1994) note that, in order to communicate effectively with patients, nurses need to pay attention to assessment skills, the handling of difficult questions or conflict, dealing with anger and denial, and providing support and supervision.

((((●))))

REFLECTION POINT 1.7
Communication

- Consider a professional colleague whom you would judge to be a truly excellent communicator. Identify the main skills and attributes this person has.

- Consider ways in which nurses can become skilled in communication. Jot down your thoughts before reading on.

The majority of authors assert that we gain these skills through training (Faulkner 1993, Faulkner & Maguire 1994, Heaven & Maguire 1996, Wilkinson 1991). How these skills are taught, however, is crucial. Audiotape or videotape feedback with role-play, incorporated into small group teaching, have been used. Heaven & Maguire (1996) contend that simple skills training is insuffi-cient to change clinical behaviour. They advocate that communication work-shops should include handling of emotions, self-efficacy and challenging nurses' attitudes and beliefs about both their communication skills and the consequences of their actions for patients. Nurses can acquire and improve their communication skills by developing their self-awareness, particularly by reflecting on their practice, by developing empathy with their patients and learning by role-modelling their peers in the clinical environment. The current evidence base would suggest that incorporating skills into a palliative care course over a period of time, gaining supervision and support to transfer skills into practice (Heaven & Maguire 2003) or undergoing a module-based certificate course in counselling skills over a year, incorporating practice and self-awareness at all stages of the programme (Johnston & Smith 2005), are the best ways of learning skills and transferring them to the workplace and sustaining them over time.

THE ROLE OF THE NURSE

DEFINING NURSING

Despite the fact that nursing has been an occupation for several hundred years, few authors or researchers have defined it successfully. It could, however, be argued that no one definition encompasses all that nurses do, particularly when we bear in mind that nurses work in a variety of settings, adopting a variety of roles. Indeed, Florence Nightingale stated that 'I use the word nursing for want of a better' (Nightingale 1980). She went on to say that 'the very elements of nursing are all but unknown'. How far have we come in defining the role of the nurse?

Nursing is a complex activity, a practice-based, eclectic discipline. Its very essence is concerned with human nature, professional caring and the building of therapeutic relationships, with the practice of nursing involving complex decision-making processes.

NURSE–PATIENT RELATIONSHIPS

Nurse–patient relationships are central to the role of the nurse in palliative care and this relationship should benefit the patient. Muetzel (1988) suggested that the three concepts of partnership, intimacy and reciprocity come together in a therapeutic encounter between nurse and patient. Muetzel believed that the nurse must be self-aware, or at least growing towards that goal, for any meaningful relationship to occur. Furthermore, according to Watson (1988), a caring relationship is formed between nurse and patient when the nurse recognises the patient as an individual and is able to empathise and establish rapport. Campbell (1984), a theologian, likens the nurse–patient relationship to a journey. Two people travel for a while together, becoming close and committed to each other, but only within defined limits. At the end of the journey they part without having formed a deep personal relationship. He called this 'moderated love'.

In a study exploring the nurse–patient relationship, Morse (1991) found that four types of nurse–patient relationship occurred. The type of relationship depended on the duration of the contact between the nurse and the patient. The four types were clinical, connected, therapeutic and over-involved relationships.

In a UK study that examined the therapeutic potential of nurses' personal involvement with patients, Savage (1995) identified the relationship between nurse and patient as a crucial element in the effectiveness of nursing care. Savage referred, in particular, to the 'closeness' between nurse and patient, a concept she identified from the 'new nursing' literature. For instance, Pearson (1991), in his description of the work at Burford and Oxford Nursing Development Unit, stated that nurses achieve successful outcomes through the establishment of 'close relationships' with their patients and by using this closeness to therapeutic effect in a planned and systematic way. This 'closeness' can be seen as similar to the connected relationship described by Morse (1991). This closeness and connectedness is also explored in the work of Perry (1996), who examined the actions and beliefs of exemplary oncology nurses in Canada. She found that nurses used dialogue in silence, mutual touch and humour in the relationships they developed with cancer patients. Significantly in Savage's study, closeness is seen, in part, as developing from the performance of intimate activities, such as bathing a patient, in the context of a continuing relationship. Interestingly, health-care professionals largely undervalue these activities.

THE PRACTICE OF NURSING

Another seminal research project that has had an influence on the way that nursing is practised, managed and taught is the work of an American nurse, Patricia Benner (1984). She identified five levels of competency in clinical nursing practice. These levels – novice, advanced beginner, competent, proficient and expert – were described in the words of nurses working in critical care units in the USA. Nurses were interviewed and observed, either individually or in small groups. Only patient care situations where the nurse made a positive difference were included.

Novice nurses were newly qualified nurses in a new clinical area, or student nurses. They were beginners who had little or no expertise of the situations in which they were expected to perform. They practised by rule-governed behaviour. Expert nurses, on the other hand, no longer relied on rules or guidelines to connect their understanding of the situation. They possessed an 'intuitive' grasp of each situation and 'zeroed in on the accurate region of the problem without wasteful consideration of a large range of unfruitful, alternative diagnoses and solutions' (Benner 1984, p. 32).

Additionally, in an Australian grounded theory study, Lawler (1991) explored the invisible aspects of nurses' work. She studied how the body is managed by nurses in their work and in particular what happens 'behind the screens'. She advocated that nursing involves not only doing things that are traditionally assigned to females in our society but also crossing 'social boundaries and breaking taboos and doing things for people which they would normally do for themselves in private if they were able' (Lawler 1991, p. 30).

Lawler also stated that the relationship a nurse has with a hospitalised patient is context and situationally related. It is unlike a 'normal' social relationship as it occurs when the patient is experiencing one of the most stressful events that they will encounter. She proposed that nurses created an 'environment of permission' for the patient in which to reconcile what has happened to their bodies. She asserted that this is made possible by the construction of a particular kind of relationship and by the use of clinical strategies, which affect both the nurse and the patient.

Lawler concluded that there was a widespread consensus that nursing is not a well-understood occupation in society generally and that a level of ignorance exists about the work of nurses. She advocated that people tend to focus on the aesthetically unpleasant or sexually related aspects of nursing practice. You only have to look at the current media portrayal of nurses to concur with this idea.

THE ROLE OF THE NURSE IN PALLIATIVE CARE

It is apparent that nursing, as an occupation, is difficult to define. This may be in part to do with the fact that much of nursing is 'hidden'. In this respect an attempt will now be made to elicit what it is that palliative care nurses do.

Care of the dying patient and the family is primarily a nursing responsibility. As patients shift from the sick to the dying role it is principally the nurse who deals with the day-to-day task of supporting and helping them and their families to live with the psychological, social, physical and spiritual consequences of their illness.

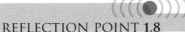

REFLECTION POINT 1.8

The dying patient

Think back to the first death you witnessed as a nurse.

- From that experience how would you prepare a student to deal with their first death in clinical practice?

- What do you consider are the most important aspects of the role of the nurse in palliative care and how would you explain this role to others?

Despite the fact that caring for the dying is and always has been a fundamental aspect of nursing, few researchers have examined this role and only one study (Johnston 2002) has examined patients' perceptions of this role and the effectiveness of palliative nursing. Much of the literature on the subject is anecdotal or descriptive. One of the difficulties in research of this nature is that few researchers have been able to articulate what it is that the experienced palliative care nurse does and how they influence patient and family outcomes.

Although research studies examining what nurses do are scant, the role of the nurse in palliative care has been defined in a variety of ways (Box 1.2).

The few studies that have been carried out on the role of the nurse in palliative care are mainly North American.

Quint (1967) was the forerunner in this field. Her original research arose out of the grounded theory sociological study carried out in San Francisco by Glaser & Strauss (1965, 1968), with Quint as a co-researcher in the team. Fieldwork from this study focused on what nurses do around dying patients in social relationship and work demands, in different ward settings. The nursing part of the investigation centred on what nursing students learn about death and *when* they learn. Quint's findings are still relevant today. Students are often inadequately prepared for dealing with death and dying and classroom teaching does not always match the reality of practice.

In a Canadian qualitative study, Degner et al (1991) identified seven critical nursing behaviours. Ten experienced palliative care nurses and ten nurse educators were asked to describe situations in which student nurses or qualified nurses had displayed very positive or very negative attitudes towards care of the dying. The following seven critical behaviours were identified:

- Responding during the death scene
- Providing comfort

Box 1.2

Definitions of the nurse in palliative care

Descriptor	Author
• Supportive	Davies & Oberle 1990, 1992, Heslin & Bramwell 1989
• Intensive caring, collaboration, continuous knowing and continuous giving	Dobratz 1990
• Fostering hope	Herth 1990
• Providing comfort	Degner et al 1991
• Providing an empathic relationship	Raudonis 1993
• Clinical, consultative with teaching, leadership and research functions	Webber 1993
• Being there and acting on the patient's behalf	Steeves et al 1994

- Responding to anger
- Enhancing personal growth
- Responding to colleagues
- Enhancing the quality of life during dying
- Responding to the family.

The authors have since used their results in their curricula content in Canada towards developing and testing a model of expert nursing practice in the care of the dying.

Williams (1982) in her American study examined the role of the professional in the care of the dying. Her subsequent conceptual framework for nurses engaged in the care of dying patients suggested that, as the patient reaches a state of terminal illness, they shift from the dependence of the sick role to a more independent and autonomous dying role. This role transition of the dying patient called for a complementary shift on the part of the doctor and nurse, the doctor's role essentially being that of curing and treatment orientation. Conversely, the nursing role was seen as caring and supportive, which became dominant when the patient was dying (Fig. 1.1).

These views could be viewed as somewhat simplistic and would not apply in specialist palliative care environments such as hospices. They do, however, go some way to describe the fact that caring for the dying, particularly in the terminal phase of someone's illness, could be seen as fundamentally a nursing responsibility.

Davies & Oberle (1990, 1992) explored the dimensions of the palliative care nurse. The purpose of their study was to describe the clinical component of the nurse's role in palliative care. Data were collected, using a grounded theory approach, from in-depth retrospective descriptions of the care given by one clinical nurse specialist to 10 patients and their families. This included 25 hours of interviews.

The nurse's role was found to be a supportive one with multiple dimensions. The researchers develped a model for palliative care nurses, which consists of six interwoven but discrete dimensions: valuing; connecting; empowering; doing for; finding meaning; and preserving integrity (see Fig. 1.2). Some of these dimensions are regarded as attitudinal, others are task-oriented, but all are regarded as playing a yital part in the support process (Davis & Oberle 1990).

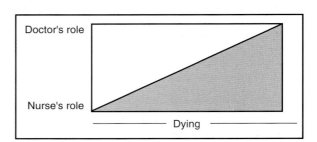

Figure 1.1 Roles in the continuum of dying.

All dimensions are regarded as playing a vital part in the support process (Davies & Oberle 1990). Davies & Oberle considered 'valuing' as a contextual dimension in that it provides the context within which supportive care can occur. In order to be supportive, the nurse needs to believe in the inherent worth of their patients and in their strengths and capabilities. 'Connecting', in essence, referred to forming a bond with the patient. 'Empowering' implied that the nurse helped patients to find or build strength within themselves. 'Finding meaning' involved helping patients make sense out of what was happening in the world of the health-care system. 'Doing for' is the aspect of nursing care that involves the provision of physical care and is not supportive unless interwoven with the patient. In other words, 'doing for' behaviours can become empowering, can help the patient to find meaning and can help to maintain the connection between the nurse and the patient. Moreover, although the four do not necessarily occur in any particular order, some degree of 'connecting' must occur before other dimensions can appear. 'Preserving integrity' is the core concept.

The authors argued that nurses must maintain their own wholeness if they are to provide support to others. A notion that was reiterated by the work of McWilliam et al (1993), who argued that preservation of integrity was a vital factor in maintaining role adaptation and intrapersonal and interprofessional conflict management for the palliative care clinical nurse specialist in Canada.

Davies & Oberle's study provides an in-depth, novel conceptual model of palliative nursing care that has since been validated in practice (Davies & Oberle 1992; Fig. 1.2).

In the second paper on their study, Davies & Oberle (1992) evaluated and tested their supportive care model. They did this by giving presentations on the model to 'numerous groups of nurses in a variety of settings' who were asked to provide feedback to the authors. The feedback indicated that the model had captured the dimensions of their own nursing roles. The authors do not give any information on the range of nurses spoken to, or details on the clinical settings. However, the authors use this as an example of the validity and rigour of the content of the model.

The key concepts here relate to the nurse as a person, as much as to being seen as central to the dimensions of nursing, thus implying that the nurse as a professional cannot be separated from the nurse as a person.

Despite its limitation in research design, i.e. using only one informant and relying on her reflections on her own practice, the findings of Davies & Oberle's research have been widely adopted, including being the basis of the curriculum model for the palliative care courses.

THE ROLE OF THE NURSE IN THE HOSPICE

Surprisingly, there are no UK studies describing the role of the hospice nurse, despite the fact that the hospice movement was founded by Dame Cicely Saunders, herself a former nurse.

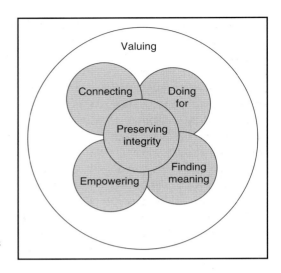

Figure 1.2 Dimensions of care (from Davies & Oberle 1992).

It has been suggested that the role of the nurse in palliative care is directly related to the setting in which nurses practise (Brockopp et al 1991, Irvine 1993, Reisetter & Thomas 1986). When hospice nurses are compared with other groups of nurses, particularly nurses from the acute setting, it has been shown that they experience less death anxiety (Bene & Foxall 1991, Payne et al 1998) and more positive attitudes towards death (Brockopp et al 1991, Field 1989, Kirschling & Pierce 1982). In addition, it has been argued that hospice nurses experience less occupational stress than nurses in other care settings (Dean 1998, Vachon 1995), although the need for support in this area of nursing is acknowledged (McKee 1995). It therefore seems pertinent to explore the literature specifically pertaining to this group of nurses in palliative care.

Dobratz (1990), an American nurse, examined the role of the hospice nurse in an extensive literature review. She identified four categories of nursing function in hospice care:

- **Intensive caring**, managing the physical, psychological, social and spiritual problems of dying persons and their families
- **Collaborative sharing**, the coordinated and collaborated efforts of the extended and expanded components of hospice care services
- **Continuous knowing**, the acquisition of the counselling, managing, instructing, caring and communicating skills/knowledge required for the specialty of hospice nursing
- **Continuous giving**, the balancing of the hospice nurses' own self-care needs with the complexities and intensities of death and dying.

This study goes some way to describing in detail what hospice nurses do. There is, however, a note of caution to be observed in generalising findings, with respect to the cultural context of the American health-care system.

Raudonis's (1993) naturalistic field study explored patients' perspectives of the nature, meaning and impact of empathic relationships with hospice nurses. Data were collected through in-depth interviews with 14 terminally ill adults receiving home-based hospice care. The findings showed that an empathic relationship with the nurse developed through a process of recipro-cal sharing in the context of caring and acceptance. This was based on being acknowledged as an individual, a person of value. The outcome of this empathic relationship between hospice nurses and their patients was mainte-nance or improvement of the patient's physical and emotional wellbeing. Understanding the patient as an autonomous person was seen as being critical for effective nursing intervention and a meaningful outcome.

This study is particularly important because the findings were elicited directly from patients. The most important aspect of the relationship for the patients was the acknowledgement of their individuality.

Hull (1991) also examined the caring behaviours of hospice nurses, as per-ceived by family caregivers in a hospice home care programme. Semi-structured interviews and participant observation were used to collect data from a sample of the families. Four areas of caring behaviours of hospice nurses were identified: 24-hour accessibility, effective communication, clini-cal competence and non-judgemental attitudes.

It is evident from reviewing the literature in relation to the role of the nurse in the hospice setting that this area is under-researched.

THE IMPACT OF DEATH AND DYING ON THE PALLIATIVE CARE NURSE

It has been argued that the care of dying patients and their families is differ-ent from ritualised general nursing practice, because it involves physical as well as emotional labour (Field 1989, James 1986, Wakefield 1999). Indeed, Wakefield found that, when nurses in a surgical ward were caring for dying patients, they were more likely to spend more time with the patient and adopt holistic care. Nurses were also observed to engage in sensitive and more sedate forms of practice, such as the use of touch, patience, empathy and ten-derness. It may be that it is these caring aspects of palliative nursing that nurses who choose to work in palliative care find attractive. It has been sug-gested that a need for emotional reward plays a part in the motivation to work in a hospice (Vachon 1995). Other reasons are a sense of calling or vocation and previous personal experience (Vachon 1995). Moreover, Rasmussen et al (1995) identified that hospice nurses were motivated by the desire to have an opportunity to form close relationships with patients and families.

It has been further identified that nursing care of the dying can be a stress-ful and demanding experience (Booth 1995, McKee 1995, Vachon 1995). There is evidence that nurses often experience feelings of inadequacy and inability to cope with pain management and symptom control (Copp & Dunn 1993). Other studies have identified that palliative nurses have a more posi-tive attitude towards death, experience less death anxiety, have a greater sense of personal control and have less fear concerning their own mortality and the death of others than nurses working in non-palliative care areas (Brockopp et al 1991, Field 1989, Kirschling & Pierce 1982, Payne et al

1998). Studies have also indicated the importance of education about palliative care in influencing nurses' attitudes to the dying (Degner & Gow 1988a, b, Hurtig & Stewin 1990).

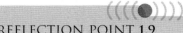

REFLECTION POINT 1.9
Attributes of the palliative care nurse

Is the palliative care nurse a special breed? Read the opinions below and debate.

My experience suggests that nurses who choose to work in specialist palliative care are often dedicated, caring people with a sense of humanity who also often possess spiritual or religious beliefs. These nurses often, therefore, avoid the 'cut and thrust' of acute areas and 'high-tech' areas and prefer instead the slower, more individualised pace of a hospice setting. I would also suggest that there is also speculation, but no evidence base, to suggest that nurses choose palliative care because of a previous experience of loss or death and the subsequent 'need to be needed'. However, until further research is undertaken, the long-term impact on nurses of being exposed to death and dying and the reasons why nurses choose to work in palliative care remain unclear.

A FRAMEWORK FOR EXPERT NURSING PRACTICE

In an in-depth qualitative study from a phenomenological perspective, Johnston (2002) explored the experience of being a palliative care nurse from the perspective of palliative nurses and dying patients.

Figure 1.3 details the framework of expert nursing practice derived from the in-depth interview data. Data were collected from 22 patients and 22 nurses from two hospitals and two hospices in Scotland using in-depth interviews and the repertory grid technique.

PATIENT DATA

Connecting

'Connecting' was a central theme for both nurses and patients (Fig. 1.3). Connecting formed the core of how the patients viewed palliative nursing and the role of the expert palliative nurse. As a term, 'connection' implies a joining together of two or more elements with a relationship formed between them. Connecting therefore was an appropriate term to link the concept of interpersonal communication with the building of a nurse–patient relationship.

Figure 1.3 places 'connecting' in the centre to illustrate that all the other theme categories coexisted, with the nurse possessing good communication skills and the building and establishing of the nurse–patient relationship. Without good communication skills and an effective nurse–patient relationship, the other components of effective palliative care and characteristics of an expert palliative care nurse could not occur. It should be noted that 'connecting' was not always effective; for example, some patients described a lack of connection in terms of being left alone or avoided. The first theme was composed of the clusters *someone to talk to, willing to listen, getting to know me* and *avoiding me.*

Being in control

The second theme category title was used because of the emphasis patients placed on being in control during their terminal illness as a mechanism for maintaining their independence and, therefore, their quality of life and well-being. 'Being in control' was composed of the theme clusters *maintaining my independence* and *fighting spirit*. Patients wanted to be cared for and wanted their families around them. Nevertheless, they still wanted to be able to control what was happening to them. Thus, 'being in control' was something they wanted both the nurses and their families to respect.

Meeting my needs

The theme category of 'Meeting my needs' was formed from the following theme clusters: *not helping me, knowing about my illness, providing comfort, being there for me* and *supporting me*. This theme category encapsulated what the patients were saying about how they wished care to be provided by nurses in palliative care. The majority of patients described the importance of the nurse 'meeting their needs', 'being there for them' and 'respecting their

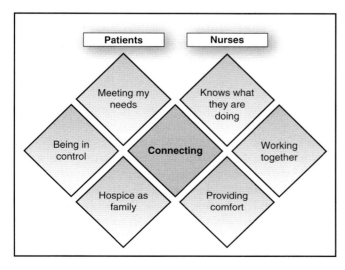

Figure 1.3 Framework of expert nursing practice (from Johnston 2002).

wishes' at some point in the interview. 'Meeting my needs', together with the theme of 'connecting', encompassing how the patients described the role of the nurse in palliative care, was not always viewed as effective by the patients and subsequently involved both helpful and unhelpful activities.

Hospice as family

'Hospice as family' was chosen by the researcher as the title of the fourth theme category in order to encapsulate the importance that hospice patients attributed to the atmosphere, safety and sanctuary of the hospice environment. Thus, this theme category was formed from the following clusters: *making me feel relaxed* and *feeling safe and secure*. The patients were of the opinion that the hospice in this respect was very different from the hospital where they had been inpatients. This therefore seems to be a concept that was unique to the hospice setting.

NURSE DATA

Connecting

'Connecting' was chosen as the title of the first theme category for the nurse data as well as the patient data. The nurses also placed much emphasis on the need for good interpersonal skills as well as on the building of therapeutic nurse–patient relationships. The theme was chosen from the theme clusters: *willing to listen, facilitating communication, providing information, barriers to communication, building rapport, spending time with patients* and *supporting the patient and their family*.

Providing comfort

'Providing comfort' consisted of the following theme clusters: *keeping patients comfortable* and *controlling pain and symptoms*. When describing issues of providing comfort, the nurses largely referred to the physical caring, or 'doing for', aspect of the nurse's role in palliative care. Many of the features of providing comfort were considered unique to the role of the nurse in palliative care, such as aspects of keeping patients comfortable, possibly because of the close relationships that many nurses formed with dying patients.

Working together

The theme category 'Working together' arose from the theme clusters *teamwork, acting as a go-between for the patient* and *the professional knows best*. The theme category title was selected to represent the number of nurses who discussed issues of teamwork and professional working practices at some point in their interviews. 'Working together' indicated that the majority of the nurses from both hospice and hospital settings were of the opinion that working as a team was an integral part of providing effective palliative care. The nurses felt that those practitioners who chose to work in isolation could not provide effective care. When there was a dispute about goals or treatment, or a breakdown in communication between the professionals, ineffective care occurred and, ultimately, it was patients who suffered.

Knows what they are doing

The theme category 'Knows what they are doing' was composed of the theme clusters *learning about palliative care, professional experience* and *personal experience*. The nurse sample was virtually unanimous in indicating that having knowledge and experience were prerequisites for being an expert palliative care nurse. A third of the nurses also mentioned that they felt that their personal experience of death and dying had made them a better nurse and more empathetic towards the dying patients they were looking after.

USING THE FRAMEWORK

So how can the framework be used? It could be used to guide practice, to form a framework on which to plan care in conjunction with the patient. It could also be used to plan and formulate educational initiatives for palliative nurses.

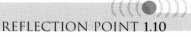

REFLECTION POINT 1.10
Using the framework

Having considered the framework set out above, think about ways you might apply it to your own practice.

THE EXPERT PALLIATIVE CARE NURSE

Figure 1.4 outlines how both nurses and patients described the 'expert palliative care nurse'.

In Johnston's study, both the nurse and the patient study sample alluded most often and most strongly to features such as having good interpersonal skills and possessing personal characteristics such as warmth, kindness and compassion. Building rapport and having a good relationship with the patient were also perceived by the study sample to be essential characteristics of a good palliative care nurse. Particularly notable aspects of this relationship were 'getting to know me as a person' and 'understanding me', as well as the patient having confidence and trust in the nurse.

The nurses asserted that a good nurse should provide emotional support for the patient and their family. The patients also stressed the importance of the nurse being there for them by spending time with them. Both nurses and patients perceived that a good nurse should provide comfort to the dying

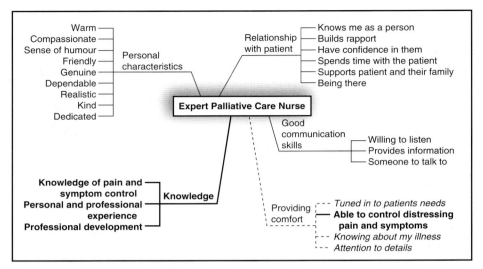

Figure 1.4 Diagram representing nurses' and patients' perceptions of an expert nurse in palliative care. Key: *** represents patients' and nurses' perceptions of an expert nurse; *** represents nurses' perceptions of an expert nurse; *** represents patients' perceptions of an expert nurse (from Johnston 2002).

patient by tuning into their needs. The nurses stressed the importance of being able to control the patient's distressing pain and symptoms. They considered that it was impossible to be a good palliative nurse or maintain one's expert status without having knowledge, experience and the ability to maintain and improve one's knowledge through continuous professional development.

Patients in previous research have alluded to the pain and symptom control role of the nurse (Bergen 1992, Cox et al 1993, Hunt 1992). It is therefore somewhat surprising that, in this study, no patients discussed the ability of the nurse to control their pain and symptoms and no patient identified controlling pain and symptoms as a feature of a 'good nurse' in palliative care. This may be because they did not see controlling pain and symptoms as a role for the nurse or it may be that they did not think of this as a feature because their pain and symptoms were under control at the time of data collection. On the other hand, patients may have perceived that controlling pain and symptoms was a medical rather than a nursing function.

This novel finding has particular implications for nursing practice, as much of the training and education in palliative nursing is related to alleviating pain and controlling distressing symptoms. Johnston is not suggesting that nurses do not still need to learn about and understand pain and symptom control in order to function effectively as specialist palliative nurses. She does, however, suggest that this training should be tempered by equal emphasis on the psychosocial role of the palliative nurse and, in particular, the role of effective communication and caring characteristics.

These findings related to the good nurse are new in that no previous studies have identified the attributes and characteristics of a good palliative care nurse from both the nurse's and the patient's viewpoint. There is however a small body of evidence from nurse informants to confirm these findings (Degner et al 1991, McClement & Degner 1995, Zerwekh 1995).

The unique findings from this study in relation to a good nurse, therefore, also include all the characteristics identified by patients, as no studies have previously asked patients for their views about what makes a good palliative nurse. This dearth of literature regarding patients' views of their nursing care reveals an important omission from previous literature. Indeed, it has already been identified that dying patients are rarely asked for their views of their care and that researchers are now identifying this problem and beginning to tackle it (Field et al 2001).

Moreover, none of the previous studies that explored the role of a good/expert palliative nurse identified that knowledge, professional development and experience were important components of the good palliative nurse, as identified in this research.

The model of a good palliative nurse, therefore, contains five separate but interwoven dimensions: personal caring characteristics, knowledge, providing comfort, nurse–patient relationship and good communication skills. The majority of these are comfort and caring dimensions, with effective communication as the key. The psychosocial dimensions, therefore, appear to be valued above technical or complex skill elements. I would therefore argue that this has significant implications for nursing practice as well as for education and training.

CLINICAL NURSE SPECIALISTS IN PALLIATIVE CARE

Various authors in recent years have examined the role of the Macmillan nurse (Bullen 1995, Cox et al 1993, Graves & Nash 1992, M Kindlen, unpublished data 1987, Sloan & Grant 1989, Webber 1993).

On the whole, the role of the Macmillan nurse is perceived favourably by both practitioners and patients and their families. This role has provided a model for clinical nurse specialists in the UK. However, it should be taken into account that their perceived role is emotive for both professionals and lay people.

While existing research has advanced the body of knowledge regarding the role of the Macmillan nurse, this has largely been from the practitioner's viewpoint. Attempts to elicit the views of patients and carers have been limited. This is partly due to ethical problems in facilitating such a study.

WHERE DO WE GO FROM HERE?

What then is the future for palliative care and nursing? With the implementation of *Agenda for Change* (Royal College of Nursing 2004) there will be new opportunities for nurses to increase their roles and responsibilities.

Other initiatives that will serve to enhance the value of nursing in palliative care include nurse practitioner posts. Traditionally, nurse practitioner roles complement the role of the doctor. For example a nurse practitioner in an accident and emergency department would take on roles such as treatment of minor injuries without reference to a doctor, thus allowing medical expertise to be applied where it is most needed (Scott 1995). In an innovative scheme in Hull, nurse practitioners were established in a hospice. Their role incorporated: being consulted about pain and symptom control; being involved in research; taking on extra responsibilities clinically, including venepuncture and making decisions about readmission of patients; and being designated liaison contacts with outside agencies (Scott 1995). Other initiatives that can enhance the role of the nurse include nurse-led clinics such as symptom control clinics in palliative care, bereavement services run by nurses and nurse-led beds in specialist palliative care units. Moreover, the recently established role of the consultant nurse can also enhance patient care.

With the development of an increasing number of specialist courses in palliative care at degree and postgraduate level, there will be more opportunities for developing specialist and advanced practitioners in palliative care.

SUMMARY

This chapter has emphasised the importance of the nursing role in palliative care and suggested ways in which that role might be enhanced in the future. It has explored the key characteristics of the role of the nurse in palliative care and explored the literature in this area. Finally, the words of Solzhenitsyn (1968) help to sum up the role of the nurse in palliative care:

How many adult human beings are there, now at this very minute, rushing about in mute panic wishing they could find a nurse, the kind of person to whom they can pour out the fears they have deeply concealed?

REFERENCES

Addington-Hall J, McCarthy M 1995 Dying from cancer: results of a national population-based investigation. Palliative Medicine 9:295–305

Anstey S 1993 Care in acute hospital units. Nursing Standard 7:51

Avis M, Jackson J G, Cox K, Miskella C 1999 Evaluation of a project providing community palliative care support to nursing homes. Health and Social Care in the Community 7:32–38

Bates T D, Hoy A M, Clarke D G, Laird P P 1981 The St Thomas' hospital terminal care support team – a new concept of hospice care. Lancet 1:1201–1203

Bene B, Foxall M J 1991 Death anxiety and job stress in hospice and medical–surgical nurses. Hospice Journal 7(3):25–41

Benner P 1984 From novice to expert: excellence and power in clinical nursing practice. Addison-Wesley, Menlo Park, CA

Bergen A 1992 Evaluating nursing care of the terminally ill in the community: a case study approach. International Journal of Nursing Studies 29:81–94

Booth K 1995 Professional support within hospices. International Journal of Palliative Nursing 1:206–210

Brockopp D Y, King D B, Hamilton J E 1991 The dying patient: a comparative study of nurse care giver characteristics. Death Studies 15:245–258

Buckman R 1993 Communication in palliative care: a practical guide. In: Doyle D, Hanks G W C, Macdonald N P (eds) Oxford textbook of palliative medicine. Oxford University Press, Oxford, p 47–61

Bullen M 1995 The role of the specialist nurse in palliative care. Professional Nurse 10:755–756

Campbell A 1984 Moderated love. SPCK, London

Cartwright A 1991 Balance of care for the dying between hospitals and the community. Perceptions of GPs, hospital consultants, community nurses and relatives. British Journal of General Practice 1:10–14

Copp G, Dunn V 1993 Frequent and difficult problems perceived by nurses caring for the dying in community, hospice and acute care settings. Palliative Medicine 7:19–25

Cox K, Bergen A, Norman I J 1993 Exploring consumer views of care provided by the Macmillan nurse using the critical incident technique. Journal of Advanced Nursing 18:408–415

Davies B, Oberle K 1990 Dimensions of the supportive role of the nurse in palliative care. Oncology Nursing Forum 17:87–94

Davies B, Oberle K 1992 Support and caring – exploring the concepts. Oncology Nursing Forum 19: 763–767

Dean R A 1998 Occupational stress in hospice care: causes and coping strategies. American Journal of Hospice and Palliative Care 15:151–154

Degner L F, Gow C 1988a Preparing nurses for care of the dying. Cancer Nursing 11:160–169

Degner L F, Gow C 1988b Evaluation of death education in nursing. Cancer Nursing 11:151–159

Degner L F, Gow C M, Thompson L A 1991 Critical nursing behaviours in care for the dying. Cancer Nursing 14:246–253

Directory of Hospice Services 2003 Available on line at: www.hospiceinformation.info/factsandfigures/ukhospices.asp

Dobratz M C 1990 Hospice nursing: present perspectives and future directives. Cancer Nursing 13:116–122

Douglas C 1992 For all the saints. British Medical Journal 304:579

Dunlop R J, Hockley J M 1990 Terminal care support teams. The hospital–hospice interface. Oxford Medical Publications, Oxford

Dunn V 1992 Palliative care problems addressed and problems created in cancer nursing changing frontiers. Proceedings of the Weekend Symposium of the 7th International Cancer Conference, Vienna

Ellershaw J Ward C 2003 Care of the dying patient: the last hours and days of life. British Medical Journal 326:30-34

Faulkner A 1993 Teaching interactive skills in health care. Chapman & Hall, London

Faulkner A, Maguire P 1994 Talking to cancer patients and their relatives. Oxford University Press, Oxford

Field D 1989 Nursing the dying. Tavistock/Routledge, London

Field D, James N 1993 Where and how people die. In: Clark D (ed.) The future for palliative care. Open University Press, Buckingham, p 6–29

Field D, Clark D, Corner J, Davis C (eds) 2001 Researching palliative care. Open University Press, Buckingham

Froggatt K 2000 Evaluating a palliative care education project in nursing homes. International Journal of Palliative Nursing 6:140–146

Froggatt K A, Hoult L 2002 Developing palliative care practice in nursing and residential care homes: the role of the clinical nurse specialist. Journal of Clinical Nursing 11:802–808

Glaser B G, Strauss A 1965 Awareness of dying. Aldine Publishing Company, New York

Glaser B G, Strauss A 1968 Time for dying. Aldine Publishing Company, New York

Gooch J 1988 Dying in the ward. Nursing Times 84(21):38–39

Graves D, Nash A 1992 A friendship that inspires hope: a study of Macmillan nurses' working patterns. Professional Nurse April:478–485

Griffin J 1991 Dying with dignity. Office of Health Economics, London

Harris L 1990 The disadvantaged dying. Nursing Times 86(22):26–29

Heaven C M 2001 The role of clinical supervision in communication skills training. Unpublished PhD thesis, University of Manchester, Manchester

Heaven C M, Maguire P 1996 Training hospice nurses to elicit patient concerns. Journal of Advanced Nursing 23:280–286

Heaven C M, Maguire P 2003 Communication issues. In: Williams L (ed.) Psychosocial issues in palliative care. Oxford University Press, Oxford

Herd E B 1990 Terminal care in a semi-rural area. British Journal of General Practice 40:248–251

Herth K 1990 Fostering hope in terminally ill people. Journal of Advanced Nursing 15:1250–1259

Heslin K, Bramwell L 1989 The supportive role of the staff nurse in the hospital palliative care situation. Journal of Palliative Care 5:20–26

Higginson I, Wade A, McCarthy M 1990 Palliative care: views of patients and their families. British Medical Journal 301:277–281

Higginson I J, Sen-Gupta G J A 2000 Place of care in advanced cancer: a qualative systematic literature review of patient preferences. Journal of palliative medicine 3:3, 287-300

Hill H C 2003 Palliative care education in nursing homes. Unpublished report, Strathcarron Hospice, New Opportunities Fund Project, Strathcarron Hospice, Denny

Hinton J 1979 Comparison of places and policies for terminal care. Lancet 1:29–32

HMSO 1992 Standing Nursing and Midwifery Advisory Committee and Standing Medical Advisory Committee. The provision of palliative care. HMSO, London

Hockley J M 1989 Caring for the dying in acute hospitals. Nursing Times Occasional Paper 55:47–50

Hockley J M, Dunlop R, Davies R J 1988 Survey of distressing symptoms in dying patients and their families in hospital and the response to a symptom control team. British Medical Journal 296:1715–1717

Hull M M 1991 Hospice nurses' caring support for caregiving families. Cancer Nursing 14:63–70

Hull R, Ellis M, Sargent V 1989 Teamwork in palliative care. Radcliffe Medical Press, Oxford

Hunt M 1992 Scripts for dying at home– displayed in nurses', patients' and relatives' talk. Journal of Advanced Nursing 17:1297–1302

Hurtig W A, Stewin L 1990 The effect of death education and experience on nursing students' attitudes towards death. Journal of Advanced Nursing 15:29–34

Irvine B M 1993 Developments in palliative nursing in and out of the hospital setting. British Journal of Nursing 2:218–224

James V 1986 Care and work in nursing the dying: a participant study in a continuing care unit. Unpublished PhD thesis, University of Aberdeen, Aberdeen

Johnston B M 2002 Perceptions of palliative nursing. Unpublished PhD Thesis, University of Glasgow, Glasgow

Johnston B M, Smith V 2005 Students' experience of counselling skills training and their perception of its impact on clinical practice. International Journal of Palliative Nursing, in press

Katz J, Komaromy C, Sidell M 1999 Research study. Understanding palliative care in residential and nursing homes. International Journal of Palliative Nursing 5:58, 60–64

Kirschling J M, Pierce P K 1982 Nursing and the terminally ill: beliefs, attitudes and perceptions of practitioners. Issues in Mental Health Nursing 4:275–286

Lamerton R 1980 Care of the dying. Penguin, Harmondsworth

Lawler J 1991 Behind the screens: nursing, somology and the problem of the body. Churchill Livingstone, Edinburgh

McClement S E, Degner L F 1995 Expert nursing behaviours in the care of the dying adult in the intensive care unit. Heart and Lung Journal of Critical Care 24:408–419

McKee E 1995 Staff support in hospices. International Journal of Palliative Nursing 1:200–210

Macleod Clark J 1983 Nurse–patient communication – an analysis of conversations from surgical wards. In: Wilson-Barnett J (ed.) Nursing research: ten studies in patient care. John Wiley, Chichester, p 25–26

Macmillan Cancer Relief 2004 About Macmillan. Available on line at: www.macmillan.org.uk/aboutmacmillan/

McWilliam C L, Burdock J, Wamsley J 1993 The challenging experience of palliative care support-team nursing. Oncology Nursing Forum 20:779–785

Maynard A 2003 The interdisciplinary team. In: Doyle D, Hanks G, Cherny N, Calman K (eds) Oxford textbook of palliative medicine. Oxford University Press, Oxford

Morse J 1991 Negotiating commitment and involvement in the nurse–patient relationship. Journal of Advanced Nursing 16:455–468

Muetzel P 1988 Therapeutic nursing. In: Pearson A (ed.) Primary nursing: nursing in the Burford and Oxford nursing development units. Croom Helm, London, p 89–116

NCHSPCS 1995 Specialist palliative care: a statement of definitions. National Council for Hospice and Specialist Palliative Care Services, London

NHS Quality Improvement Scotland (QIS) 2004 Available on line at: www.nhshealthquality.org

Nightingale F 1980 Notes on nursing: what it is and what it is not. Churchill Livingstone, Edinburgh

Norum J 1995 Cancer patients dying at home: care providers' experience. Journal of Cancer Care 4:157–160

Parkes C M 1985 Terminal care: home, hospital or hospice. Lancet 1:155–157

Payne S A, Dean S J, Kalus C 1998 A comparative study of death anxiety in hospice and emergency nurses. Journal of Advanced Nursing 28:700–706

Pearson 1991 Taking up the challenge: the future for therapeutic nursing. In: McMahon R, Pearson A (eds) Nursing as therapy. Chapman & Hall, London, p 192–208

Perry B 1996 Influence of nurse gender on the use of silence, touch and humour. International Journal of Palliative Nursing 21:7–14

Quint J C 1967 The nurse and the dying patient. Macmillan, New York

Rasmussen B H, Norberg A, Sandman P O 1995 Stories about becoming a hospice nurse: reasons, expectations, hopes and concerns. Cancer Nursing 18:344–354

Raudonis B M 1993 The meaning and impact of empathic relationships in hospice nursing. Cancer Nursing 16:304–309

Reisetter K, Thomas B 1986 Nursing care of the dying: its relationship to selected nurse characteristics. International Journal of Nursing Studies 23:39–50

Royal College of Nursing 2004 Agenda for change. Available on line at: www.rcn.org.uk/agendaforchange

Saunders C 1991/2 The evolution of the hospices. Free Inquiry 12:19–23

Saunders C 1993 Introduction – history and challenge. In: Saunders C, Sykes N (eds) The management of terminal malignant disease. Edward Arnold, London, p 1–14

Savage J 1995 Nursing intimacy: an ethnographic approach to nurse–patient interaction. Scutari Press, London

Scott G 1995 Challenging conventional roles in palliative care. Nursing Times 91(3):38–39

Seale C F 1991 A comparison of hospice and conventional care. Social Science and Medicine 32:147–152

Seale C F 1992 Community nurses and care of the dying. Social Science and Medicine 34:375–382

Sloan D, Grant M 1989 Evaluating a Macmillan nursing service. Senior Nurse 9:20–21

Solzhenitsyn A 1968 Cancer ward. Penguin, Harmondsworth

Spiller J A, Alexander D A 1993 Domiciliary care: a comparison of the views of terminally ill patients and their family caregivers. Palliative Medicine 7:109–115

Stedeford A 1994 Facing death: patients, families and professionals, 2nd edn. Sobell Publications, Oxford

Steeves R, Cohen M Z, Wise C T 1994 An analysis of critical incidents describing the essence of oncology nursing. Oncology Nursing Forum Supplement 218:19–25

Thorpe G 1993 Enabling more people to die at home. British Medical Journal 307:915–918

Townsend J, Frank A O, Fermont D, et al 1990 Terminal cancer care and patients' preference for place of death: a prospective study. British Medical Journal 301:415–417

Vachon M L S 1987 Occupational stress in the care of the critically ill, the dying and bereaved. Hemisphere, Washington, DC

Vachon M L S 1995 Staff stress in hospice/palliative care: a review. Palliative Medicine 9:91–122

Wakefield A B 1999 Changes that occur in nursing when a patient is categorised as terminally ill. International Journal of Palliative Nursing 5:171–176

Walsh M, Ford P 1989 Nursing rituals: research and rational actions. Butterworth-Heinemann, Oxford

Watson J 1988 Nursing: human science and human care: a theory of nursing. National League for Nursing, New York

Webber J 1993 The evolving role of the Macmillan nurse. Unpublished paper, Cancer Relief Macmillan Fund, London

Wilkinson S 1991 Factors which influence how nurses communicate with cancer patients. Journal of Advanced Nursing 16:677–688

Williams C A 1982 Role considerations in care of the dying patient. Image 14:8–11

World Health Organization 2005 WHO definition of palliative care. Available on line at: www.who.int/cancer/palliative/definition/en/

Zerwekh J V 1995 A family caregiving model for hospice nursing. Hospice Journal 10(1):27–44

CHAPTER TWO

Education and development in palliative care

Jacqueline S Nicol, Noreen Reid

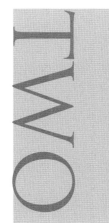

CONTENTS

Education is a diverse and wide-ranging topic. Its focus should remain dynamic in order to meet ever-changing expectations. Readers are invited to consider palliative care education in its very broadest sense. We believe that individual health practitioners have a responsibility to be involved in education in either delivery and/or as a recipient.

CHAPTER AIMS

In reading this chapter, readers are encouraged to:

- Acknowledge responsibility for their own learning
- Recognise the relationship between personal/professional development and legislation
- Learn to access educational opportunities and resources for funding these
- Understand and apply different approaches to learning and teaching
- Implement formal and informal learning strategies in the workplace.

As a specialty, palliative care is relatively young; however, in recent years, in response to professional demand and government recommendations, momentum has been gathering to formalise the standard of palliative care education. The report *Higher Education in the Learning Society* (Dearing 1997) was produced to determine the future development of higher education. This report emphasises the key role of higher education in helping deliver the Learning Age.

Education is a dynamic activity that should evolve to comply with government initiatives linked to maintaining standards of care. Such initiatives include the NHS Knowledge and Skills Framework (Department of Health 2003), which supports career progression and personal development, and the Agenda for Change report (Department of Health 2004), which harmonises pay systems and terms and conditions of NHS employees. The environment of care is also constantly changing, involving new and expanding roles. It is vital to develop professional knowledge and competence to meet these demands. If individuals do not display commitment to ongoing education for altruistic reasons, then the fact that skills and knowledge are now to be directly linked to rate of pay may well provide the necessary catalyst.

LEARNING IN THE WORKPLACE

The importance of workplace learning in health care is highlighted in the NHS lifelong learning strategy (Department of Health 2001a). To date the focus for many organisations remains firmly fixed on formal education and training rather than exploring alternative options (Dowswell et al 1998). Given the issues related to releasing staff to attend education sessions, and the cost not only of the education itself but also of the replacement staff, employers should consider a combination of approaches to staff development. In his publication *Developing Effective Workplace Learning in UK Hospices: Findings, Issues and Challenges*, Clarke (2004) reports that, although many of the 120 hospices surveyed used a mix of both formal and informal learning methods, only 52% had policies in place to support informal education initiatives. He speculates that such policies would encourage the use of informal methods.

PROMOTING A POSITIVE LEARNING CLIMATE

The learning climate within organisations can create a barrier to the delivery of education. Clarke (2004) suggests that senior managers should be given the responsibility for staff development as this will not only raise the profile of education but also support its assessment. One means of determining the learning needs of an individual is to utilise the annual staff appraisal process.

NHS Quality Improvement Scotland (QIS) (2002) states that all employees should have a personal professional development plan that actually documents gaps in training/education. An action plan with achievable targets is produced as an outcome of this process. These plans are helpful in cost-effective planning of an organisation's education strategy. Invariably managers have the responsibility for the budget and so are best placed to prioritise the needs of individual practitioners and the department.

The literature related to informal learning supports the premise that installing particular organisational conditions can have the effect of improving the quality of learning outcomes (Clarke 2003, Lahteenmaki et al 2001). There is also an issue with the assessment of education content and delivery within hospices as currently there is no standardisation (Audit Commission 2001). This is an ongoing problem often included on the agenda of those organisations responsible for maintaining the standards in the field of palliative care (SPPC 2004).

POLICY AND STANDARDS

The Nursing and Midwifery Council (NMC) links continuing professional development to the registration renewal process under the post-registration education and practice (PREP) standards. These represent an important part of lifelong learning linked to professional practice (Nursing and Midwifery Council 2002a). By encouraging professional development in line with the PREP standards, employers will not only help nurses meet registration requirements but also support the principles of clinical governance. The NMC do have some concerns about the quality and nature of the assessments that students receive in achievement of NMC standards and they are currently developing a standard to address this issue (Nursing and Midwifery Council 2002b). Clinical governance provides the cornerstone of good practice. It is a framework that unites a range of quality initiatives, including clinical effectiveness, evidence-based practice, reflective practice, quality improvement processes and workforce development (Quinn 2000). As Naysmith (2004) reminds us, clinical governance is simply 'a term for doing the right thing in the right way at the right time' (p. 329).

In the UK, there are two main national bodies that debate and define standards and areas of excellence within the field of palliative care. They are the National Council for Hospice and Specialist Palliative Care Services (NCHSPCS) for England, Wales and Northern Ireland, and the Scottish Partnership for Palliative Care (SPPC) for Scotland (NCHSPCS 1996, SPPC 2004). These organisations contribute to national thinking and policy in relation to palliative care. They also include guidance on access and delivery of education. The SPPC, in conjunction with the Clinical Standards Board for Scotland (CSBS), has produced the *Clinical Standards for Specialist Palliative Care*. This document is the end result of a consultative process determining generic and disease specific standards of care. Standard 4 relates specifically to professional education and recommends a variety of levels of multiprofessional education opportunities at specified levels according to the role. Standard 3.b.7 recommends that specialist units should be able to demonstrate that they are working towards all nurses having a degree or postgraduate qualification in palliative care (CSBS 2002). The document does acknowledge that 'specialist' qualifications at degree and postgraduate level have only recently been available and accessible in Scotland (p. 43). It is important to point out, however, that both the NCH-SPCS and the SPPC collaborate to develop and maintain a UK perspective across palliative care.

As of 2003, the CSBS is now known as NHS Quality Improvement Scotland (NHS QIS). In England and Wales, the equivalent body to NHS QIS is the National Institute for Clinical Excellence (NICE). Northern Ireland is not covered by guidance from NICE but is currently establishing clinical and social care governance arrangements for health and social services. It is evident, therefore, that there are several differences throughout the UK; however, all are committed to excellence in palliative care through the professional education and development of practitioners.

RANGE AND LEVEL OF PROVISION

There are different levels of education available, the appropriateness of the level being determined to some extent by the organisational position held by the nurse/health-care professional. For example, nurses/health-care professionals working in specialist palliative care units or hospices, or those employed in key resource positions, will require tertiary level education. However, the learning needs of those employees who are working in non-specialist posts but who apply a palliative approach to the care of their patients may adequately be met by specifically targeted short course or study day education. There are many organisations involved in the delivery of such education programmes, one example being Marie Curie Cancer Care. Among its many recommendations, the Marie Curie Cancer Care education strategy (Marie Curie Cancer Care Education 2004) promotes the delivery of education programmes for medical and allied health professionals rather than solely the nursing workforce. This acknowledges and addresses the multiprofessional profile of palliative care service delivery. The National Health Service University (2004) is a new kind of learning organisation available in nine regions of England and offering learning opportunities to staff at all levels in health and social care, which aims to improve patient care. Another new initiative is the transnational palliative MSc for health professionals in Britain and France; this is an exciting prospect for multiprofessionals to undertake a part-time MSc and to become familiar with two different health-care systems and languages (Hoban 2004).

FINDING THE RIGHT COURSE

So – where can practitioners find information about the provision of palliative care education?

It may be advisable to explore local options in the first instance, since many hospices now have education departments. The Hospice Information Service (HIS; www.hospiceinformation.info/training.asp) offers a quarterly e-mail service – eChoices – that lists information about upcoming conferences and training opportunities.

The Scottish Partnership for Palliative Care (www.palliativecarescotland. org.uk) publishes a comprehensive list of accredited and non-accredited courses available throughout Scotland.

In 2002, the HIS records displayed 13 degree-level programmes in palliative care, several other degree courses with the option to specialise in palliative care, and many diploma and stand-alone modules. A variety of on-line courses are now available in response to practitioners' difficulties in directly accessing palliative care education. When embarking on any educational programme, however, it is imperative to select the most appropriate one to address individual needs.

BOX **2.1**

Funding options for palliative care courses

For registered nurses
- Margaret Parkinson scholarship awards for post-registration nurses
  c/o Awards Officer RCN
  20 Cavendish Square
  LONDON W1G 0RN

- www.macmillan.org.uk

- The Nightingale Fund Council
  108 Brancaster Lane
  PURLEY
  Surrey CR81HH

All health professionals
- Help the Hospices: tel: 02075202911; www.helpthehospices.org.uk

International students
- www.ukcosa.org.uk/pages/advice.htm#finance

- www.educationuk.org

The charities Macmillan Cancer Care and Marie Curie Cancer Care have both supported many educational initiatives. It could be argued that, without these charities' provision, together with free provision from some independent hospices, the range of programmes on offer today might never have been developed. Short courses may produce some income to offset the delivery costs; however the provision of degree programmes generates little income while requiring substantial resources. Practitioners are therefore required to self-fund courses, apply for sponsorship from their employers or apply to charities.

Box 2.1 lists a selection of funding options.

THE CHANGING ROLE OF THE EDUCATOR

Throughout their career as health professionals, providing education is an integral component of any professional's role. While it is an expectation of the role, formal training seldom supports it. It cannot be assumed that a good clinician will make a good teacher and, while they are very valuable for clinical updates, peer group tutorials should not be a substitute for formal education provided by qualified teachers.

As organisations' and students' expectations change, so too does the role of the educator. In the 1980s, there was a major reshaping of nurse education when it moved from schools of nursing into the tertiary system. There are standards laid down across the UK regarding the basic requirements of the staff managing education departments involved in cancer and palliative care. In Scotland, the standards (CSBS 2002) state that staff should have access to an educator, specialist palliative care library, Internet facilities and an evidence-based programme of education for professionals. They also advise that the education unit should have links with an institution of higher education and contribute to multidisciplinary preregistration, undergraduate and postgraduate education in palliative care.

Hospices may employ nurses in the position of an educator; however, there are several advanced nursing practice roles that have emerged over the last 10–15 years, an example of which is the Lecturer Practitioner role. As the name suggests, the Lecturer Practitioner positions, although based in education, do have a clinical practice component that varies depending on the needs of the organisation. The professional requirement of this all-encompassing role covers a wide spectrum. According to Fitzgerald (1989), such nurses should have mastery of practice, education, management and research. They must have the ability not only to develop their own personal skills and knowledge but also to lead a team of nurses. This new role provides nursing with a prime opportunity to bridge the theory–practice gap. The underpinning rationale for this, according to Hewison & Wildman (1996), is that teachers should be based in practice areas where both student nurses and trained staff will be accessible.

APPROACHES TO LEARNING

According to the literature there are three main teaching modes; individualised learning, group learning and mass instruction. The method chosen should not be arbitrary but rather appropriate for the content. The programme aims, objectives and learning outcomes should be taken into account before the choice of instructional method is made (Ellington et al 1993). Kolb (1982) presents the learning process as a cycle that incorporates four stages. The first stage of *planning* the learning experience maintains that the learner should always be involved with the planning. Jeffery (2002) supports this theory in his description of adult learning. *Exploration* of the learning experience is the second stage. This involves the students being involved in dictating the points of guidance that facilitate the learning. The authors that support the third stage of *reflection* include Conway (1994) and Spalding (1998). This encourages the students to look back on an experience and, through reflection, to consider if a change in their behaviour or actions could have improved or altered the outcome. The fourth and final stage provides an opportunity to present the theories that underpin practice. This process should be at the forefront of the minds of educators and trainers when they prepare teaching sessions. Evidence suggests that educators in medical faculties would benefit from revisiting teaching methodologies, and that the need for more effective teaching is clear (Soriano & Bensinger 2004, Stratos et al 2004).

Personality has an effect on the learning approach adopted and the response to teaching methodologies. Personality is a complex topic summarised by Krahe (1992) as having three components. In his work, Krahe states that 'personality' reflects uniqueness, is stable and enduring, and is determined by intrinsic forces. This has relevance to education, as the personality of students will influence their learning style and the student–teacher relationship. When designing and planning teaching material at any level, all the above dimensions should be considered. Building rapport with individual students by creating a non-threatening yet stimulating learning environment is fundamental if the learning process is to be effective.

LEARNING METHODS

In 1993, Race & Brown documented four ingredients of successful learning experiences: they are wanting, doing, feedback and digesting:

- The first ingredient of 'wanting' refers to **motivation**. The literature alludes to the adult desire for, and enactment of, self-direction (Jeffery 2002). Beaty et al (1996) explore this further by considering the reasons for students enrolling in courses, divided into 'intrinsic' and 'extrinsic'. An example of intrinsic motivation would be a nurse recognising a deficit in personal knowledge and sourcing an educational endeavour that will address the issue. Extrinsic motivation could be an adult learner studying as a requirement of their employment rather than through choice. If this is in fact true then, although the literature differentiates between adult and non-adult learning, an adult's level of commitment may be no different from that of a non-adult learner. Teachers should assess each student as an individual and be cautious of making assumptions.

- The '**doing**' and '**feedback**' elements are closely associated. Adults are competency-based learners who appreciate application of their newly acquired skills. Badly given feedback can demotivate and destroy confidence and enthusiasm. Poorly managed feedback can be more damaging than no feedback at all.

- '**Digesting**' relates to a sense of ownership and synthesis of the information. This, however, is a higher-level skill and as such can be difficult to achieve. It takes practice and is highly regarded in the assessment process of adult learning.

LEARNING TO LEARN

Prior to embarking on a course of study, many students are unaware of the skills necessary to complete the programme successfully. For example, a university may recommend that applicants have basic computer skills as a prerequisite to enrolment, but some students embark on courses underestimating the significance of this advice. This misunderstanding can lead to a delay in the student learning and participation in class activities, which may in turn result in decreased motivation and enjoyment of the learning experience. There are a variety of study-skills courses available, including distance learning and on-line options: a selection of on-line resources is listed in Box 2.2. The content of such courses includes planning study, reading critically and referencing technique, all of which can help equip students in the necessary study skills.

BOX 2.2

On-line study skills resources

- www.bradford.ac.uk/acad/civeng/skills/essays.htm
- www. sussex.ac.uk/langc/skills/
- www.bbc.co.uk/learning/returning/betterlearner/studyskills/index.shtml
- http://osiris.sunderland.ac.uk
- http://nulis.napier.ac.uk/StudySkills/

There is, however, some controversy about the level of responsibility that the tertiary education facilities should take in ensuring that students fulfil skills prerequisites. Some are of the opinion that it may be acceptable to assume that, in adult education, the students themselves shoulder this responsibility. As Knowles's (1984) landmark work reminds us, one of the principles of adult learning is to involve the learners in diagnosing their own needs.

SELF-AWARENESS AND LEARNING

For an individual to fulfil personal learning needs, it is important to have a degree of self-awareness. Self-awareness develops as a result of experiences gained and, to some degree, on what we think others think and feel about us. The whole concept of self-awareness is complex and changes over time. It relates not only to our personal life but also to how we behave and perform in the work environment. In 1969, Luft published what became known as the 'Luft Johari window'. It offers a mechanism for conceptualising self-awareness. Burnard further developed this work in 1990 when he produced a simplified version of Luft's concept of self-awareness. Burnard's approach involves three hypothetical 'zones'. The first zone involves turning our attention towards the outside world and our behaviour – think of this in terms of 'wakefulness'. The second zone asks us to look inward and focus our attention on our thoughts and feelings. The third zone asks us to use our imagination and/or daydream. Burnard suggests that, by adopting this model, nurses, as a result of a heightened awareness of their focus of attention and the shifting between the three zones, will improve skills of both observation and interpretation. This model can be applied to all health professionals.

SURFACE LEARNING OR DEEP LEARNING?

Individuals have differing approaches to studying and learning. In 1996, Marton & Saljo reported the results of their research into determining how students approached a learning activity. A group of students were asked to read an article and were interviewed later to ascertain differing learning styles. The authors concluded that the participants fell into one of two groups, adopting either a deep or a surface approach. The distinction between the two was the *intention* of the students. Those who adopted a deep approach began the task with the intention of understanding the article, assimilating the information, based on their own experience, and evaluating the supporting evidence. The other group concentrated on memorising important points, guided by the questions they thought might subsequently be asked. Entwistle (1981) continued to build on this seminal work and included the strategic approach. He maintains that in this approach the students concentrate their efforts on passing the assignments and/or gaining the highest marks possible.

None of these approaches should be viewed negatively; each may be appropriate depending on the task at hand or the context of the education activity. It is, however, important that students and teachers have an awareness of the different approaches and that, for the most part, teaching methods are implemented that promote a deep approach.

REFLECTION POINT 2.1

Learning approaches

Think about some learning or study that you have undertaken in the past.

* Which learning approach did you adopt – deep, surface or strategic?

* Why did you adopt this approach?

* How did it make you feel about yourself and the learning experience?

* Did the assessor know that you had adopted this approach?

* If so, what did they feel about your choice?

* Will you adopt the same approach to the next learning experience with which you are involved?

Having some awareness of your own preferred learning style can help you to survive the learning experience and perhaps even enjoy it. As a result you will grow personally and professionally.

LEARNING FROM EACH OTHER

In practical terms, it is not always suitable or feasible for nurses to enter into tertiary education, one of the main inhibitors being fiscal concerns. It should be remembered that, within nursing, education has always taken place in the workplace, be it in mentoring colleagues new to a specialty or facilitating nursing students. There are many teaching strategies and approaches that can be implemented within peer groups. However, it is perhaps presumptuous to assume that all health professionals have either the inclination or the skills to perform such a task. Individuals should endeavour to find an approach that suits both their personality and their skills.

Setting up a learning network is one initiative that some may find helpful (John 2004). For example, for an individual working in the acute care setting, meeting regularly with other professionals who have an interest in palliative care practice can not only help to improve practice but can also make it fun. The group may consider utilising the local palliative specialist team or hospice as a resource. Journal clubs offer another forum for the creation of a multiprofessional learning environment. Both these activities involve sharing ideas and practice experiences related to the care of the dying. An informal learning environment will be created and this can evolve into a more formal and structured format if that better meets the learning needs of the group. In this type of learning each person takes responsibility for personal learning: no one person takes overall responsibility. Taking the lead in organising such a network will provide nurses with a set of organisational and professional skills that can be added to their PREP.

Stiles (2004) reminds us that nurses, no matter how experienced, are all learners and by developing themselves can inspire others in the art of nursing and, as a result, can improve patient outcomes.

In a professional role that entails responsibility for peer group education, it may be helpful to think in terms of Benner's model of skill acquisition in clinical practice. Benner (1984) based her model on work carried out by Dreyfus & Dreyfus (1980) and documented the results of her research in her book *From Novice to Expert*. Level 1 is directed by rule-governed behaviour. However, as experienced nurses know, blind adherence to principles does not necessarily result in good practice. Stages 2–5 progress from advanced beginner to competent, proficient through to expert. This framework can provide a fundamental guide to inexperienced teachers and help in forming realistic learning outcomes and expectations.

The remainder of this chapter discusses some peer-assisted learning techniques. With managerial support, any health professional can introduce one or more of the examples given.

DEVELOPMENT THROUGH REFLECTIVE PRACTICE

Reflection in learning is not a new idea and can in fact be traced back to the educational philosopher John Dewey (1933). Reflective practice as a means of critically reviewing practice has been gaining momentum in nurse education since the work of Schon in the 1980s. It is generally thought to be a good process, encouraging practitioners to review their performance and, by doing so, to improve their practice. As a result of this belief, reflection has been incorporated into many different levels of nurse education (Hannigan 2001). O'Connor et al (2003) found that the terms 'reflection' and 'reflective practice' were used interchangeably; therefore, throughout this section, the terms will be used synonymously.

In their requirement that practitioners should maintain a personal professional profile, the Nursing and Midwifery Council (NMC) incorporates written reflection into its PREP requirements (Nursing and Midwifery Council 2004a). However, reflective practice in nursing is not without its critics. Cotton (2001) and Hannigan (2001) maintain that there is no robust research to support the hypothesis that reflective practice improves patient care and they recommend further research in this field. An opposing viewpoint is offered by Markham (2002) and Teekman (2000). While welcoming the critical analysis approach to reflection, they conclude that, although not directly related to improved practice and patient outcomes, the increase in self-awareness as a result of the reflective process could lead to an improvement of performance in a broad sense as it provides individuals with an insight into their personal behaviours, strengths and weaknesses.

Although several approaches to reflection have evolved in recent years (Boud et al 1985, Gibbs 1988, Johns 1992), they are similar in that they all encourage practitioners to critically review their behaviours, beliefs and ideas in relation to practice (Quinn 2000). Johns (2000, p. 34) aptly describes critical reflection as 'a window through which the practitioner can view and focus self within the context of her own lived experience in ways that enable her to confront, understand and work to resolving the contradictions within her practice between what is desirable and actual practice'.

ANALYSIS OF CRITICAL INCIDENTS

By reflection, actions can be revisited in a constructive manner, resulting in improved performance, clinical expertise and patient outcomes. The word 'critical' appears frequently in the literature relating to reflective practice. This is somewhat unfortunate as it can have negative connotations for some individuals. Should we therefore consider renaming the critical incident 'a significant event' to address these negative connotations? The concept of reflection may be embraced with a more positive response if negative language is rejected. Because the majority of authors use the term 'critical' We shall continue to use this terminology but acknowledge the potential for practitioners to be confused as to its meaning.

Using a critical incident technique provides a framework for the reflective process (Quinn 2000). Benner (1984) goes on to describe reflection as the description of an incident that was critical to the practitioner. The process involves thinking about what the practitioner was feeling and thinking before and after the incident. Wood (1998) takes this process a step further by including the identification of implications for practice. If the process is used appropriately, it can involve review of both good and bad practice outcomes, although it must be said that the culture within health care usually tends to dwell on our failings rather than our successes, so, with that in mind, some words of caution. When learning to use the reflective process, consider beginning with a successful practice outcome. Consider what components of your action or inaction contributed to making the outcome good and through analysis of the incident determine whether some change in your behaviour could have changed the outcome for the better.

Using a reflective cycle can illustrate the process and is shown in Figure 2.1.

Being open to new ways of thinking and a commitment to becoming the best practitioner you can be are prerequisites to using the reflective process (Cranton 1994). To use the reflective process effectively, you must be capable of self-analysis, brave enough to challenge your own behaviour or that of colleagues, and able and willing to adapt and change. Practitioners may find this threatening and difficult but, if the skills can be learned with support from educators and experienced colleagues, it will become easier with practice (Appleton & Duke 2000, Williams 2001).

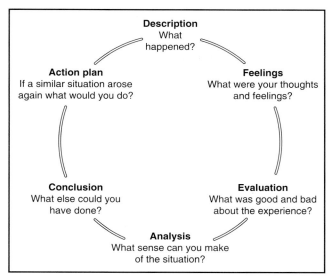

Figure 2.1 Gibbs's reflective cycle (Adapted from Gibbs 1988).

AU: Authors cred is ok?

1st step	**Description** – Describe what happened in factual terms.
2nd step	**Feelings** – What were you thinking and feeling? This stage can be difficult as it involves being totally honest with yourself. It may also bring forth some very strong emotions, so be gentle with yourself.
3rd step	**Evaluation** – Consider what was both good and bad about the experience. In most cases, there are some positive occurrences even in an otherwise negative incident.
4th step	**Analysis** – Try to make some sense of the event.
5th step	**Conclusion** – What else could you possibly have done to improve or change the outcome?
6th step	**Action plan** – If you found yourself in the same situation again, would you change your behaviour?

REFLECTION POINT 2.2

Gibbs's cycle of reflection

- Take some time to think of a particular significant event that has occurred in your palliative care practice (remember, this is something that is personal to you)

- Using Gibbs's cycle of reflection, reflect on the significant event you have identified

- Having now used the process, have you seen any benefits from using structured reflection in this way?

- Would you consider it to be worthwhile incorporating it into your regular practice?

Perhaps, to consolidate our thoughts on reflection, we should consider the words of Conway (1994). She described reflection as providing 'an ideal vehicle for uniting the art and science of nursing' (p. 117). Andrews (2000) supports this. When, as a third-year occupational therapy student, she documented the impact of the process on her learning experience, she found it had guided her in her clinical reasoning and resulting patient interventions. Reflective practice can be of value to practitioners as they continue to grow and develop into a more rounded individual, with an increased therapeutic effect on patient outcomes.

DEVELOPMENT THROUGH CLINICAL SUPERVISION

Within the health-care professions there are many instances in practice where practitioners question their judgement and require support. This is addressed in a variety of ways, for example chatting over issues with colleagues while having a break. Clinical supervision is a forum where two parties, a supervisor and supervisee/s, can meet in a more formal setting. So what do we mean by the term clinical supervision? According to the Department of Health (1993), clinical supervision is described as a formal process of professional support and learning. It enables practitioners to develop competence and accountability for their own practice, thus improving patient outcomes. The two parties, agreeing to meet at a prearranged time, achieve this. The supervisee is responsible for bringing issues to the meeting for discussion. These may be of a clinical nature or personal issues arising from the workplace. The supervisor facilitates the supervisee, using reflection, to come to their own conclusions and not, as the term might imply, advising the supervisee. It should be highlighted that the emphasis should not be on negative situations but rather on issues of significance to the supervisee that warrant further deliberation. Documentation can be kept to a minimum but should include time and date of meetings and be stored in a confidential file.

The NMC (Nursing and Midwifery Council 2004b) advocates the importance of establishing clinical supervision as a mechanism to support clinical governance in the interests of maintaining and improving the standard of patient care. It is therefore interesting to note that, in many health disciplines, clinical supervision, while deemed best practice, is not mandatory. NMC (Nursing and Midwifery Council 2004b) recommendations underscore the value of supervision but as yet this has not been widely embraced by the National Health Service, perhaps as the potential cost of funding such a venture is prohibitive.

The term 'clinical supervision' can have ambiguous connotations. The word 'supervision' implies observation and direction (Oxford 1999) whereas, in reality, clinical supervision refers to providing a safe environment within which to explore issues of concern to the individual practitioner through a process of self-awareness and reflection. Acknowledging that clinical supervision is best developed at a local level, the NMC (Nursing and Midwifery Council 2004b) does not therefore advocate any one particular model. It does, however, define a set of principles to underpin the process.

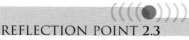

REFLECTION POINT 2.3

Clinical supervision

Begin by accessing and reading the section pertaining to clinical supervision on the NMC website (www.nmc-uk.org). Having reflected on this, consider:

- If you are already involved in clinical supervision, are these underlying principles being used in your area of practice?

- If you are not currently involved in clinical supervision but intend to become involved as either a supervisor or a supervisee, would you consider adopting the principles as outlined by the NMC (Nursing and Midwifery Council 2004b)?

If clinical supervision is to be successful, it is crucial that the purpose of supervision is clearly understood by both the supervisor and the supervisee (Fowler 1996). Supervisees should be encouraged to choose their supervisor, not necessarily from within the organisation. However, there will be cost implications if the person selected is external. It is suggested that, since the supervisor should not have a hierarchical relationship with the supervisee, peers may be best suited to fill the role (Goorapah 1997). Keeping in mind that the supervisor is a facilitator and not an advisor, Duarri & Kendrick (1999) suggest that the main attributes for a supervisor are empathy, being non-judgemental and being genuine, with active listening skills and with the ability to challenge constructively. For the interaction to be effective there must be a contract between the two parties that includes agreement and commitment to confidentiality, time, place and duration of meetings, and maintenance of records. It should be acknowledged that the supervisee is responsible for instigating appointments.

This process relies on mutual respect and commitment, so either of the parties can end the contract at any time.

Models of clinical supervision

Clinical supervision can contribute to lifelong learning by being accessible to registered practitioners throughout their careers. A great deal of nursing literature views clinical supervision as a way of giving support to nurses while offering them a way of learning from their experiences (Butterworth et al 1997, Department of Health 1994, Magnusson et al 2002, Nursing and Midwifery Council 2004b).

A number of different models of clinical supervision can be used (Severinsson 1996). The models are somewhat dependent on the style adopted by the supervisor and in general terms range from one-to-one supervision to group supervision. One-to-one supervision is more often the preferred choice, perhaps because of the sense of vulnerability experienced when first embarking on this process. However, in 2003, Jones discussed the benefits experienced by hospice nurses of group clinical supervision. These included learning from each other and recognising how others saw and valued them as colleagues. It is important to note that carefully chosen membership is vital in ensuring the safety of members and the coherence of the group. The facilitator should possess the skills to ensure that those less vocal have the opportunity to express their views. One important factor we cannot ignore is the cost implication of one-to-one versus group clinical supervision.

Clinical supervision can be very useful as a learning tool – why not consider approaching your colleagues and manager to implement the process?

DEVELOPMENT THROUGH MENTORSHIP

One area of concern in the nursing arena is that, in practice, individuals are often nominated by managers to provide mentorship for colleagues regardless of whether or not they have the necessary skills. Some organisations, for example tertiary education institutions, provide compulsory mentorship training programmes (Earl 2002). In its report *Preparation of Mentors and Teachers*, the Department of Health (2001b) makes recommendations for the preparation of mentors for their role. Unfortunately this is not always adhered to in practice.

So what exactly do we mean by mentorship? Mentoring relationships are established in response to an individual embarking on a role or activity that is new to them. Mentorship has come to the fore in recent years, perhaps because of the emphasis on promoting evidence-based care and issues of accountability at organisational and individual levels, hence the reason why competency frameworks are often linked to mentorship programmes. In contrast to clinical supervision, in mentorship the mentored do not necessarily choose their mentor, as the line manager may well nominate them. They should, however, have the option of selecting an alternative person for the role should this be deemed necessary; for example if there is a clash of personalities. As in clinical supervision, mentorship is founded on mutual respect, trust and good communication between the two parties. The mentored should be willing to be frank and honest in their deliberations and contribute feedback to enhance the learning experience. They should be encouraged to keep a reflective journal of their progress. This can be used to support their professional development as per PREP guidelines (Nursing and Midwifery Council 2002b). Participation in well-prepared mentorship programmes can equip practitioners to survive and to blossom in a new role where they feel valued and supported.

Making mentorship work

Mentorship is integrated into everyday practice and as such can take the form of formal meetings and/or ongoing guidance throughout practice. Quinn (2000) includes teaching, supervision, guidance, counselling, assessment and evaluation in the range of domains attributed to the role of the mentor. Within mentorship, documentation of the interaction is mandatory.

The relationship involves a minimum of two people and is often a voluntary partnership entered into in a spirit of collegiality. Mentorship differs from clinical supervision in that clinical supervision is not an advisory process.

While in clinical supervision the supervisee takes a leading role, in mentorship the mentor determines the process. Both parties commit at the beginning to the development of a learning relationship. However, for mentorship to be successful, several ground rules should be agreed. They include:

- Confidentiality
- A clear definition of professional issues raised
- Mentorship must be a two-way process/partnership based on trust
- Information should not used in other ways, for example for appraisal (Jeffery 2002).
  The role of the mentor falls into three domains:
- **Educational** – learning opportunities can be created by helping the mentored in the specialised area
- **Supportive** – by taking the mentored in hand, the mentor's experience will familiarise them with the expectations of their role in the organisation
- **Managerial** – being responsible in part for the progress and development of the mentored within the department.

In an effort to amalgamate these three aspects of the role, Channell (2002) coined the mnemonic 'WORLD' to encapsulate the three domains, as follows:

- **W**orking clinically
- **O**bserving practice
- **R**esearching a topic
- **L**earning pack
- **D**epartmental visit.

Mentors should be more experienced in the specialist area than the mentored. They can then become a sounding board; a safe person to ask for advice directly related to the specialist subject matter and, at times, to absorb frustrations in an empathetic and non-judgemental manner. This process involves encouraging nurses to fulfil their potential and to work effectively through the use of reflection (Jeffery 2002). The preparation for the role of mentor should facilitate the necessary skills to achieve these objectives. Accordingly, Watson (2000) recommends that support for mentors should be practical as well as psychosocial and educational.

It is acknowledged that, although being a mentor is a challenging role, it can bring job satisfaction while also enhancing the individual's practice development. The satisfaction is to some extent dependent upon organisations promoting to their staff a sense of being valued. Sadly, in practice, some organisations are found wanting in this respect (Duffy et al 2000). Organisations should be aware that the code of professional conduct (Nursing and Midwifery Council 2002c) places emphasis on maintaining mentorship competency. It is useful to remember that fellow mentors can provide an excellent source of support (McCarty & Higgins 2003) and this need not necessarily be instigated by the organisation; rather, the mentors themselves can take ownership of the support process.

DEVELOPMENT THROUGH PRECEPTORSHIP

Although there is some overlap of the role of preceptor and mentor and although the terms are sometimes wrongly used interchangeably, there are distinct differences. So what role does preceptorship have in the delivery of education in the workplace? Think of preceptors as being part of a 'buddy' system providing informal support and orientation to the work environment.

The preceptor is shadowed for a variable time while involved in their normal work. Those new to the role observe the interactions on decisions made by the preceptor. Time is then set aside to discuss the practice observed. The meeting offers an opportunity for the preceptor to provide a rationale for the approach taken and explain why specific decisions were made. If a buddy/preceptorship system is being implemented, documentation of the meetings may or may not be required. Preceptorship benefits both parties, encouraging reflective practice for the preceptor, who is justifying practice decisions to the observer, while the observer has the opportunity to witness the experienced practitioner in action.

COMPETENCY-BASED LEARNING

The *Lack of Competence* discussion paper (Nursing and Midwifery Council 2003) led to guidelines being introduced that monitored competence as well as misconduct in nurses and midwives. O'Dowd (2003) reminds us that, although some practitioners were apprehensive about this landmark development, the guidelines provided a means for employers to address poor practice and intractable incompetence rather than just deal with isolated incidents. To complete the competencies, the staff member works through a series of activities and tasks, at their own pace but usually within a specified timeframe. This move to competency recording provided an opportunity to bridge the theory–practice gap within the nursing profession (Conway 1994). This gap has been acknowledged for many years; however, a new dimension arose in the UK through the separation of those delivering health care from those providing education for nurses (Hewison & Wildman 1996). Over the years, a variety of approaches have been taken to address this problem, including involvement of nurse tutors in clinical areas and the appointment of Lecturer Practitioners. Clinical competency frameworks are currently being implemented within palliative care practice.

COMPETENCY FRAMEWORKS

The Royal College of Nursing (RCN), the professional body for nurses, midwives and health visitors, has produced competency frameworks for a number of specialties, including the Palliative Care Competency Framework (Royal College of Nursing 2002). By logging on to the RCN website (www.rch. org.uk) you will be able to access these using the search feature: Palliative + care + framework. As the focus on competency frameworks has gathered momentum, specialist organisations such as hospices adapted these generic guidelines to meet the specific needs of their own institutions. Although implementation of Palliative Care Competency Frameworks differs between specialist units, it is mandatory that they comply with current government frameworks for maintaining standards of care, for example the NHS Knowledge and Skills Framework (Department of Health 2003). Also, the competency framework that is used must cover the following seven domains: clinical practice/job knowledge and skills; communication skills; loss, grief and bereavement; education; quality assurance; management and leadership; and, finally, research and development.

A recent initiative in spiritual care and chaplaincy has been the development of national standards and a competency framework for chaplaincy and spiritual care. In 2004, Marie Curie Cancer Care took the lead in launching Spiritual and Religious Care Competencies for Specialist Palliative Care, in partnership with other palliative care organisations. These spiritual competencies consist of levels of attainment across the whole spectrum of staff and volunteers who have patient/family/carer contact. The four domains are structured to encompass different levels of staff/volunteer contact. These range from level 1, which includes all staff and volunteers who have causal contact with patients and their families, to level 4, which relates to staff or volunteers whose primary responsibility is the spiritual and religious care of patients, visitors and staff (Marie Curie Cancer Care 2004). In Scotland, although the CSBS does not have a separate standard for spiritual care, it is incorporated throughout the document (CSBS 2002). In England, the spiritual competencies are recommended in workforce development by the NICE guidelines (NICE 2004).

MEASURING COMPETENCE

Judging competence has always been an integral part of maintaining a high standard of care. The competency frameworks are merely a means of formalising this process. Perhaps the term 'competency' is somewhat ambiguous. In this context, it brings together attributes such as knowledge, attitudes, values and skills. It is the coherence and the application of these attributes within specific practice situations that are being judged (Manley & Garbett 2000).

The level at which competency is measured is dependent on the role of the individual within the organisation. A self-directed learning package allows the learner greater control over the learning process while working through a variety of tasks and activities (Tennant 1997) and the practitioner's performance in terms of qualities, knowledge and abilities is judged against predetermined criteria (Milligan 1998). To maintain the integrity of the competency measurement process, it is imperative that the assessors have achieved a higher level of competence than those being assessed.

Throughout the framework, for all grades of staff, mentorship is an integral component. This can be provided in a variety of ways; for example, the lecturer/educator can take the lead as academic mentor while a ward sister or senior registered nurse provides clinical mentorship. The lecturer/educator is also responsible for writing and updating the content in collaboration with senior clinical staff.

Mentoring is the formation of a learning relationship between teacher and learner, in which both parties have responsibilities. The learner must be willing to be honest in discussing personal practice and should keep a record of professional development. The teacher supports the student by providing a safe environment that facilitates reflective practice (Jeffery 2002). Part of the process is also to provide the student with feedback. In individualised learning, supervision from the teacher is critical to success. The competencies feedback is a two-way process, with the learner contributing to the process. Individualised learning is dependent upon the student's ability to work independently. Motivation is also necessary to work through the programme.

THE THEORY–PRACTICE LINK

Competency frameworks provide a mechanism to assess application of theory to practice. Specific tasks and/or formal education supported by clinical activities can integrate theory-based knowledge with clinical skills. This encourages staff to explore the rationale that underpins their practice. Table 2.1 provides an extract from a competency framework in current use.

PROBLEM-BASED LEARNING

Historically, nurse education and universities have relied heavily on teacher-led approaches to learning. However, in recent years, there has been a shift towards more student-focused learning, thus encouraging a more active role in learning (Morris & Turnbull 2004). An example of a student-led approach is problem-based learning (PBL). You may see the term 'enquiry based learning' (EBL) in literature. EBL and PBL approaches to learning are fundamentally the same, the main difference being that EBL does not require a 'problem' as such to initiate the process.

Problem-based learning is an approach to learning in which a stated problem is the stimulus for students to use their cognitive skills to gain knowledge of the concepts and issue(s) identified. PBL alters the roles of teachers and students, with students assuming a greater responsibility for researching the subject matter in order to address the problem. Students are given a problem

TABLE 2.1

Example of a competency framework

Knowledge	Skills	Behaviour
Attend a study day on symptom management		
Read Twycross R, Wilcock A 2001 Symptom management in advanced cancer, 3rd edn (Radcliffe Medical, Oxford), Chapters 3, 4 and 5		
Read protocols on management of constipation and mouth care		Self-awareness Motivation
Measure: complete quiz and discuss results with mentor		
Understands the theory behind the use and management of syringe drivers		Confidence Judgement Accountability
Measure: complete the 'Setting up a syringe driver' tutorial available on-line at www.helpthehospices.org.uk	**Measure:** The mentor will demonstrate setting up and monitoring a syringe driver. Following this observation, the student will carry out the procedure, explain the rationale for their method and discuss the ongoing care needs.	

From Highland Hospice 2003 Level 2 Nurse Competency Framework. Adapted from RCN Palliative Care Competency Framework (2002).

to consider before they have all the information necessary to solve it. They work alone or in teams to define the nature of the problem, identify additional resources needed, and find viable solutions. Teachers may act as facilitators by asking questions and monitoring the students' progress (Major 1999). However, when employing PBL in its purest sense, the teacher adopts a 'hands off' approach, acting as a facilitator only when the students are communicating the results of their findings. It is not uncommon for students to question the role of the educator in this process, and rightly so, since this mode of learning differs so vastly from the traditional style in which the teacher gives information and answers questions. In contrast, with PBL, the emphasis is on the teacher guiding and coaching the problem-solving process.

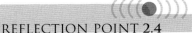

REFLECTION POINT 2.4
Problem-based learning

Have you ever had the opportunity to use the problem-based learning approach as a student? What advantages and disadvantages do you consider that this approach to learning might have?

For example, if your multiprofessional team is caring for a patient with complex needs, consider presenting their history and current situation as a case study at a team meeting:

- Ask the team members to identify any knowledge/skills deficit they might have and to suggest possible resources necessary to form a viable patient management plan

- This process will not only build on existing knowledge and enhance coherence of the team, but also improve your skills as a facilitator and could potentially improve patient outcomes

- This is also a great opportunity to consider patient management, drawing on the perspective of different disciplines within the team.

ON-LINE AND BLENDED LEARNING

Recently, there has been an explosion of Internet use in both the home and work environment. Schoolchildren are exposed to information technology (IT) from a very young age and many adults are using the Internet for on-line shopping, banking, etc. It seems natural, therefore, that education should embrace IT for learning. Chickering & Ehrmann document the advantages of on-line learning, suggesting that on-line learning facilitates total flexibility that is not only accessible '24/7' but is also available worldwide (Chickering & Ehrmann 1996).

CHALLENGES AND BENEFITS OF ELECTRONIC LEARNING

This mode promotes an active, student-based learning or assignment-based approach and fosters cooperation skills. It can also increase interactions between students and teacher, allowing the learner to participate in both formal and informal web-based learning communities. This mode of teaching accommodates different approaches to learning, although there is some debate in the literature surrounding the extent to which surface as opposed to deep learning is facilitated by on-line education programmes (Ellington et al 1993). For some students, a classroom can appear intimidating and not an environment where they feel able to vocalise thoughts or, if the class has several vocal students, there may not be the opportunity to participate in discussions because of being overshadowed. The on-line environment allows less vocal or more reflective learners to contribute using the medium of the electronic discussion board.

Dearing (1997) confirms that education technology is crucial to the future of higher education. In his report there is, in fact, hardly a chapter that does not mention what Dearing has chosen to call C & IT (communications and information technology). Computer-assisted learning (CAL) is the term used to discuss a wide variety of electronic teaching applications. They include retrieval of on-line reports, databases and publications, the use of on-line notice boards as a communication tool and the posting of courseware on the World Wide Web.

FULLY ELECTRONIC OR BLENDED LEARNING?

Two broad classifications used in on-line learning are enhanced face-to-face learning (blended learning approach) and instruction that is entirely on line. A blended approach (sometimes referred to as hybrid or complementary) consists of both face-to-face and on-line interactions. Dearing (1997) endorses this type of flexibility to promote the effectiveness of higher education in teaching and learning. However, many experienced health-care professionals are apprehensive about CAL, preferring the face-to-face environment, possibly because their own education history was embedded in the traditional classroom setting. The entirely on-line approach has advantages as well as disadvantages.

Advantages include:

- It can deliver learning at any time in virtually any place
- It can increase the number of interactions between the learners and the facilitator
- It can make use of resources already available on the Internet.

Disadvantages include:
- Technical limitations – lack of access to appropriate hardware or connections
- Expense involved in establishing the learning environment
- Training implications for both learners and facilitators.

It should be acknowledged that teaching and learning are social processes based on basic communication that includes telling, asking, responding and discussion. To allow for this to happen on-line, interactions can either be synchronous (real time) or asynchronous (communication without the need for a common time). Decisions about whether to use wholly on-line or blended learning methods will be made by the programme designer on the basis of factors such as the programme aims, the learning platform and the subject content. The key to learning is sharing knowledge through interactions with others and this can readily be achieved within a variety of learning environments (McDermott 1999).

The significance of student support should not be underestimated for successful on-line learning. Giving feedback is always an important component of the teacher's role but nowhere more so than in on-line education, where it is perhaps the strongest link. The advantage with computer-based learning is that students get a response while they still remember exactly what the feedback relates to (Ellington et al 1993). To date, there is little evidence about the experience of on-line learners (Kenny 2002). When students first embark on this as a new mode of learning, they may well need time to adjust and, if not supported, may feel a sense of isolation and not being part of a programme, or lack motivation. This could result in a high attrition rate. One strategy is to build a sense of belonging through a 'virtual classroom community'.

Educators need to help health-care professionals to embrace this new modality. CAL should be positively promoted as it opens up opportunities for learning and facilitates this on a global level. This is perhaps most beneficial to practitioners working within isolated or rural settings since it allows them equitable access to education and information in palliative care. Those who manage health care have a responsibility to equip practitioners with the skills to use computers in the workplace.

Educational establishments and teachers need to recognise the huge and daunting learning curve that novice web learners have to undertake, especially at the beginning of the on-line course. It is essential to ensure that advance planning and preparation are in place to combat attrition and ultimately enhance the learning experience for the participants (Atack & Rankin 2002). Before embarking on an on-line course, participants have an obligation to become aware of hardware and software requirements, web connections and required computer skills and to familiarise themselves with the issues they may face, whether they are home or work learners, well in advance of the commencement of the course. Most institutions will offer an induction day to help orientate participants.

The presence of an on-site facilitator can be very reassuring. We cannot assume that all who wish access to education have the necessary IT equipment and there are significant resource implications if they are to acquire this. In the UK, we are fortunate in that many higher education facilities have IT laboratories, and libraries have computers available for students to use. In areas where there is relative IT deprivation, students could perhaps access Internet cafes where these are available. Differences in infrastructure to support on-line learning can result in inequities in access to learning.

In the 21st century, new technologies touch every facet of our lives; education is perhaps the last frontier for some health-care professionals. Ward (2001) highlights the dearth of nurses' skills in effectively using the Internet. As authors, we acknowledge that the main limitation to using CAL effectively is the deficit in technical skills in both teachers and students. By improving these skills, we can develop a workforce that is modern, highly professional and marketable to employers. With many clinical guidelines, key government documents and research evidence now available electronically, the need for a more computer-literate profession is now urgent.

REFLECTION POINT 2.5

On-line learning

The super-highway is the new road to learning and development. Things are changing fast! Consider the following questions:

- Do you currently have the necessary skills to embark on an on-line education programme?

- Whose responsibility is it if you need to improve your IT skills?

- If the next education course you are interested in has an on-line option, would you consider taking it?

- What range of feelings does the thought of learning on-line evoke in you?

- You are a health-care professional with a real interest in caring and improving patient outcomes. If engaging in on-line education is one option offering easy access to current programmes, why not take the chance to pick up the gauntlet and join the worldwide community of e-learners.

Ongoing education is a viable option – even with your busy lifestyle. Go for it! To get you started, why not check out these websites?

- www.bbc.co.uk/webwise: an absolute beginner's guide to the keyboard, mouse and Microsoft Windows

- www.vts.rdn.ac.uk/tutorial/nurse: a 'teach yourself' tutorial aimed at nurses

- www.elearningguild.com/

- www.e-learningguru.com/

CONCLUSION

This chapter introduced you to some new terms and some ideas about how you can develop in your everyday practice. Hopefully you will have acquired a better understanding of how you, as an individual, can integrate some of these ideas into your own plans for learning and development. Do remember that it is important to choose a teaching approach and learning style that suits you. Education is integral to every nurse's role and, as such, should continue to evolve in response to the ever-changing expectations of students and to new developments in clinical practice, technology and education. With this in mind, teachers should constantly be seeking out new and innovative methods of delivering content.

We now invite you, the reader, to rise to the challenge. Talk to your colleagues and managers. Make a start in establishing a positive learning climate that encourages and supports learning and development within your own working environment. You might even consider using some of the strategies discussed throughout this chapter. We leave you with this quote:

An education isn't how much you have committed to memory, or even how much you know, it's being able to differentiate between what you do know and what you don't.

Anatole France (1844–1924), French novelist

REFERENCES

Andrews J 2000 The value of Reflective Practice: a student case study. British Journal of Occupational Therapy 63:96–99

Appleton J, Duke S 2000 The use of reflection in a palliative care programme: a quantitative study of the development of reflective skills over an academic year. Journal of Advanced Nursing 32:1557–1568

Atack L, Rankin J 2002 A descriptive study of registered nurses' experience with web based learning. Journal of Advanced Nursing 40:457–465

Audit Commission 2001 Hidden talents: the education, training and development of healthcare staff in NHS Trusts. Audit Commission, London

Beaty L, Gibbs G, Morgan A 1996 Learning orientations and study contracts. In: Marton F, Hounsel I D, Entwisle N (eds) The experience of learning, 2nd edn. Scottish Academic Press, Edinburgh

Benner P 1984 From novice to expert: excellence and power in clinical nursing practice. Addison-Wesley, Menlo Park, CA

Boud D, Keogh R, Walker D 1985 Reflection: turning experience into learning. Kogan Page, London

Burnard P 1990 Learning human skills: an experiential guide for nurses, 2nd edn. Heinemann, Oxford

Butterworth T, Carson J, White E, et al 1997 Clinical supervision and mentorship. It is good to talk: an evaluation study in England and Scotland. School of Nursing, Midwifery and Health Visiting, University of Manchester, Manchester

Channell W 2002 Helping students to learn in the clinical environment. Nursing Times 98(39):34–35

Chickering A, Ehrmann S 1996 Implementing the seven principles. AAHEBulletin.com. Available on line at: www.aahe.org/technology/ehrmann.htm

Clarke N 2003 The relationship between workplace environment and different learning outcomes. Paper presented at the University of Greenwich Work and Employment Research Unit Seminar Series, December

Clarke N 2004 Developing effective workplace learning in UK hospices: findings, issues and challenges. University of Greenwich, London

Clinical Standards Board for Scotland 2002 Clinical standards: specialist palliative care. NHS Quality Improvement Scotland, Edinburgh

Conway J 1994 Reflection, the art and science of nursing and the theory–practice gap. British Journal of Nursing 3:114–118

Cotton A 2001 Private thoughts in public spheres: issues in reflection and reflective practices in nursing. Journal of Advanced Nursing 36:512–519

Cranton P 1994 Understanding and promoting transformative learning. Jossey-Bass, San Francisco, CA

Dearing R 1997 Higher education in the learning society. Report. DH, London

Department of Health 1993 A vision for the future. National Health Service Management Executive, London

Department of Health 1994 Clinical supervision for the nursing and health visiting professions. CNO Professional Letter 94, 11 February. DH, London

Department of Health 2001a Working together – learning together. A framework for lifelong learning in the NHS. DH, London

Department of Health 2001b Preparation of mentors and teachers. DH, London

Department of Health 2003 The NHS knowledge and skills framework. Scottish Executive, Edinburgh

Department of Health 2004 Agenda for change. Scottish Executive, Edinburgh.

Dewey J 1933 How do we think: a restatement of the relation of reflective thinking to the educative process. Heath, Lexington, MA

Dowswell T, Hewison J, Hinds M 1998 Motivational forces affecting participation in post-registration degree courses and effects on home and work life: a qualitative study. Journal of Advanced Nursing 28:1326–1333

Dreyfus S, Dreyfus H 1980 A five stage model of the mental activities involved in directed skill acquisition. Unpublished report supported by the Air Force Office of Scientific Research, University of California, Berkley, CA

Duarri W, Kendrick K 1999 Implementing clinical supervision. Professional Nurse 14:849–852

Duffy K, Docherty C, Cardnuff L et al 2000 The nurse lecturer's role in mentoring the mentors. Nursing Standard 15(6):35–38

Earl S 2002 Postgraduate Certificate in Teaching and Learning in Higher Education. Guidelines for mentors. Napier University, Edinburgh

Ellington H, Percival F, Race P 1993 Handbook of education technology, 3rd edn. Kogan Page, London

Entwistle N 1981 Styles of learning and teaching. John Wiley, Chichester

Fitzgerald M 1989 The lecturer-practitioner: action researcher. Unpublished thesis, University of Wales, Cardiff

Fowler J 1996 How to use models of clinical supervision in practice. Nursing Standard 10(29):42–47

Gibbs G 1988 Learning by doing: a guide to teaching and learning methods. Oxford: Further Education Unit, Oxford Polytechnic, Oxford

Goorapah D 1997 Clinical supervision. Journal of Clinical Nursing 6:173–178

Hannigan B 2001 A discussion of the strengths and weaknesses of reflection in nursing practice and education. Journal of Clinical Nursing 10:278–283

Hewison A, Wildman S 1996 The theory–practice gap in nursing: a new dimension. Journal of Advanced Nursing 24:754–761

Highland Hospice 2003 Nurse competency framework (level 2). Highland Hospice, Inverness

Hoban V 2004 Franco-British palliative care MSc is underway. Nursing Times 100(33):147

Hospice Information Service 2005 eChoices. Available on line from: www.hospiceinformation.info/training.asp

Jeffery D 2002 Teaching palliative care – a practical guide. Radcliffe Medical, Oxford

John C 2004 How to set up a learning network. Nursing Times 100(30):48–49

Johns C 2000 Becoming a reflective practitioner. Blackwell Science, Oxford

Johns P 1992 Reflective practice and nursing. Nurse Education Today 12:174–181

Jones A 2003 Some benefits experienced by hospice nurses from group clinical supervision. European Journal of Cancer Care 12:224–232

Kenny A 2002 Online learning: enhancing nurse education? Journal of Advanced Nursing 38:127–135

Knowles MS 1984 Andragogy in action: applying modern principles of adult learning. Jossey-Bass, San Francisco, CA

Kolb D 1982 Experiential learning: experience as the source of learning and development. Prentice Hall, Englewood Cliffs, NJ

Krahe B 1992 Personality and social psychology: towards a synthesis. Sage, London

Lahteenmaki S, Toivonen J, Mattila M 2001 Critical aspects of organisational learning research and proposals for its measurement. British Journal of Management 12:113–129

Luft J 1969 Of human interaction. National Press, Palo Alto, CA

McCarty M, Higgins A 2003 Moving to an all graduate profession: preparing preceptors for their role. Nurse Education Today 23:89–95

McDermott R 1999 Why information technology inspired but cannot deliver knowledge management. California Management Review 41:103–117

Magnusson A, Lutzen K, Severinsson E 2002 The influence of clinical supervision on ethical issues in home care of people with mental illness in Sweden. Journal of Nursing Management 10:37–45

Major C 1999 Connecting what to know and what we do through problem based learning. AAHE Bulletin 51(7):7–9

Manley K, Garbett B 2000 Paying Peter and Paul: reconciling concepts of expertise with competency for a clinical career structure. Journal of Clinical Nursing: 9:347–359

Marie Curie Cancer Care 2004 Spiritual and religious care competencies for specialist palliative care. Marie Curie Cancer Care, Edinburgh

Marie Curie Cancer Care Education 2004 Marie Curie Cancer Care education strategy (2004–2007). Marie Curie Cancer Care, Edinburgh

Markham T 2002 Response to: 'Private thoughts in public spheres: issues in reflection and reflective practices in nursing'. Journal of Advanced Nursing 38:286–287

Marton F, Saljo R 1996 Approaches to learning. In: Marton F, Hounsell D, Entwisle N (eds) The experience of learning, 2nd edn. Scottish Academic Press, Edinburgh

Milligan F 1998 Defining and assessing competence: the distraction of outcomes and the importance of educational process. Nurse Education Today 18:273–280

Morris D, Turnbull P 2004 Using student nurses as teachers in inquiry-based learning. Journal of Advanced Nursing 45:136–144

National Health Service University 2004 www.nhsu.nhs.uk

Naysmith A 2004 Clinical governance in specialist palliative care. International Journal of Palliative Nursing 10:329–332

NCHSPCS 1996 Education in palliative care. National Council for Hospice and Specialist Palliative Care Services, London

NICE 2004 Guidance of cancer services: improving supportive and palliative care for patients with cancer, the manual. National Institute for Clinical Excellence, London

Nursing and Midwifery Council 2002a Supporting nurses and midwives through lifelong learning. NMC, London

Nursing and Midwifery Council 2002b Employers and PREP. NMC, London

Nursing and Midwifery Council 2002c Code of professional conduct. NMC, London. Available on line at: www.nmc-uk.org

Nursing and Midwifery Council 2003 NMC News, winter (4). NMC, London. Available on line at: www.nmc-uk.org/nmc/main/publications/$NMCNews

Nursing and Midwifery Council 2004a The PREP handbook: protecting the public through professional standards. NMC, London

Nursing and Midwifery Council 2004b Clinical supervision. Available on line at: www.nmc-uk.org/nmc/main/advice/clinicalSupervision.html

O'Connor A, Hyde A, Treacy M 2003 Nurse teachers' constructions of reflection and reflective practice. Reflective Practice 4:107–119

O'Dowd A 2003 Judging competence. Nursing Times 99(9):22–24

Oxford 1999 The Concise Oxford dictionary, 10th edn. Oxford University Press, Oxford

Quinn F 2000 The principles and practice of nurse education. Nelson Thornes, Cheltenham

Race P, Brown S 1993 500 Tips for tutors. Kogan Page, London

Royal College of Nursing 2002 A framework for nurses working in specialist palliative care. Competencies project. RCN, London. Available on line at: www.rcn.org.uk

Scottish Partnership for Palliative Care 2004 SPPC Annual Conference held at Dunblane Scotland September 2004. Available on line at: www.palliativecarescotland.org.uk

Severinsson E 1996 Nurse supervisors' views of their supervisory styles in clinical supervision: a hermeneutical approach. Journal of Nursing Management 4:191–199

Soriano R, Bensinger L 2004 Becoming a medical teacher: a novel elective teaching medical students how to teach. Journal of the American Geriatrics Society 52(Suppl 1):S89

Spalding N 1998 Reflection in professional development: a personal experience. British Journal of Therapy and Rehabilitation 5:379–382

Stiles M 2004 Teaching others new skills can aid your own learning. Nursing Times 100(26):66–67

Stratos G, Bergen M, Skeff K 2004 Embedding faculty development in teaching hospitals: moving beyond the status quo. Journal of General Internal Medicine 19:286–287

Teekman B 2000 Exploring reflective thinking in nursing practice. Journal of Advanced Nursing 31:1125–1135

Tennant M 1997 Psychology and adult learning, 2nd edn. Routledge, London

Twycross R, Wilcock A 2001 Symptom management in advanced cancer, 3rd edn. Radcliffe Medical, Oxford

Ward R 2001 Internet skills for nurses. Mental Health Practice 4:31–38

Watson S 2000 The support that mentors receive in the clinical setting. Nurse Education Today 20:585–592

Williams B 2001 Developing critical reflection for professional practice through problem based learning. Journal of Advanced Nursing 34:27–34

Wood S 1998 Ethics and communication: developing reflective practice. Nursing Standard 12(18):45–47

CHAPTER THREE

Holistic care

Christine M Pearce, Anthony Duffy

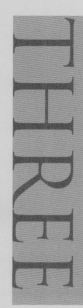

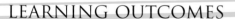

LEARNING OUTCOMES

This chapter will assist the reader to:

- Explore the meaning of holism within the context of palliative care practice
- Briefly review key policy and professional developments that support an holistic approach to palliative care
- Review the broad principles and aims of holistic assessment in palliative care
- Discuss the contribution of the multiprofessional team to holistic palliative care provision.

Everywhere the whole, even the least and most insignificant apparently, is the real wonder, the miracle which holds the secrets for which we are groping in thought and conduct. Here is the within which is the beyond.

Smuts 1927

WHAT IS HOLISM?

The word 'holism' is commonly used within health-care settings but where does it come from and what does it mean? The word 'whole' comes from the Greek *holos* meaning entire or whole and the Greek word derived from the Indo-European root *solo*, meaning firm, sound or correct (Aronson 2003).

When applying the concept of holism to states of health, Illich (1975, cited in Buckley 2002) held that health can be influenced by an individual's ability to adapt to changing environments, to ageing, to times of suffering and to the expectation of death. This implies that individuals have the potential to influence their own lives and that holistic care should consider the whole human experience. Using the diagram illustrated in Figure 3.1, Illich advocated that holism should be conceived as a number of facets, which form important elements of the human response in health and illness.

Central to this model is the idea that personal/inner resources are as important as external ones and that there is a link between the body and the mind. However, this link has not always been readily accepted and this has led to many decades of controversy and argument in health care. This issue will be looked at in detail later.

HOW DOES HOLISTIC CARE RELATE TO QUALITY OF LIFE?

Quality of life can be understood as 'an individual's subjective satisfaction with life and is affected by all the dimensions of personhood – physical, psychological, social and spiritual' (Twycross 1999, p. 4).

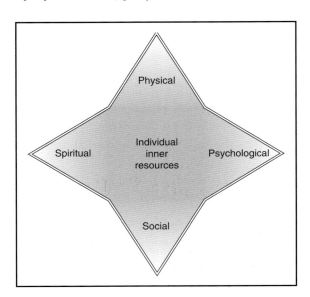

Figure 3.1 Facets of holism (with permission from Illich 1975).

It is apparent that all the elements of personhood that influence a patient's global assessment of quality of life are the same aspects of personhood that need to be considered by the holistic health-care practitioner. Ill health can be caused by a virus, disease or cancer but because people are holistic beings the physical illness can also have detrimental effects upon psychological, social and spiritual wellbeing. When nursing a person back to health, all aspects of that person's humanity must be considered. A healthy individual is no longer perceived to be someone in whom physical disease is absent (Sarafino 1998). Quality of life is a better outcome measure of good nursing care than eradication of disease. This concept is especially important in palliative care, where often there is little hope of physical cure but there is great benefit to be gained by addressing other aspects of the illness such as social isolation, psychological distress and spiritual pain. The framework of holism can be directly applied to patient care in any setting and delivering holistic care can help the person who is experiencing life-threatening illness to maintain the best possible quality of life up to and including the point of death.

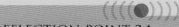

REFLECTION POINT 3.1
Facets of holism

Think for a few moments about all the personal things that you believe contribute to your general health and wellbeing (your quality of life). Make a list of these things so you can refer back to them as you read on.

After you've made your list, look again at Illich's facets of holism and consider how your list relates to this model. You may have chosen such things as independence and the right to make your own choices in life. In any form of illness these and many more elements of perceived quality of life are challenged and when the illness is life-threatening the challenges are greater still.

WHY IS HOLISTIC CARE SO IMPORTANT IN PALLIATIVE CARE?

In the previous section the relationship between holistic care and the promotion of quality of life was discussed. Holistic care is a central concept of palliative care. This can be seen in the internationally accepted definition of the World Health Organization (WHO) as to what palliative care entails:

an approach that improves the quality of life of patients and their families facing the problem associated with life-threatening illness, through the prevention and relief of suffering by means of early identification and impeccable assessment and treatment of pain and other problems, physical, psychosocial and spiritual.

World Health Organization 2003

Palliative care obtained its holistic focus from the modern hospice movement from which it developed. Hospice care took its philosophy and direction from the work of Dame Cicely Saunders, who insisted that each patient was assessed as a 'whole person' who possessed unique perceptions, beliefs and needs (Aranda 1999, Kabel & Roberts 2003). It aims to offer expertise and support based on trust and mutual respect for patients and families and relates to the importance of acknowledging and working alongside the whole person as they experience the changes brought about by life-threatening illness. Palliative care is an active approach to managing the whole patient and family (Higginson & Addington-Hall 1999) and, as such, embraces all that is important to the patient throughout the course of the illness and for the family in their bereavement.

REFLECTION POINT 3.2
Concerns of the critically ill

If you were to become seriously ill you would obviously have many concerns about your health but what other things would you worry about as your illness progressed?

You may have identified some important factors about the ways in which you respond to issues of health and illness. You may have expanded ideas about how much the social aspects of our lives are affected by illness, how debility can diminish our self-esteem, and our feelings of self-control. You may also have gained some further insight into your use of coping strategies.

HOW DO YOU TREAT ILLNESS IF NOT HOLISTICALLY?

Holism and Cicely Saunders's philosophy of care is based upon a belief that all aspects of a person must be considered during the treatment of illness and the promotion of quality of life. However, such an approach has not been readily accepted in the past and directly challenged the medical model that dominated health care in the UK in the 20th century. This model, often called *biomedicine*, conceptualised illness as a dysfunction of the corporeal body. The mind was considered to be something quite separate and, as such, had no influence upon the body's state of health (Ogden 2000). This mind–body divide, or *cartesian dualism*, is often attributed to the writings of the Renaissance mathematician René Descartes (Sarafino 1998), although the separation of the mind from the body was never Descartes's intention and is increasingly regarded as a misreading of his work (Duncan 2000, Engebretson 1997, Kirkeboen 2001, Paley 2002).

Sullivan (1986) argues that the characteristics of biomedicine developed because of the way in which disease was studied. Knowledge was primarily derived from observations made during autopsies where the nature and extent of disease took precedence over the experience of illness. This approach means that the objective evidence of disease and treatment can be valued to the exclusion of subjective evidence. The strong influence biomedicine still has upon clinical practice is evident in the fact that only objective studies based upon quantitative and parametric data can be regarded as being 'gold standard' when trying to determine best practice in palliative care (NICE 2004).

Stated simply, the sort of medical and nursing care a patient with cancer would receive if cared for under the biomedical paradigm could be excellent in many areas but potentially poor in many others. Seeking to promote homeostasis by curing people of disease when the body becomes upset by the presence of antigens, the biomedical approach requires the patient to submit their diseased body to the care of health-care experts for treatment. The view that the mind had no influence upon physical health meant that it was not usually considered necessary for the surgeon, oncologist or radiotherapist to ask about how the illness was making the patient feel. It was the patient's responsibility to seek help, such as talking to a priest or trusted friend, when difficult thoughts made life unbearable. If the mind became too distraught, the patient could be referred to a psychiatrist. Using the biomedical model, mental ill health is conceived as due to chemical imbalances in the central nervous system and is treated with drugs. Sometimes surgery on the body was performed to treat mental or behavioural problems. For example, many women received hysterectomies to promote calmness of mind and happiness (Duin & Sutcliffe 1992).

For several decades after the creation of the National Health Service (NHS) in 1948, the biomedical model of care was very much to the fore, as can be seen by this era of health care being identified with the phrase 'nanny state' (Clark et al 1997). Boasting that it would care for the British population from the cradle to the grave, two main NHS objectives were to eliminate infectious diseases and to prevent or find cures for the other killers such as cancer (Rivett 1998).

Although care of the dying was never ignored, greater attention and resources were spent on preventative medicine and curing acute illnesses than on palliative care (Clark & Seymour 1999, Whynes 1997). Indeed, caring for the incurable is not a need easily addressed by the biomedical model of care, which can result in dying patients being offered futile treatments that may have no therapeutic benefits (Clark 2002). In addition, research in the 1970s and 1980s demonstrated that the practical, emotional and social needs of the dying were not being met within the NHS (Higginson 1993).

The biomedical fight against disease has been highly successful in many areas, especially in certain cancers such as breast cancer and childhood leukaemia (Rivett 1998). Unfortunately, the mental wellbeing of patients was often overlooked. This may be regarded as acceptable if you believe your role is to fight disease and the mind has no influence upon health and illness. However, the holistic approach asks us to consider the patient not just as a diagnosis but as a person who may require our help with issues other than just the physical. Is there any justification or evidence to suggest that palliative care practitioners are correct in asking nurses to consider a patient as an ill person rather than just a diseased body?

((((●))))

REFLECTION POINT 3.3

The patient as an ill person

Reflect upon the assessment method you are asked to use in your clinical practice area when an ill person is encountered for the first time. How many of the questions you ask are focused upon the physical effects of the illness and how many focus upon other aspects of the patient such as their psychological wellbeing, spiritual health or social comfort?

WHY SHOULD WE FOCUS ON THE PERSON AND NOT JUST THE ILLNESS?

For holism to be accepted as the main paradigm of care it has to demonstrate that the biomedical model, despite its great successes, is flawed because it focuses upon fighting somatic disease almost to the exclusion of promoting health and quality of life. One way to do this is to demonstrate that there is no such thing as cartesian dualism. One fascinating area of scientific study that seeks to demonstrate the body–mind link is psychoneuroimmunology (PNI). PNI has conducted psychological studies into how life events are evaluated as stressors and investigated how stress alters the effectiveness of the body's immune system (Ogden 2000).

To preserve a healthy homeostasis, our bodies need to be constantly checking for the presence of 'invaders' and, once detected, to be able to destroy these bacteria or viruses by the activation of specific lymphocytes (Tortora & Grabowski 2003). With regards to cancer, the human body constantly maintains immunological surveillance so as to detect mutated cells. Once these are identified, the body can create specific T cells that attack and destroy cancer before it can establish itself as a threat to normal physical function (Tortora & Grabowski 2003). Several physical attributes, such as ageing, have long been identified as reducing the effectiveness of the body's immune function (Tortora & Grabowski 2003) – thus leading to a greater incidence of cancer in this population – but for a long time it was not believed that the immune system interacted with the central nervous system (Ogden 2000).

However, PNI research suggests that thoughts, feelings, emotions, personality and beliefs can all influence health and the course of disease and it has worked to demonstrate this link over the last three decades. Poorly managed stress and depression have been demonstrated to lower T-cell count and certain people, such as those who feel that they have little control over events that influence them, have personalities that appear to increase the likelihood of them getting cancer and, once present, can accelerate the speed at which cancer develops (Baum & Posluszny 1999, Cohen et al 2000, Ogden 2000). The pathway of interactions between the mind and the body is becoming clearer and more defined (Reiche et al 2004), allowing for some simple (but very non-biomedical) interventions to be suggested that may promote not only comfort but also physical resistance to cancer and its progression. Some examples of this are laughter, so to enhance mood (Bennett et al 2003), the use of complementary therapies (Goodfellow 2003) and the involvement of patients in clinical decision-making so to promote a sense of control over events (Brosschot et al 1998).

The biomedical approach has been accused of medicalising the dying process, resulting in patients dying unnatural deaths (Biswas & Ahmedzai 1993, Illich 1975 cited in Clark 2002), although this same medicalisation has also been praised for greatly improving symptom management in palliative care (Clark 2002). Certainly, one of the great achievements of Cicely Saunders was the improvements she achieved in the medical management of symptoms in terminal care (Rivett 1998).

However, nursing literature often states that you cannot effectively manage the symptoms of advanced disease without also understanding how the experience and the meaning of each symptom is affecting the patient (Haworth & Dluhy 2001). It is becoming evident that nursing care of terminally ill and cancer patients will not be of a high standard unless the patient is cared for holistically. For example, recent research demonstrates that the management of pain in advanced cancer patients is greatly improved when psychological, social and spiritual elements are addressed in conjunction with the physical causes of discomfort (Ashby & Dowding 2001). The introduction of nursing models has been credited with making nursing care more patient-centred and holistic (Archibald 2000). However, it is interesting that the dominant nursing model of the 1980s and early 1990s paid great attention to 'activities of daily living' and evaluated physical ability to self-care far more than it investigated the meaning of the illness for the patient's life. It may be argued that nursing models suggested the introduction of holistic care rather than espousing it. Return to your answers for Reflection point 3.3: how holistic do you think the nursing model you currently use is?

The holistic paradigm of care should not be regarded as the correct approach to effective patient care replacing an incorrect biomedical approach. There is nothing wrong with biomedicine. It is just limited in its perception of patient care. It is released from its shackles by the integration of holistic principles into the processes of assessment, choice of intervention and evaluation of care. This encourages the health-care professional to see the patient as a person and not just a disease. It also encourages professionals to realise that they have a duty to care for the whole family unit and not to attempt to exclude spouses and siblings in the belief that 'they are not my concern'.

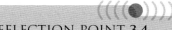

REFLECTION POINT 3.4
Factors influencing quality of life

Return to Reflection point 3.1 and reflect upon those factors that you think contribute to your sense of wellbeing and quality of life. How often do you think things go wrong and what stress does that make you feel? Have you ever considered that difficult or adverse life-events might affect your body's ability to fight cancer or other illnesses?

WHO SAYS THAT NURSES SHOULD PROVIDE HOLISTIC CARE?

The WHO definition of palliative care (World Health Organization 2003) clearly states what attributes must be addressed so as to ensure good nursing practice and the best patient outcomes when caring for people diagnosed with a life-threatening illness. It is clear that best practice is synonymous with holistic care. This link has been reinforced recently in England and Wales with the publication of a report by the National Institute for Clinical Excellence (NICE) designed to give guidance to service providers to ensure patients with cancer, with their families and carers, receive the level of support and care required to cope effectively with the cancer diagnosis, its treatment at all stages and changes in prognosis (NICE 2004). All aspects of personhood are considered and recommendations are made to help identify best practice.

The NICE (2004) guideline can be seen as the latest development from a 10-year investigation into what patients and care providers want from their health service. In a major survey of public, carer and patient perceptions of health care in England, in preparation for the NHS Plan (Department of Health 2000a), it was clear that most people wanted NHS services to be more patient-centred so that the recipient of care was treated as a person as well as a collection of symptoms (Office for Public Management 2000). This survey also revealed that medical professionals who have a biomedical rather than a holistic approach are regarded as patronising (Office for Public Management 2000). Although the public and patients' perceptions of nurses' attitudes were not investigated, it could also be assumed that nurses who fail to care for their patients holistically may also be negatively labelled. This can cause barriers to communication and trust between patient and nurse, which may have adverse consequences for quality of care.

The NICE guideline also reinforces the belief that good holistic care cannot be provided only by doctors and nurses. All the major national English and Welsh government cancer-related publications over the last 10 years have identified that the highest standard of care may only be achieved through the adoption of multiprofessional and multidisciplinary team working (Department of Health 2000b, Expert Advisory Group on Cancer 1995, National Assembly for Wales 2001). It is clear that nurses who want to provide good palliative care to their patients must not only regard the patients and their families holistically but must also be prepared to communicate effectively and work in collaboration with other professional groups, such as social workers, physiotherapists and occupational therapists, to ensure that the patient's holistic needs are met.

Patients with cancer are not alone in their need to be cared for in a holistic way. Good evidence exists to suggest that people with other progressive conditions such as Parkinson's disease and human immunodeficiency virus (HIV) infection, and children with inherited disorders, have needs that can be met by the holistic approach used within palliative care (Farrell & Sutherland 1998, Goldman 1998, Kutzen 2003, Lee et al 2004, McPherson 2004, World Health Organization 2003). In England, there is already a concerted effort to include palliative care principles in coronary heart disease care within the NHS (Department of Health 2000c). The holistic palliative care approach can be applied to all health and social care settings if it is based on a comprehensive assessment of need.

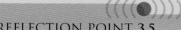

REFLECTION POINT 3.5
Guidelines in holistic care

Can you identify a guideline or protocol in your local practice area that encourages you to consider the patients' holistic needs and not just focus upon an aspect of physical care?

HOW DOES A PALLIATIVE CARE NURSE APPLY HOLISTIC PRINCIPLES TO PATIENT CARE?

As in all care settings the overriding principles of assessment, planning, implementation and evaluation apply. What must the nurse do to make these holistic in nature and application?

HOLISTIC ASSESSMENT IN PALLIATIVE CARE

Although it is acknowledged that assessment is the key to effective care planning, ongoing evidence tells us that professionals are not eliciting patients' problems or concerns (NICE 2004). In the previous quote from WHO, the emphasis on 'impeccable assessment' is clear and supports the view that without timely, comprehensive and sensitive assessment, quality palliative care cannot be achieved.

The National Institute for Clinical Excellence (NICE 2004) emphasises the need to undertake assessment at key points throughout the course of the patient's illness. Based within the context of self-help and informal support, this emphasises the nature of continuous assessment and evaluation and offers models of assessment and support for use by all levels of health-care professional, such as the model of professional psychological assessment and support, in which a range of psychological skills and expertise are identified and linked to both the appropriate professional group and relevant assessment target (NICE 2004, p. 7).

Further support for this argument comes from end-of-life care initiatives such as the Gold Standards Framework (Thomas 2003) and the Liverpool Care Pathway for the Dying Patient (Ellershaw & Wilkinson 2003). All these documents reiterate the importance of systematic and consistent assessment of patient and family needs from the point of diagnosis and at intervals throughout the course of the illness.

But how can we apply holistic principles in the assessment of a person facing life-threatening illness? Some of the themes in current published articles on holistic nursing refer to the concepts of 'personhood' and 'person-centredness' (Ford & McCormack 2000, Kabel & Roberts 2003, Kelly 1999, McCormack 2003, Olsen 1997, Wurzbach 1999). What do these terms mean?

REFLECTION POINT 3.6

Personhood

A person becomes who they are as the result of many influences over time.

In Reflection points 3.1 and 3.2 you were asked to consider issues related to your own health and illness. The way in which you responded to those questions has everything to do with you as a person, your personal experience, upbringing and a host of other factors.

- What do you think are the influences that have made you a unique person?

By working through the above reflection point you will have gained further insight into the development of your own personhood. Personhood as a concept is defined by Armstrong & Fitzgerald (1996, cited in Kabel & Roberts 2003) as 'one's identity as a social person'. They go on to suggest that the boundaries of personhood vary between cultures. In reflecting, you may have identified some of the following factors: your current health status, beliefs, personality, gender, values, age, life experience, financial status, cultural heritage, intellect/education, social status and stage in the life cycle (Gross 2004).

These broad categories are predictable in the main but will be quite different in detail, meaning and effect for each of us. It is the detail that can help us to understand the complexities of what personhood means to an individual and how we can use sensitive assessment skills to promote and sustain well-being.

Let us find out what such categories have to offer in the form of a holistic assessment tool for use in clinical practice. To achieve this we will select a clinical case scenario as an example.

CASE STUDY 3.1
Joe

Mr Joseph Franklin was 79 when he was referred by his hospital consultant to the local palliative care team, for assessment and management of chronic obstructive pulmonary disease (COPD) at home.

Mr Franklyn, or Joe as he liked to be called, had spent many years as a steel worker in the north-east of England but following the death of his wife some 2 years earlier had moved to Essex to be near his only daughter and her family.

Joe had been managing by himself for a year after his bereavement but had found the physical effort of cooking, cleaning and shopping an increasing burden. Since moving to Essex, Joe had been admitted to hospital on a number of occasions for the management of breathlessness and repeated chest infections but was increasingly reluctant to accept further hospital inpatient care, preferring to stay in his bungalow with his daughter providing as much of his care as possible, given her own family commitments.

At first glance there might seem to be few issues that require attention. Joe has a daughter to look after him and, although his pulmonary function is poor and breathlessness is a problem, he appears to be managing well on the whole. Let us use the factors above and see if they help us to learn more about Joe.

Person-centred assessment

Assessment focus	Assessment findings
Health status – physical and psychological	Joe's health had always been good until the onset of COPD at around the age of 58. Joe's lung disease had now advanced and was exacerbated by coexisting problems of anaemia and arthritis. His vision was becoming weaker but his hearing was good. Joe had smoked from the age of 11 years and accepted that this had contributed to his current health status.
	In terms of nutrition, before moving to Essex Joe had survived on processed supermarket meals and baked beans, with little in the way of fresh vegetables and fruit.
	Joe's sleep pattern was poor: he found it difficult to sleep sitting up in bed, so he often spent the night sitting in an armchair.
	Joe's main concern now was his breathlessness, weakness and lack of interest in life. He had never felt like this before.

Continued

CASE STUDY **3.1**—CONT'D

Gender	Joe describes himself as 'a man's man' and attributes this to his upbringing and work experience in the steel works. Joe's wife was similarly traditional in her upbringing and never expected Joe to cook or undertake domestic chores. As his illness developed Joe had been cared for devotedly by his wife until her sudden death 2 years ago. Joe had been an active trade union man, and as such had been a member of close and supportive employment and social groups.
Experience	Joe had seen his father die early as a result of an industrial accident, and his younger brother die from lung cancer in the late 1960s. In both cases his memories of their medical and nursing care were bad ones, leaving him anxious and mistrustful of health services. Joe's recent experience of the health service was based on investigations and management of his COPD and, although this was relatively straightforward and involved mainly outpatient care his views of the health service hadn't really changed.
Intellect/education	Although Joe had left school early to join his father in the steel industry, he had always read widely and enjoyed furthering his education later in life by taking a course on politics when he retired.
Beliefs	Joe was a committed atheist, with a healthy respect for human strength and human rights. Joe's health beliefs were clear: when he became aware of the risks associated with smoking he could have stopped but, since he didn't drink to excess or gamble, he believed it was a pleasure for which he was prepared to take health risks – 'you've gotta die from something'.
Values	Joe had valued his long marriage and the companionship it provided. He and his wife shared a love of music, the countryside and political views. Joe had been an active member of the Labour Party for many years until recently, when his deteriorating health had curtailed his involvement.
Financial status	Joe had never earned a great deal but felt that he had a pension sufficient for his needs.
Social status	Until 4 years ago Joe and his wife Eileen had been popular members of various clubs, but this had stopped as a result of his advancing illness and his wife's death. His move to Essex had left him isolated, with the exception of visits from his daughter and her family.

Personality	Joe had always been an optimistic person with energy and motivation. He had been able to withstand difficulties, and coped with life's crises in a forthright way, preferring honesty to kindness. Now Joe was expressing uncharacteristic feelings of fatigue and defeat.
Age	Joe had survived active service during the war and accepted risk-taking as a part of life.
Cultural heritage	Joe was proud of his family's working class history and long links with the steel industry, and he had been proud to fight for his country. Joe's family had all been 'God-fearing folk' and their home had been strict but loving.
Stage in the life cycle	Joe had lived a long and active life. He had brought up one child with whom he had a good relationship. Joe retired at 60 because of his lung disease but continued to be active until his wife's death. As a widower, Joe was finding the loss of his wife of 57 years difficult to bear. He loved his daughter, son-in-law and grandson, but felt that his life had little quality left.

By employing these broad categories as a guide it is possible to develop quite a comprehensive picture of Joe as a person, and to establish the things that are important to him.

This kind of assessment can be carried out over a few days: the sensitive approach and discussion necessary to discover such information requires good communication skills and the desire to form a therapeutic relationship based on mutual respect and trust.

In addition to gaining insight into an individual's personhood, it is essential to obtain information about that person's experience within the context of a specific illness. In this case another guide to assessment – the 'total pain concept' adapted from the work of Cicely Saunders (1990)–can be used to good effect (Fig. 3.2).

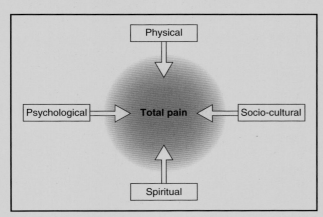

Figure 3.2 Palliative care approach to symptom management: total pain concept (with permission from Saunders 1990).

The total pain concept can help us to assess pain and other symptoms in the light of their relationship to a range of emotions and practical issues. Use of the model gives us an opportunity to look behind the obvious problems and to appreciate how the different elements of symptom distress are interdependent. A person's experience of pain, for example, is exacerbated by anxiety. If you can discover what is making the patient anxious, your interventions for the management of pain will be enhanced.

This model asks us to look beyond the physical and examine what is worrying the patient. It acknowledges the effect that emotions such as anxiety, anger and depression have on the perception of symptom distress, and it gives expression to the complexity of the individual patient's experience.

REFLECTION POINT 3.7
Using the total pain concept

- Given the picture of Joe as a person that you formed from the earlier assessment process, how do you think you can develop and expand your holistic assessment of Joe using the Saunders model?

- Using the total pain concept, take each section and think about the kinds of skills you will need to employ to assess Joe's needs effectively.

The use of any model of assessment requires the application of certain core principles. Assessment must be:

- Based on a relationship of trust and mutual respect
- Centred on analysis of patients' and relatives' changing needs
- Communicated within the multiprofessional team
- Documented to create a timely and effective plan of care.

REFLECTION POINT 3.8
Tools to inform assessment practice

When you are next at work, investigate the basis of assessment practice in your clinical area, and identify tools that may be in use to inform assessment practice.

Assessment principles will help us to be alongside the patient and family and to provide care in a sensitive and dynamic way.

Whatever the basis of assessment practice in your clinical area, assessment is rarely the responsibility of one health-care professional alone and, depending upon the stage of a patient's illness, they may be receiving health and social care from a wide range of agencies.

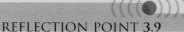

REFLECTION POINT 3.9

The palliative care team

Think about a patient you have cared for recently and, using the total pain concept as a guide, identify all the people who were in any way involved in providing palliative care and support to the patient and family.

You may have identified some of the following:

- Hospital consultant
- Complementary therapist
- Art/music therapist
- Day services staff
- Marie Curie nurse
- Counsellor.

Each of the professionals involved in a patient's care will plan their intervention on the basis of an assessment of need, and may elicit information in a number of different ways. These findings, when communicated effectively within the care team, will add to our understanding of the whole person and how best to support both patient and family.

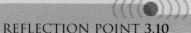

REFLECTION POINT 3.10

Patient assessment

Think for a few moments about assessment of patients in your own clinical area. Make some notes about the kind of assessment detail that is recorded – by whom and where?

You may find that the majority of assessment outcomes are entered into patients' medical and nursing notes and relate to physical elements of care more than any other. You may also find that these notes are almost exclusively written by medical and nursing staff. But, with the range of people involved in the assessment and delivery of care, is this appropriate?

The National Institute for Clinical Excellence's key recommendation 3 tells us that:

each multidisciplinary team or service should implement processes to ensure effective interprofessional communication within teams and between them and other service providers with whom the patient has contact. Mechanisms should be developed to promote continuity of care, which might include the nomination of a person to take on the role of 'key worker' for individual patients.

NICE 2004

Assessment, therefore, is as much a team responsibility as an individual one but, as you found earlier in your reflective exercise, the multiprofessional team can be large and complex.

MULTIPROFESSIONAL TEAM WORKING

The provision of comprehensive and quality palliative care for any patient demands a wide range of expertise, which can only be achieved within the multiprofessional team. A team is an active, constantly changing, dynamic force in which a number of people come together to discuss objectives, assess ideas, make decisions and work together towards a common goal (Heller 1998). The multiprofessional membership of a team will be governed by the needs of the patient and family, and may be as minimal as the general practitioner (GP), the specialist palliative care nurse (SPCN) and the district nurse (DN) delivering care in the patient's own home, or as complex as the hospice palliative care consultant (HPCC) and nursing staff, psychologist, speech therapist, dietitian and physiotherapist extending care in a hospice setting. As the team membership increases, so does the risk of team difficulties in communication and the application of quality care. To avoid such difficulties the principles of effective teamwork must be observed. Effective teamwork principles include the following elements.

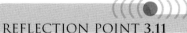

REFLECTION POINT 3.11
Effective multidisciplinary teams

Take a moment to reflect upon a team that you have been part of; what were the things that made your team effective?

You may have identified many of the following elements:

- **Team membership**: Team members are selected on skills/strengths appropriate to the agreed goals
- **Direction**: Each member of the team understands where they are going
- **Goal orientation**: The goals are set based on discussion of the options, and are clear to all members of the team
- **Decision-making**: All relevant members of the team are involved in agreed decisions

- **Communication**: Each member of the team listens, understands and contributes to the team's work
- **Information**: Available facts are revealed within the team and checked
- **Participation**: Each individual team member is involved in the work
- **Atmosphere/culture**: Individuals are interested and committed to team goals
- **Time**: Available time is planned and used well. (Adapted from Hayes 1997 and Heller 1998.)

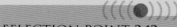

REFLECTION POINT 3.12
Effect of team difficulties on holistic care

Think about the last time you met with your professional team, and using the above principles, consider the effect of any identified deficits in team working on holistic patient care.

To illustrate how effective teamwork principles can enhance holistic palliative care, let us look at the case of Celia, a 74-year-old retired musician.

CASE STUDY 3.2
Celia

Celia was a 74-year-old single woman, who had enjoyed a busy and rewarding career as a concert pianist. Celia had always been accustomed to being in control of her life and her work and, although she had many friends, she was a very private lady. Celia had ignored a developing lump in her breast for more than 3 years, and it was not until she had fallen at home and was examined at her local Accident & Emergency Department that the breast lump was investigated and found to be malignant. Further investigations identified widespread bony metastases and a small left-sided pleural effusion.

The consultant oncologist asked the palliative care team to visit and, together with Celia, they discussed the diagnosis, treatment options and care.

Celia was generally well for her age and only her confidence had been damaged by the recent fall; she felt strongly that she did not want to undergo radical treatment regimes that could reduce her quality of life. She had greatly enjoyed her life and wanted to remain as well as possible and in her own home for as much as possible of the time that was left. She decided that, for her, palliation of symptoms as they arose was the best direction. The teams ensured that Celia had as much information as she needed and time to consider her choice, and when it was clear that her decision was made, palliation became the focus of care. Celia was transferred to the hospice for a period of 2 weeks, during which time she underwent palliative radiotherapy to reduce the tumour bulk,

Continued

CASE STUDY **3.2**—CONT'D

symptom control and assessment of her daily routines when at home to establish an energy conservation programme that would suit her diminishing energy reserves.

The complementary therapy nurse visited Celia to provide aromatherapy and massage, and to teach Celia relaxation techniques that she could use when at home.

The physiotherapist saw Celia each day to encourage gentle rehabilitation and, at her request, Celia's own vicar was contacted to discuss her spiritual and practical needs concerning her eventual death.

The hospice team collaborated with the primary care team to plan her discharge home and, with Celia's permission, involved her closest friend and neighbour in those plans.

Following discharge home, contact with the hospice was maintained by regular visits from the hospice's 'Hospice at Home' staff, who also provided expert advice and support for the community staff when necessary.

From this case study it can be seen that, based upon Celia's expressed needs and with effective communication between the individuals concerned, an appropriate holistic plan of care was developed to provide the best possible opportunities for quality of life. This is in concordance with key recommendation 4 (NICE 2004): 'Mechanisms should be in place to ensure the views of patients and carers are taken into account in developing and evaluating cancer and palliative care services.'

It is however often practically very difficult to develop assessment and care documentation that contains contributions from all those involved in care delivery. A recent development that goes a long way towards offering a solution to this difficulty is the Liverpool Care Pathway for the Dying Patient, developed by John Ellershaw (2002). This pathway is designed to be a record of planned care to which all members of the multiprofessional team are invited to contribute. It is based on comprehensive multiprofessional assessment and records both achievements and variances of expected care outcomes. The pathway provides us with a dynamic and responsive method for delivering quality palliative care.

Although originally designed for use within the hospital environment, the pathway can be adapted to other care settings.

Teamwork is essential if assessment and care delivery are to be effective, and holistic assessment is the ideal to promote quality nursing outcomes. The health service aims to deliver 24-hour care for patients in need, but can holistic assessment and management be achieved in the out-of-hours context?

Community patients and their carers continue to express feelings of uncertainty and anxiety in relation to out-of-hours care (King et al 2004). In this qualitative study, although carers reported feeling generally well supported by out-of-hours services, problems were identified associated with poor provision of information and inadequate communication with carers, difficulties in accessing night-sitter services and the inflexibility of services.

The Macmillan Gold Standards Framework developed by Dr Keri Thomas (2000, 2003) seeks to address these problems by offering a set of standards aimed at helping primary care teams to:

- Work as a team and ensure continuity of care
- Plan in advance for developments in a patient's illness
- Provide patients with the best symptom control
- Give support to patients and carers.

We have investigated some important evidence relating to principles of holistic assessment. Perhaps a brief case scenario that synthesises some of these elements and indicates their relevance to care management will help to illustrate the reality of such an approach.

Case study 3.3
Anne Jenner

Anne had been diagnosed with poorly differentiated cancer of the right breast 10 months before. She was a 38-year-old mother of two girls aged 7 and 9. A year earlier, Anne's mother had died from breast cancer. Anne's husband Peter was a self-employed engineer, whose job had occasionally taken him abroad for periods of up to 3 months at a time. Peter had lost his mother and aunt to breast cancer during the previous 9 years. Since diagnosis, Anne had been treated conservatively with surgery and radiotherapy. Further investigations had identified some secondary disease in the bone, and a small pleural effusion that had resolved after her radiotherapy treatment.

Anne was referred by her oncologist to the community palliative care team, who carried out a comprehensive assessment over the course of three visits. Relevant outcomes were used to plan the care management in the following way.

Assessment focus	Assessment findings	Care management
Assessment of health status (physiological needs)	On taking a clinical history Anne was reporting: • Bone pain – generally well controlled with a low dose of oral morphine and non-steroidal anti-inflammatory drugs • Sleep loss due to increasing breathlessness • Anxiety • Poor appetite • Constipation	Anne was prescribed laxatives and encouraged to eat the kind of foods that she knew helped in the past, which for Anne were dried prunes or pears, and live yoghurt. Anne was referred to the oncologist for assessment of her recurring breathlessness, which was the result of a further plural effusion and subsequent chest infection. This was treated by

Continued

CASE STUDY 3.3—CONT'D

Assessment focus	Assessment findings	Care management
	• The development of nodules behind her right knee and above her right third rib Anne spoke openly about her symptoms and considered that her two most distressing symptoms were constipation and breathlessness.	pleural aspiration and continual drainage via an ambulatory drainage system for management at home and to prevent further accumulation of fluid. A course of antibiotics successfully treated the chest infection. Anne's sleep pattern was largely restored following improvement in her breathing.
Assessment of health-care beliefs	Anne had been active and questioning in her approach to the diagnosis and treatment of her illness and had sought information from a range of sources, including Internet information sites, other health-care professionals and a friend who had been living with breast cancer for more than 5 years. Anne had acted on dietary advice, clear in the understanding that it was not a cure but could improve her general condition and ability to cope with the recommended forthcoming chemotherapeutic treatment. Anne's main concern at this time was for her two daughters, who she understood were at higher risk of developing cancer because of the direct relationship. Anne asked for information about who to consult about their future health.	In discussion with Anne it became evident that she was worried about the proposed chemotherapy treatment plan. A second visit was made to spend time with Anne and Peter to share information and explanation about the options and potential outcomes of chemotherapy. The written material Anne had been given at the hospital was clarified, and she was offered an additional appointment with the oncologist if she wished.
Cultural assessment	Anne and Peter were intelligent and articulate people. They had enjoyed an active social life, at	Anne was given time to talk about her hopes and fears. She found great comfort in her faith

	Christian faith and church activities: Anne had been a youth leader until the beginning of her cancer treatment. She had discussed her illness and possible death with her minister, and found support and strength in her beliefs. Anne and Peter's marriage was strong, but Peter's recent family bereavements had left him anxious and fearful about his wife and his daughters' future. Anne wanted to plan how she would prepare her husband and children for her death, but was unsure of the right way to go about it. Anne believed in the power of the mind to overcome hardship.	the centre of which was their and the friendship of her church. Anne was encouraged to express her desires about preparing her husband and children for her death, and some practical but supportive suggestions were made, such as creating a family history record of facts known previously only to Anne, making a note of certain items that the children should have after her death and their background, talking to Peter about the value she placed on him and their marriage.
Personality	Anne had a strong and optimistic nature, although she was realistic when faced with facts.	Anne's personality was a normally positive one, but the SPC nurse planned support should she experience moments of doubt.
Gender	Anne was concerned about the nature of her family history and the health of her two daughters.	Anne was encouraged to ask questions about the risk of cancer to her daughters, and it was suggested that she talk to her oncologist about it at her next appointment, also to discuss it with her GP, who would be able to monitor their health and refer for specialist advice if necessary.
Financial status	Peter anticipated problems related to loss of earnings as Anne's treatment and conditions continued.	A social assessment was made by the palliative care family support worker, who was able to advise about services and benefits that would be appropriate.
Age	In discussion, Anne expressed feelings of being cheated out of a future with the people	The SPC nurse discussed the merits of setting relatively small but achievable goals for the

Continued

CASE STUDY **3.3**—CONT'D

Assessment focus	Assessment findings	Care management
	she loved. She had many hopes and plans but acknowledged that these were now unlikely to come about. Anne had particularly wanted to go to Paris and visit the art galleries there.	foreseeable future; a weekend away somewhere together as a family, a visit to the theatre or cinema; shopping for clothes with her daughters. These activities would offer a sense of achievement for Anne and a store of happy memories for Peter and the children.
Stage in the life cycle	Anne expressed great sadness at the thought of missing her children's future development, and the chance to enjoy retirement with Peter. She admitted to feeling angry with God at times, although with the help of her minister this hadn't lasted long.	The SPC nurse spent time listening to and supporting Anne, and referred Anne to helpful publications that might help the whole family to adjust to their changing situation.

EVALUATION

The evaluation of holistic care must be carried out by the continual review of outcomes for both the patient and family. Only if care is measured and critically appraised can we hope to provide quality holistic care for patients whose situation is increasingly complex. Evaluation can be formal and quantitative in the manner of clinical audit, or qualitative by investigating patient satisfaction.

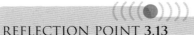

REFLECTION POINT 3.13

Evaluating holistic care

From the previous reflective exercises and your current thoughts on holistic palliative care, write some short notes on how your new knowledge and ideas will inform your future practice and make a plan to share this with your professional colleagues.

We have acknowledged that patients who require holistic palliative care often have complex needs. The society in which we live is also becoming more complex in terms of the global movement of people, and this increase in migration of people worldwide presents us with an ever-expanding diversity of needs within our own population.

CAN HOLISTIC CARE BE EFFECTIVELY PROVIDED TO ALL PEOPLE WITH A LIFE-THREATENING ILLNESS IN A MULTICULTURAL SOCIETY?

Diversity refers to differences in national origin, race, ethnicity, age, gender, religion, sexual orientation, education, ability/disability, economic and social status, and other related elements of individual cultural groups.

The Oxford English Dictionary (1996) defines culture as 'the customs, civilisation, and achievements of a particular time or people' and 'the way of life of a particular society or group'. This suggests that everyone has a cultural heritage, and that culture is not confined to an individual's colour or religion. Nurses, for example, have a cultural heritage relating to care of the sick and dying.

In the fourth edition of their book *Transcultural Concepts in Nursing Care* (2003), Andrews & Boyle use the term 'cultural competence', a concept that refers to 'a complex integration of knowledge, attitudes and skills that enhance cross-cultural communication and appropriate/effective interactions with others' (American Academy of Nursing 1992, cited in Andrews & Boyle 2003). They go on to explain that cultural competence is a process rather than an outcome, which requires the nurse to work effectively within the context of an individual family or community.

Green-Hernandez et al (2004) expand on the theme of cultural competence by offering a set of nursing competencies that can be measured. They propose that cultural competence is demonstrated when the nurse:

- Shows respect for the inherent dignity of every human being irrespective of their age, gender, religion, socioeconomic class, sexual orientation and ethnic or cultural group
- Accepts the rights of individuals to choose their care provider, participate in care or refuse care
- Acknowledges personal biases and prevents these from interfering with the delivery of quality care to persons of other cultures
- Recognises cultural issues and interacts with persons from other cultures in culturally sensitive ways
- Incorporates cultural preferences, health beliefs and behaviours, and traditional practices into the care management plan

- Develops appropriate educational materials that address the language and cultural beliefs of the patient
- Accesses culturally appropriate resources to deliver care to patients from other cultures
- Assists patients to access quality care within a dominant culture.

WHAT RELEVANCE HAS TRANSCULTURAL NURSING TO HOLISTIC PALLIATIVE CARE?

Accompanying the rise in multicultural identities is an expectation that cultural beliefs, values and lifestyles will be understood and respected by health-care providers. Palliative care has led the field in holistic nursing for many decades, and yet ethnic minority access to health-care services in general remains patchy even in areas of rich ethnic mix (Rhodes et al 2003) and access to palliative care services though improved still falls short of the ideal (Higginson 1999, Hill & Penso 1995)

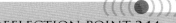

REFLECTION POINT 3.14
Cultural diversity

- Spend a few moment thinking about where you live and work. What cultural groups can you identify?
- Reflect for a moment on your knowledge concerning the needs of these different cultural groups.

  If you live in a city or urban area, you may have identified many different cultural groups, e.g. Asian, African/Caribbean, Polish, Jewish. Each group may have quite specific health-care needs, particularly if facing a life-threatening illness.

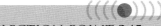

REFLECTION POINT 3.15
Assessment criteria and cultural diversity

Think now about the health-care setting in which you work.

- Do you have a dedicated assessment criterion that takes into account cultural diversity?
- If not, how do you think your current assessment protocol can be changed to incorporate such considerations?

Earlier in this chapter we examined two useful models of assessment of need; now we can expand these thoughts to incorporate cultural aspects of care. The following framework, adapted from the Transcultural Nursing Assessment Guide (Andrews & Boyle 2003), offers a clear and comprehensive framework by means of which we can assess some of the issues necessary for the development of a plan of care sensitive to and inclusive of cultural needs.

In Box 3.1 are some broad headings that may help you to expand a few of the things you might already have considered.

These and many other lines of enquiry used during assessment within the palliative care setting can significantly enhance the quality of person-centred care planning and delivery and demonstrate cultural competency.

When you read Chapter 11, on ethics in holistic palliative care, you will find many of these elements drawn together in the form of principles that you can develop further and apply within your own clinical area.

SUMMARY

In this chapter we have investigated the theory and meaning of holism and the whole person in terms of health and illness. We have examined the role of holistic assessment in the development of culturally sensitive holistic care. The importance of multiprofessional teamwork has been reviewed, and the need for cultural competence, illustrated by examples of nursing competencies in support of the theory.

Finally, the management and evaluation of appropriate care has been examined, with examples of good practice, such as the Global Assessment Factors assessment format and the Liverpool Care Pathway for dying patients.

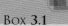

Box 3.1

Transcultural Nursing Assessment Guide (Andrews & Boyle 2003)

Epidemiological, physical and developmental considerations: are there any specific genetic or acquired conditions that are more prevalent in a specific cultural group (e.g. sickle cell disease)?

Education   **Cultural expression**
Communication   **Social networks**
Cultural values and cultural variations   **Cultural identity/affiliation**
Religious affiliation   **Health beliefs and practices**
Nutrition

With this information and a will to apply the very best of evidence to the care of patients with life-threatening illness, nursing interventions will be a true reflection of quality, sensitive, timely holistic care.

REFERENCES

American Academy of Nursing 1992 Expert Panel on Culturally Competent Nursing Care: Culturally competent health care. Nursing Outlook 40(6):277–284.

Andrews M, Boyle J 2003 Transcultural concepts in nursing care, 4th edn. Lippincott Williams & Wilkins, Philadelphia, PA

Aranda S 1999 Global perspectives on palliative care, 4th edn. Cancer Nursing 22:33–39

Archibald G 2000 A post-modern nursing model. Nursing Standard 14(34):40–42

Armstrong M J, Fitzgerald M H 1996 Culture and disability studies: an anthropological perspective. Rehabilitation Education 10(4):247–304.

Aronson J 2003 When I use a word. British Journal of Medicine 326:392

Ashby M E, Dowding C 2001 Hospice care and patients' pain: communication between patients, relatives, nurses and doctors. International Journal of Palliative Nursing 7:58–67

Baum A, Posluszny D M 1999 Health psychology: mapping biobehavioural contributions to health and illness. Annual Reviews in Psychology 50:137–163

Bennett M P, Zeller J M, Rosenberg L, McCann J 2003 The effects of mirthful laughter on stress and natural killer cell activity. Alternative Therapies in Health and Medicine 9:38–45

Biswas B, Ahmedzai S 1993 The medicalisation of dying. In: Clark D (ed.) The future for palliative care. Open University Press, Buckingham

Brosschot J F, Godaert G L R, Benschop R J et al 1998 Experimental stress and immunological reactivity: a closer look at perceived uncontrollability. Psychosomatic Medicine 60:359–361

Buckley J 2002 Holism and a health-promoting approach to palliative care. International Journal of Palliative Nursing 8:505–508

Clark D 2002 Between hope and acceptance: the medicalisation of dying. British Medical Journal 324:905–907

Clark D, Seymour J 1999 History and development. In: Reflections on palliative care. Open University Press, Buckingham, ch 4

Clark D, Malson H, Small N et al 1997 Half full or half empty? The impact of health reform on palliative care services in the UK. In: Clark D, Hockley J, Ahmedzai S (eds) New themes in palliative care. Open University Press, Buckingham

Cohen L, Marshall Jr G D, Cheng L et al 2000 DNA repair capacity in healthy medical students during and after exam stress. Journal of Behavioural Medicine 23:531–544

Department of Health 2000a The NHS plan: a plan for investment, a plan for reform. DH, Leeds

Department of Health 2000b The NHS cancer plan: a plan for investment, a plan for reform. DH, London

Department of Health 2000c National service framework for coronary heart disease: executive summary. DH, London

Duin N, Sutcliffe J 1992 A history of medicine. Simon & Schuster, New York

Duncan G 2000 Mind–body dualism and the biopsychosocial model of pain: what did Descartes really say? Journal of Medicine and Philosophy 25:485–513

Ellershaw J 2002 Clinical pathways for care of the dying: an innovation to disseminate clinical excellence. Journal of Palliative Medicine 5:617–621

Ellershaw J, Wilkinson S 2003 Care of the dying. Oxford University Press, New York

Engebretson J 1997 A multiparadigm approach to nursing. Advances in Nursing Science 20:21–33

Expert Advisory Group on Cancer 1995 A policy framework for commissioning cancer services. Department of Health and the Welsh Office, London

Farrell M, Sutherland P 1998 Providing paediatric palliative care: collaboration in practice. British Journal of Nursing 7:712–716

Ford P, McCormack B 2000 Keeping the person in the centre of nursing. Nursing Standard 14(46):40–44

Goldman A 1998 ABC of palliative care: special problems of children. British Medical Journal 316:49–52

Goodfellow L M 2003 The effects of therapeutic back massage on psychophysiologic variables and immune function in spouses of patients with cancer. Nursing Research 52:318–328

Green-Hernandez C, Quinn A, Denman-Vitale S et al 2004 Making nursing care culturally competent. Holistic Nursing Practice 18:215–218

Greer S, Moorey S 1997 Adjuvant psychological therapy for cancer patients. Palliative Medicine 11:240–244

Gross R 2004 Psychology: the science of mind and behaviour, 4th edn. Hodder & Stoughton, London

Haworth S K, Dluhy N M 2001 Holistic symptom management: modelling the interaction phase. Journal of Advanced Nursing 36:302–310

Hayes N 1997 Successful team management. Thomson Business Press, London

Heller R 1998 Managing teams. Dorling Kindersley, London

Higginson I 1993 Quality, costs and contracts of care. In: Clark D (ed.) The future for palliative care. Open University Press, Buckingham

Higginson I 1999 Evidence-based palliative care. British Medical Journal 319:462–463

Higginson I, Addington-Hall J 1999 Palliative care needs to be provided on basis of need rather than diagnosis. British Medical Journal 318:123

Hill D, Penso D 1995 Opening doors: improving access to hospice and specialist palliative care services by members of the black and ethnic minority communities. National Council for Hospice and Specialist Palliative Care, London

Illich I 1975 Medical nemesis: the expropriation of health. Marian Boyars, London

Kabel A, Roberts D 2003 Professionals' perceptions of maintaining personhood in hospice care. International Journal of Palliative Nursing 9:283–289

Kelly L 1999 Evaluating change in quality of life from the perspective of the person: advanced practice nursing and Parse's goal of nursing. Holistic Nursing Practice 13:61–70

King N, Bell D, Thomas K 2004 Family carers' experiences of out-of-hours community palliative care: a qualitative study. International Journal of Palliative Nursing 10:76–83

Kirkeboen G 2001 Descartes' embodied psychology: Descartes' or Damasio's error? Journal of the History of the Neurosciences 10:173–191

Kutzen H 2003 The positive outcomes of HIV palliative care consultations: five meaningful cases. HIV Clinician 15:1–5

Lee M, Walker R, Prentice W 2004 The role of palliative care in Parkinson's disease. Geriatric Medicine 34:51–54

McCormack B 2003 A conceptual framework for person-centred practice with older people. International Journal of Nursing Practice 9:202–209

McPherson G 2004 Children with cancer and their families believed and expected suffering was necessary to overcome cancer. Evidence-Based Nursing 7:29

National Assembly for Wales 2001 Improving health in Wales. NHS Cymru, Cardiff

NICE 2004 Improving supportive and palliative care for adults with cancer; the manual. National Institute for Clinical Excellence, London

Office for Public Management 2000 Shifting gears: towards a 21st century NHS. DH, London

Ogden J 2000 An introduction to health psychology. In: Health Psychology: a textbook, 2nd edn. Open University Press, Buckingham, ch 1

Olsen D 1997 Development of an instrument to measure the cognitive structure used to understand personhood in patients. Nursing Research 46:78–84

Paley J 2002 The Cartesian melodrama in nursing. Nursing Philosophy 3:189–192

Reiche E M V, Nunes S O V, Morimoto H K 2004 Stress, depression, the immune system and cancer. Lancet Oncology 5:617–625

Rhodes P, Nocon A, Wright J 2003 Access to diabetes services: the experiences of Bangladeshi people in Bradford, UK. Ethnicity and Health 8:171–188

Rivett G 1998 From cradle to grave: 50 years of the NHS. King's Fund, London

Sarafino E P (ed.) 1998 An overview of psychology and health. In: Health psychology: biopsychosocial interactions, 3rd edn. John Wiley, New York, ch 1

Saunders C 1990 Hospice and palliative care – an interdisciplinary approach. Edward Arnold, London

Smuts J C 1927 In: Holism and science, Encyclopaedia Britannica. Available on line at: www.tocmed.com/Nature/Smuts_3.html

Sullivan M 1986 In what sense is contemporary medicine dualistic? Culture, Medicine and Psychiatry 10:331–350

Thomas K 2000 Out-of-hours palliative care – bridging the gap. European Journal of Palliative Care 7:22–25

Thomas K 2003 The Gold Standards framework in community palliative care. European Journal of Palliative Care 10:113–115

Tortora G J, Grabowski S R (eds) 2003 The lymphatic and immune systems and resistance to disease. In: Principles of anatomy and physiology, 10th edn. John Wiley, New York, ch 22

Twycross R 1999 Introducing palliative care, 3rd edn. Radcliffe Medical, Oxford

Whynes D 1997 Costs of palliative care. In: Clark D, Hockley J, Ahmedzai S (eds) New themes in palliative care. Open University Press, Buckingham

World Health Organization 2003 Definition of palliative care. Available on line at www.who.int/cancer/palliative/definition/en/

Wurzbach M E 1999 The moral metaphors of nursing. Journal of Advanced Nursing 30:94–99

CHAPTER FOUR

Symptom management

Noreen Reid, Paula McCormack

CONTENTS

INTRODUCTION

Symptom management is a fundamental aspect of palliative care (World Health Organization 2003). It is the primary therapeutic goal of service delivery and is aimed at subjective wellbeing (De Conno & Martini 2001). Although it is estimated that 90% of patients who access palliative care services have a diagnosis of cancer (Bruera & Portenoy 2001), governments worldwide are now committed to ensuring that palliative care is available to all who need it, including patients diagnosed with incurable non-malignant diseases (Armstrong 2001, Scottish Executive 2001, World Health Organization 2003). The aims and principles of symptom management can be applied to all patients requiring palliative care services regardless of diagnosis. Irrespective of the symptom, a generic framework can be utilised in symptom management in advanced disease.

The large and diverse number of symptoms that occur within palliative care cannot be addressed in a book chapter of this length, so we have decided to focus on those symptoms that, in our professional experience, have caused significant problems for patients and have an adequate evidence base underpinning the management plan. In this chapter, therefore, only some of the commonly reported symptoms will be considered in depth.

The aims of this chapter are to enable the reader to:

- Appreciate the value of adopting a multiprofessional approach to the management of symptoms
- Recognise contributory factors that determine the impact of the symptom(s) on the individual patient
- Identify appropriate nursing interventions that contribute to the comfort of the patient and family
- Explain the pharmacological management of the symptoms discussed in this chapter.

KEY PRINCIPLES OF SYMPTOM MANAGEMENT

When considering symptom management, Regnard & Kindlen (2002) remind us that several key issues should influence any decision. First, in implementing any intervention or treatment related to the management of symptoms, the preferred choice of the patient should be at the forefront of the minds of practitioners. This includes agreeing to non-treatment as an option. Second, open communication involving not only patients and family members but also all relevant health professionals will facilitate informed decision-making. Third, listening to the patient's own story, including past and present life experiences, will assist the professional to understand the impact of symptoms from the patient's perspective (Chochinov 2002, Steinhauser et al 2000).

The impact of any physical or psychological symptom on the individual patient manifests itself in a degree of suffering; however, it should be noted that the severity of unrelieved symptoms is not necessarily directly related to suffering. Suffering may be more concerned with a sense of hopelessness and futility, experienced by the essence of the person rather than the body per se. It can be exacerbated by the disruption of personal identity (Kissane 2000). Aranda (2003) alerts us to the fact that as health professionals we may find it less traumatic to focus on the occurrence of the symptom rather than on the experience of the individual patient. Kearney (2000) reminds us that by look-ing on the patient as an individual, caregivers can create an environment that facilitates inner healing, thus reducing suffering. Symptom management in palliative care is much more than using evidence-based interventions, it also involves fostering hope and showing by our actions and words that we con-sider patients to be worthwhile even if they themselves do not (Regnard & Kindlen 2002). Achieving this involves a degree of giving of oneself in facili-tating a therapeutic relationship with the patient (Kabel & Roberts 2003, Ramfelt et al 2002).

Symptoms are multidimensional in nature and therefore symptom manage-ment is best achieved by adopting a multiprofessional approach. An interdis-ciplinary therapeutic model encompassing all dimensions of care is considered the most appropriate unit of care (Bruera & Portenoy 2001). This model allows members to share information through discussion and working together to formulate goals. The task at hand determines who takes the leadership role, rather than the most senior member of the team assuming leadership. The interaction between team members is integral to successful outcomes as the team, rather than an individual practitioner, is the vehicle for action (Waller & Caroline 1996). We would encourage the reader to explore this model in more detail.

One must be cautious when discussing symptom incidence and prevalence data because patient cohorts, symptom checklists and study methodologies differ. However, when consulting literature related to hospice admissions, several core symptoms continue to emerge regardless of diagnosis. They are fatigue, pain, dyspnoea and constipation (Donnelly et al 1994, Weitzner et al 1997). Discussing symptom prevalence in both malignant and non-malignant diseases, Faull & Woof (2002) concurred with the previous authors in that the same symptoms are reported albeit with different prevalence depending on the diagnosis. It has been noted by several authors that patients may not be forthcoming in discussing symptoms and may need to be prompted (Passik et al 2002, Regnard & Tempest 1998). It is therefore important that clinicians take time and use skilled communication techniques to elicit information by gentle enquiry.

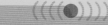

REFLECTION POINT 4.1

The multidisciplinary team

Take some time to reflect on your own practice. Identify a patient with whom you were recently involved for symptom management.

- Given that symptoms are often multifactorial, did you involve the multiprofessional team in the management?

If not, identify professionals from different disciplines whose expertise you could use in the future should the need arise.

- Did you consider the symptom from a holistic perspective? Was the degree of suffering, rather than just the clinical manifestation, explored?

As clinicians we may focus primarily on physical evidence and minimise the total impact on the patient's life. Do you need to enhance your communication skills? If so, consider attending an advanced communication skills workshop aimed at teaching the skills needed to address difficult situations specific to palliative care.

- Was the patient included as part of the decision-making team?

Having given patients time to digest information it is the role of health professionals to support patients in their choices. This can be difficult, given the paternalistic nature of health care.

THE PROCESS OF SYMPTOM MANAGEMENT

National and local best practice guidelines for symptom management are readily available and should be followed (Lothian Palliative Care Guidelines Group 2002, SIGN 2000). However, as palliative care involves a very wide-ranging patient cohort, attention should always be paid to disease specific guidelines (SIGN 1998, 2004).

Given that symptoms in advanced disease are not only multifactorial but are often interrelated, no symptom should be assessed and treated in isolation (Aranda 2003). Symptom management should never be ad hoc; rather, a systematic approach should be adopted. This can be addressed by adherence to five main principles: evaluation, explanation, management, monitoring and attention to detail (Twycross & Wilcock 2002, p. 6).

Helpful hint

Mnemonics can be useful. **EEMMA** will remind you of the key points to cover when managing symptoms.

EVALUATION

Establishing the cause of the symptom involves taking a history, including general trends and recent changes. Attention should be paid to the effectiveness of interventions that have already been implemented. A physical examination should be performed and investigations carried out if appropriate, given an individual's prognosis and goals of care (Clinical Standards Board for Scotland

2002; as of 2003, now known as NHS Quality Improvement Scotland). Because of the complexity of determining the cause of a symptom in a palliative care patient it can be helpful to think in three broad categories. Is the symptom due to the disease itself, the treatment, concurrent medical conditions or a combination of all three? Regardless of the cause a decision must be taken as to whether the symptom is reversible, treatable or a terminal event for the patient. A comprehensive explanation of the management plan should be given to the patient and family. If the patient is dying, appropriate terminal event symptom management should follow this.

It is documented that patient-reported evaluation of the symptom is mandatory and assessment instruments have a role to play (McMillan & Moody 2003). Several authors remind us that self-reporting instruments are most accurate, as staff and family members tend to over- or underestimate the intensity of symptoms (Kutner et al 2001, Sutcliffe-Chidgey & Holmes 1996). Such instruments should be used to supplement professional judgement and aid assessment. However, the role of assessment tools remains controversial, as practical application is problematic, especially because of patient and staff burden. As with any intervention in palliative care, the benefit of using the tool must outweigh the burden to the patient.

Many tools, although comprehensive, are cumbersome and their use requires time and effort from both patient and health professional (Cooley et al 2002). Although there are recommendations for use in practice (SIGN 2000), the simpler and briefer the tool the more applicable (Serlin et al 1995). There are several examples of such simple tools. Verbal Rating Scales are category scales consisting of various words placed in rank order at equal intervals along a line. The words describe the intensity of the symptom using descriptors, for example 'mild', 'moderate' or 'severe'. However, some patients may find it difficult to verbalise their experience of a distressing symptom because the choice of words may not really accurately describe the experience. An alternative is the Visual Analogue Scale. When using this scale the patient is asked to draw a mark at some point on a 10 cm line. Again, this measures the intensity of the symptom. The left end of the line indicates the least degree of the symptom and the right side indicates the worst degree of the symptom (Hawthorn & Redmond 2001). A plethora of general and disease-specific instruments exists (Keedwell & Snaith 1996, Melzack 1993, Stone 2002); however, their validity and generalisability across the broad cohort of patients accessing palliative care services remain fraught with difficulty (De Conno & Martini 2001, De Rond et al 1999). What is important is that practitioners choose a measurement tool that best suits the patient and measures the dimension of the symptom that is being assessed.

EXPLANATION

Explanation about care and treatment options is vital to the delivery of effective care and empowers patients and carers to be involved as equal partners in the decision-making process. Information about the disease process and significance of symptoms should be provided to patients when they need it, and not at a time convenient for the professionals involved in the care (Scottish Executive 2001). It is also important that the information is provided in a sensitive manner. International literature reports dissatisfaction from patients and carers with the manner in which information is imparted (Friedrichsen et al 2001, Jenkins et al 2001). It is also documented that poor communication skills in relation to information giving can have a detrimental effect on patient outcomes (Wilkinson 1999).

MANAGEMENT

Management builds on the assessment process. The first stage is to identify the cause and determine what is reversible or treatable. Health professionals should work in partnership with the patient. The patient's priorities must be considered and realistic goals set in conjunction with the patient and then documented in the management plan. Treatment interventions should be tailored to meet the needs of the individual (Regnard & Kindlen 2002). It should be remembered that team cohesiveness is crucial to achieving successful outcomes. All professionals involved should be working towards the same goals and giving the same information to the patient and family. This is especially important if the symptom is irreversible and as such may lead to a 'terminal event' for the individual. In order to achieve this cohesiveness and be efficient, it may be useful for the interdisciplinary team to incorporate elements of collaborative practice (Dudgeon 1994, Ingham & Coyle 1999).

MONITORING

Monitoring will not only determine the efficacy of interventions but also facilitate regular reassessment of the severity of the symptom and impact on the patient. The outcomes of the review should be discussed and documented following the same process discussed above. It can also be helpful to have a contingency plan in place. For example, if the first intervention, plan A, is not effective, then initiate plan B. This can have the effect of empowering the patient and again limiting any time-wasting.

ATTENTION TO DETAIL

This can perhaps have the most significant ramifications for the patient if done badly. Throughout the process of symptom management, the missing of details by health professionals can have dire consequences. Crucial time can be wasted by not actively listening to the patient at the initial assessment stage, by prescribing but not ascertaining the practical availability of medications and assessing side-effects, and by failing to ask the right questions to elicit the correct information when monitoring interventions. As health professionals, it is easy to forget just how precious time is to many patients and families involved with palliative care services. Most importantly, these things may result in patients and families losing faith in the team and lead to an increase in psychological distress and a feeling of hopelessness (Fleming 1997).

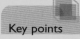

Key points

- Meticulous assessment and multiprofessional input will increase the chances of getting it right first time

- Involve the patient in a decision-making partnership by exploring the symptom experience together

- Never give up hope or underestimate the effect that showing that you truly care about the patient will have on treatment outcomes.

The remainder of this chapter will focus on the management of a selection of symptoms in some detail. However, no discussion on symptom management can be all-encompassing and readers are advised to consult some of the works referenced throughout the chapter in order to enhance their knowledge base. Also, despite their importance, there are symptoms not discussed in this chapter – fatigue, anorexia, cachexia and delirium, to name but a few. Restrictions imposed by chapter length mean it will not be possible to include them.

BREATHLESSNESS (DYSPNOEA)

Although health professionals often use the terms 'breathlessness' and 'dyspnoea' interchangeably, Hough (2001) reminds us that the definitions differ. Breathlessness is an awareness of breathing while dyspnoea is difficulty in breathing when carrying out an activity that would under normal circumstances not induce such difficulty. In practice, perhaps dyspnoea relates more to the symptom whereas breathlessness more clearly defines the subjective experience on which management should be based.

INCIDENCE

Breathlessness is an indicator of poor prognosis, occurring in 70% of patients in the last 6 weeks of life (Waller & Caroline 2000). Klinkenberg et al (2004) state that it contributes to the symptom burden in 50% of patients in the last week of life. This is inclusive of patients with a diagnosis of lung cancer, chronic obstructive pulmonary disease (COPD) and cardiac failure (SIGN 2004, Ward 2002). Lung cancer is the most common cancer in Scotland and Scotland leads international statistics in both incidence and mortality, while COPD is a common condition affecting 1.5% of the general population (SIGN 2004). Paes (2004) reminds us that each year in the UK there are 60 000 deaths from cardiac failure. Considering the presence of dyspnoea as a risk factor for morbidity in cancer patients, Edmonds et al (2000) acknowledged the broad diagnostic group that report this symptom. The diagnoses of their sample of 756 patients included gastrointestinal, respiratory, genitourinary, breast and other malignancies. Given these statistics, health professionals working in palliative care will almost certainly be involved in the management of this symptom.

In their studies measuring symptom distress related to treatment options in lung cancer patients, Cooley et al (2002) and Tanaka et al (2002) remind us of the importance of considering psychosocial factors. It is well documented that anxiety is one of the correlating factors of breathlessness and, as with any symptom, tiredness and the meaning of the symptom to the patient, possibly resulting in depression, can make the impact of the breathlessness worse (Bruera et al 2000, Twycross & Wilcock 2002). Also, on a more fundamental level, breathing is a basic physiological need and the sense of loss of control that breathlessness brings must be, understandably, very frightening.

PATHOPHYSIOLOGY

The control of normal breathing can be voluntary or involuntary. Voluntary breathing allows for activities such as eating and talking while involuntary breathing is regulated by oxygen delivery and acid–base balance. The mechanism of breathlessness is more complex and has several components. Breathlessness arises from discrepancies between peripheral sensors in the lung, respiratory muscles and chemoreceptors. This results in an imbalance between respiratory drive and respiratory load. There is also a conscious awareness of the effort needed to breathe and, as with any subjective experience, the higher centres in the brain trigger an emotional response. Anxiety is particularly damaging, as it creates a cycle of muscle tension that in turn increases the effort necessary to boost the respiratory rate (Hough 2001, Wilcock 1997).

EVALUATION

When determining the cause of the symptom it should be noted that patients with a diagnosis of cancer have a high incidence of general medical conditions that may be contributing to the breathlessness, including pulmonary embolism and pneumonia. Clinical experience also supports the considerable overlap in the symptoms of lung cancers and chronic airways disease (SIGN 2004, Waller & Caroline 2000). This can make identifying the cause(s) difficult. In cancer, although the tumour mass itself may, for example, be causing obstruction of the bronchus, cancer-related problems may also be causing an exacerbation, such as fatigue, muscle weakness, chest tumours or phrenic nerve palsy (Back 2001). Breathlessness may be the result of the cancer treatment itself, for example chemotherapy causing anaemia or radiation therapy resulting in radiation fibrosis of the lung; hence the importance of a thorough physical examination, history-taking and always weighing the benefit of any intervention compared with the burden of treatment for the individual.

Numerous assessment tools are available for the measurement of breath-lessness, the tools often measuring only one facet of this complex symptom. Andrewes (2002) and Van der Molen (1995) concur with this viewpoint in saying that no one tool assesses every aspect of breathlessness. In practice a Visual Analogue Scale can provide a simple, self-reporting tool that is sensitive and reliable in measuring breathlessness (Birks 1997, Corner et al 1995).

EXPLANATION

Following a comprehensive assessment and evaluation, an explanation of probable causes, non-pharmacological and pharmacological interventions and planned outcomes is especially important given the level of anxiety/depression associated with breathlessness. Krishnasamy et al (2001) reiterated the point that the individual patient's perspective of the experience of breathlessness should be taken into account when planning care. Where possible, time should be allocated for discussion and patients and family members encouraged to ask questions. Breathing is physically hard work and this can become very problematic in palliative care patients as research shows that fatigue is reported as a major distressing symptom by a high percentage of this patient cohort, between 50 and 100% (Faull & Woof 2002, Twycross & Wilcock 2002).

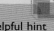

Helpful hint

Given the link between breathlessness and anxiety/depression, it should be noted that both nurses and doctors under-report depression in cancer patients (Hotopf et al 2002, Passik et al 2000). With this in mind, if a patient presents with breathlessness always consider the possibility that they may also be suffering from anxiety/depression and include appropriate management strategies in their plan of care. Refer to the section on depression for more information.

MANAGEMENT

Strategies for the management of breathlessness are often aimed at treating the cause, for example antibiotics for a chest infection, radiotherapy for intrathoracic disease or pleural aspiration for effusion. If, however, this is not a viable option then symptomatic treatment will be necessary. In the past, treatment of breathlessness was dictated, for the most part, by pharmacological strategies; however, there is now a move towards a more holistic approach to management (Syrett & Taylor 2003). Nurse-led clinics for the management of breathlessness are considered by many health professionals as the way forward (Bredin et al 1999, Loftus & Weston 2001, Moore et al 2002) in delivering this approach to care.

Non-pharmacological

When handling the patient, all communication should be clear and unambiguous so as to minimise the anxiety component. Anxiety will only exacerbate the problem by increasing oxygen consumption. Any handling should be fully explained and carried out in a slow efficient manner, allowing for a rest between each stage of the procedure. Interactions with the patient that require verbal responses should be limited, and the use of closed questions encouraged. Questions that require a 'yes' or 'no' response will keep the effort required to a minimum. As with any distressed patient, platitudes should not be used, rather the distress that the patient is experiencing should be acknowledged. Eating and talking may also increase breathlessness, so measures should be taken to minimise the effort required during mealtimes. Breathless patients benefit from unconfined spaces and fresh air. Being cared for near an open window may be favourable. A fan also reduces the sensation of breathlessness by affecting nerve receptors in the trigeminal nerve distribution (Manning 1995); hence the reason that a slow fan positioned directly on the patient's face may be preferable to an oscillating fan. It may be helpful to provide visitors with this information so that the demands they make on the patient are kept to a minimum.

Good nursing care with advice and assistance from the physiotherapist will facilitate correct positioning and posture that may help reduce the ventilation/perfusion mismatch. Sitting upright in a supported position or leaning slightly forward resting arms on a table may be of benefit. Respiratory muscle and peripheral muscle training may also have a role in reducing breathlessness, as does general exercise training if the patient's general condition permits (Hough 2001, Paes 2004). The skill and expertise of the physiotherapist can be invaluable in re-educating the patient in breathing techniques. Fatigue will exacerbate the distress caused by the symptom, so ensuring a restful night's sleep is of paramount importance. Breathless patients often have problems sleeping not only because of the effort required to breathe but also because of the fear and anxiety that each breath may be their final one. Sleeping on a reclining chair in a semirecumbent position may facilitate ease of breathing. If the patient is fearful, the presence of someone at the bedside or the use of a night light may be of some help.

Several authors concur that a proactive approach to managing breathlessness is most appropriate (Hately et al 2001, Hoyal et al 2002) rather than waiting for an acute exacerbation of the symptom to initiate a response from the health professional. By educating patients in coping techniques well in advance of the terminal phase of disease, they can be empowered to regain some level of control over the symptom, thus reducing the associated fear and anxiety. Breathing techniques and relaxation training are important in improving oxygenation to the lungs. Such techniques may also include the use of aromatherapy. However, a practitioner familiar with the special needs of palliative care patients should initiate this therapy, as different oils can have either a positive or negative effect on respirations. The principle behind therapeutic hypnotherapy is the same as deep relaxation, in that the metabolic rate decreases. This may be of benefit if patients have an anxiety component to their symptom. Acupuncture can be useful as it works directly on reducing the perception of breathlessness (Back 2001, Hoban 2003, Hough 2001, Paes 2004). In response to this evidence, Macmillan Cancer Relief (2003) have produced a variety of aids for patients; these include compact disk packs and printed booklets. The products are designed for healthcare professionals to use with patients and for patients to use independently to help manage their own breathlessness.

A trial of oxygen is recommended if the patient is hypoxic; however, its use should be tailored to the individual and an assessment made of its efficacy (Back 2001, Booth et al 2004, Paes 2004). Although oxygen is not addictive, patients may come to rely upon it. One should not underestimate the placebo effect of this treatment option. Although an expensive placebo for long-term use, in palliative care this should not prohibit its use. It should be noted that, in practice, a medical practitioner must prescribe oxygen therapy.

Occupational therapy can provide simple adaptations that may minimise the burden of the symptom on the patient (Paes 2004). One distressing aspect reported by patients in relation to breathlessness is its effect on their activities of daily living. Again, this relates to loss of control and independence and as such has a direct relationship with quality of life, which is the very essence of symptom management in palliative care (Hough 2001, McMillan & Brent 2002). Taking time to help patients accept the limitations of their disease is an essential component of care.

Pharmacological

- **Bronchodilators** are recommended for trial with any patient with advanced disease suffering from breathlessness (Back 2001, Twycross et al 2003).

- **Steroids** can also be helpful, particularly for patients with COPD or lymphangitis; however, their precise role needs to be further defined (Le Grande & Walsh 1999, Lothian Palliative Care Guidelines Group 2002).

- **Nebulised furosemide** may be effective in relieving breathlessness even in the absence of left ventricular failure. Further research is currently underway to determine its exact mode of action (Back 2001, Minowa et al 2002, Nishino et al 2000). Although not supported by scientific evidence, anecdotal evidence suggests that **nebulised saline** may also be of benefit in this group of patients (Twycross et al 2003).

- Some recent research supports the use of **cannabinoids** in low doses to alleviate breathlessness (Back 2001, Twycross et al 2003).

- **Opioids** are well established in the management of breathlessness. Although the use of nebulised opioids became popular in the late 1990s, evidence does not support their efficacy when compared with systemic administration (Davis & Sheldon 1999). In 2004, the Cochrane Collaboration reviewed 18 studies and concluded that, although there was evidence to support the use of oral and parenteral opioids, no such evidence was available to support a statistically significant improvement in breathlessness when using nebulised opioids (Jennings et al 2004).
- The use of **sedation** in the management of breathlessness can be controversial. Sedation will always relieve breathlessness but is incompatible with an active life. Therefore, if sedation is used, the goals of care should be clearly defined and expected outcomes set in conjunction with the patient (Booth 1998).
- The efficacy of **psychostimulants** in the treatment of depression is well documented (Dein 2002, Homsi et al 2000). Given their rapid onset and better side effect profile when compared with other groups of antidepressant medications, they may have a role in treating the depression associated with breathlessness. They should, however, be used with caution in a breathless patient as they may in fact increase the level of anxiety. Both anxiety and panic attacks are common in breathlessness and can be alleviated by self-administration of a **benzodiazepine** (Back 2001, Le Grande & Walsh 1999, Lothian Palliative Care Guidelines Group 2002).

MONITORING AND ATTENTION TO DETAIL

Regular contact with the patient, including assessment of physical status, will facilitate monitoring of the symptom. This process will determine the progress of the disease, review of the effectiveness of current interventions and appraisal of the psychological status and the appropriateness of the coping strategies being used. Finely honed interpersonal skills are as important as practical advice. Patients experiencing breathlessness report that management plans based not only on physical but also on psychological interventions, with an emphasis on education of the patients in implementing coping strategies, result in a decreased sensation of breathlessness, improved performance status and greater emotional wellbeing. Thus the impact of the symptom on the patient is minimised (Bredin et al 1999, Hoyal et al 2002).

SUMMARY

When considering breathlessness, health professionals should remember that the physiological changes and emotional perception are inseparable. Empowering the patient through education is an integral component of the management plan.

COUGH

INCIDENCE

Cough is commonly reported by palliative care patients, being more prevalent in those with a diagnosis of lung cancer (Beckles et al 2003, Kvale 2003). In patients with advanced disease, prevalence is estimated to be 50–80% (Twycross & Wilcock 2002). Respiratory problems including cough are also common in patients with neurodegenerative disorders. Contributing factors in this patient cohort include immobility, aspiration, poor cough reflex and progressive weakness of the intercostals and diaphragmatic muscles (O'Brien 2001).

PATHOPHYSIOLOGY

Cough is caused by mechanical and/or chemical stimulation, i.e. an irritant affecting C-fibre receptors in the airway and/or other structures causing a response from vagus, trigeminal and phrenic nerves (Twycross & Wilcock 2002). For example, in neurodegenerative disorders changes affecting the brain stem may interfere with the function of the higher centres which, in a healthy person, would facilitate the voluntary induction or suppression of a cough.

EVALUATION

Identifying and treating the cause of the cough prior to initiating symptomatic measures can be difficult as it is often multifactorial. A patient suffering from multiple sclerosis may have a cough stimulated by the pooling of saliva in the hypopharynx, particularly troublesome at night. Administration of an anticholinergic agent may decrease the production of saliva and thus control the nocturnal coughing. Side effects of other drug therapy, for example ACE inhibitors, may be the causative factor. It may be possible to discontinue the medication or substitute an alternative drug (Twycross & Wilcock 2002). Even in a patient with a malignancy there may well be coexisting non-malignant causes of the cough. These include acute or chronic infection, an irritant, airway obstruction, parenchymal disease, recurrent aspiration, interstitial disease, vocal cord palsy or drug-induced cough (Davis 1997). Cough can trigger breathlessness and vice versa. In debilitated patients a chronic cough can lead to rib fractures, insomnia, fatigue and exacerbation of pain and vomiting (Davis 1997, Woodruff 1999).

There are no symptom-specific assessment tools for this symptom; rather, the type, frequency and, most importantly, the impact on the patient's life should be assessed. It is important to establish if the cough is 'wet' or 'dry', as this will to some extent determine the management plan. The aim of treatment of a wet cough is to facilitate an easy, effective cough that clears the mucus, while suppression is the aim of treatment if the cough is dry and the cause cannot be treated (Back 2001, Davis 1997).

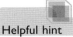

Helpful hint

Coughs may be more troublesome nocturnally, resulting in poor sleeping patterns for both the patient and others. Sleep disturbances exacerbate fatigue and can have a detrimental effect on physical and mental wellbeing and quality of life (Beck et al 2004). It is important to explain to the patient that the potential distress the symptom can cause is being taken seriously.

MANAGEMENT

Non-pharmacological

It should be noted that coughing could have some benefits, for example helping to clear excessive bronchial secretions, particularly in patients with a diagnosis of COPD. The physiotherapist can assist by teaching patients skills that will enable them to cough more effectively and with less effort (Hough 2001). A change in position or posture can also be effective, especially prior to administration of medications to facilitate expectoration. Postural drainage and steam inhalations should also be considered.

Pharmacological

There is a wide variety of medications that should be employed, depending on the factors contributing to the cough and the aim of treatment given the patient's prognosis. In general terms, if the cough is wet, antitussives (cough suppressants) should be avoided unless sleep deprivation is causing concern.

Wet cough:

- **Nebulised saline** may be helpful, particularly if tenacious secretions are a contributory factor. This inexpensive and safe treatment is often underused in palliative care.
- If aspiration pneumonia is a contributing factor, **antibiotic therapy** will decrease the formation of phlegm (Faull & Woof 2002). Even if the patient is dying, antibiotics should be considered if the cough is causing pain and distress to the patient. However, in the palliative care setting, although it is easy to commence drug therapy, it can be difficult to discontinue it. Ceasing medications in a dying patient may well pose an ethical dilemma in that it may be thought to hasten death.
- **Bronchodilators** will help if asthma is problematic or the patient has a diagnosis of COPD (Davis 1997).
- **Expectorants** are claimed to promote expulsion of secretions; however, there is no evidence to support the belief that any medication can help to facilitate expectoration. There may be a placebo effect of preparations that contain syrup or glycerol. Anecdotal evidence suggests that the soothing effect is beneficial.
- **Mucolytics** do reduce sputum viscosity and so aid expectoration (Royal Pharmaceutical Society 2004).

Dry cough:

- **Antitussive** measures including opioids act on the brain-stem cough reflex, thus suppressing the cough (Twycross & Wilcock 2002). If patients are already taking opioids for pain control it may be worth increasing the dose by an increment or two (Back 2001).

- Evidence supports using **nebulised local anaesthetics**. This intervention works by anaesthetising sensory nerves involving the cough reflex; however, caution should be employed as there is a risk of bronchospasm. Patients should be nil by mouth for 1 hour after administration (Twycross et al 2003). It should be noted that there is some controversy in the literature about the effectiveness of nebulised local anaesthetics if a conventional rather than an ultrasonic nebuliser is used (Ahmedzai & Davis 1997).

MONITORING AND ATTENTION TO DETAIL

The type, frequency and impact of the cough will change with time. Staff should reassess the symptom both during the daytime and at night and explain the rationale of the interventions to the patient. Cough can be extremely debilitating and irritating to patients and its impact on quality of life should not be underestimated.

PAIN

INTRODUCTION

Pain is a complex phenomenon defined initially in 1986 by the International Association for the Study of Pain as being 'an unpleasant sensory and emotional experience associated with actual or potential tissue damage, or described in terms of such damage' (IASP 1994). This definition is widely accepted and favoured as underpinning the Scottish Intercollegiate Guideline on Pain (SIGN 2000). Chronic pain associated with cancer is quite distinct from the more straightforward acute physiological pain. Its unrelenting nature can impact on all aspects of a person's life, including activities of daily living, mood, sexual and social relationships, sleep patterns, thought processes and the existential domain (Strang 1998). If the pain is unrelieved the sufferer can become withdrawn, unable to focus and their whole personality can appear to be changed as their quality of life diminishes. For nurses working with palliative care patients the management of pain must therefore be a priority.

While specialists in palliative care are now being asked to widen their scope to address conditions other than cancer, advances in knowledge have most significantly been with cancer pain, which is therefore the focus of this section.

INCIDENCE OF PAIN

A diagnosis of cancer is commonly thought to be synonymous with pain because it is such a significant symptom, but in reality two-thirds of patients with cancer suffer pain while one-third do not experience any pain at all (SIGN 2000). The statistics show that pain becomes moderate to severe in 40–50% of patients and it varies according to the primary site. It can become very severe or excruciating in 25–30% of cases (Bonica 1990).

PHYSIOLOGY

The nurse's understanding of the differing types of pain is fundamental to appropriate management as the intervention will depend on the nature of the pain and the pain pathways. Although very complex, our understanding of pain pathways has increased in recent years and this has been helped not only by the development of new drugs for pain relief but also by the use of drugs previously employed for other conditions.

Twycross & Wilcock (2002) identify three types of pain response.

Physiological pain is the least intricate and occurs when the nociceptive system warns of impending injury to the body, providing direct pain information to the brain. There is a close correlation between the intensity of the stimulus and the intensity of the pain.

In more long-standing, **chronic pain**, certain changes have been found to take place in the pain pathways, which can lead to increased pain responses. Nociceptors may become sensitised after an injury so that they become increasingly sensitive with each application of a noxious stimulus, thus giving a greater response (hyperalgesia). The central processing of sensation from peripheral afferent nerves may also be altered so that fibres that are normally nociceptors and responsive to touch now send messages that are interpreted as pain. This leads to the development of the 'wind up' phenomenon. Preclinical studies have shown that the N-methyl-D-aspartate (NMDA) receptor is involved in the sensitisation of the central neurones (Woolf & Thompson 1991).

Neuropathic pain: One of the commonest causes of complex pain is current or past damage to the nerve fibres, which can follow damage to the peripheral nerves or injury to the spinal cord or brain. This type of pain does not require the presence of an identifiable noxious stimulus and is due to aberrant processing of information in the peripheral or central nervous system. Commonly, there is reorganisation of central processing. In the cancer patient neuropathic pain is often associated with tumour compression, infiltration of peripheral nerves, nerve roots, or the type of spinal cord pain that occurs as a result of neurological injury. It is usually qualitatively different from other types of pain and is typically described as being 'lancing', 'a constant dull ache with a vice-like quality' or as 'paroxysms of burning and/or electric-shock-like sensations'. Descriptions of the pain sensations are useful as they can aid with diagnosis (Payne & Gonzales 1999).

Somatic pain

Pain that arises in the skin, muscle, periosteum or fascia is called somatic pain. This type of pain is usually well localised; for example, bone metastases are associated with somatic pain. It may be described as sharp, burning, constant, aching and gnawing.

Visceral pain

Visceral pain results from infiltration, compression, distension or stretching of the thoracic or abdominal viscera, usually as a result of primary or metastatic tumour growth, e.g. pancreatic cancer, liver or lung metastases. Pain of this nature is poorly localised, is described as intense, deep, dull and aching and is often accompanied by nausea.

EVALUATION

Assessment of pain

The latest World Health Organization (WHO) definition of palliative care refers to the requirement for 'impeccable assessment' of pain and other problems (World Health Organization 2003) and there is general consensus that sound assessment is fundamental to the successful management of pain and other symptoms (Doyle et al 2004, SIGN 2000, Twycross 1995). Nurses are extremely well placed to play a fundamental role in pain assessment by virtue of the time they spend with the patient and the relationship built; however, pain management is best achieved when all the health professionals involved in the care of the patient use their collective skills to tackle the problem. Despite the best team endeavours, there is no reliable way for health professionals to accurately measure pain objectively because pain is a completely subjective experience. Numerous studies have shown that observer and patient assessments are not highly correlated (Field 1996, Grossman et al 1991) and that the accuracy of clinical assessments cannot be assumed. Hence the often quoted definition 'Pain is whatever the experiencing person says it is, existing whenever the experiencing person says it does' (McCaffery 1997). The patient therefore must be the main assessor of the pain, working in tandem with the health-care team.

A number of validated pain questionnaires are available to measure pain based on the patient's responses, for example the McGill Pain Questionnaire (Melzack 1993) and the Wisconsin Brief Pain Questionnaire (Daut et al 1983). Both are intended to measure the sensory, affective and evaluative dimensions of the pain experience. In practice, such tools in their lengthiest form can be complex, demanding and place an unacceptable burden on frail patients and staff's time and so they are used mostly for research purposes. Briefer versions have been developed, for example the Memorial Pain Assessment Chart (Fishman et al 1987), but many palliative care areas have devised their own pain assessment charts based on these tools but in a shorter form.

The SIGN guidelines (2000) offer a useful framework for the evaluation of pain, which can be incorporated into a pain tool. They suggest that a comprehensive assessment should include a detailed history of:

- Site and number of pains
- Intensity and severity of pains
- Radiation of pain
- Timing of pain
- Quality of pain, e.g. burning, stabbing
- Aggravating and relieving factors
- Aetiology of pain
- Type of pain
- Analgesic drug history
- Presence of any clinically significant psychiatric disorder.

It can also be useful to know to what extent pain is impacting on the patient's activities of daily living, such as eating, sleeping or moving, and the effects on the patient's mood. The inclusion of a body diagram within the chart provides a useful visual aid of the exact sites where the pain is being experienced and this can be very helpful in complex situations. The areas affected can then be labelled as a, b, c, etc., since patients may have more than one pain with differing aetiologies. Grond et al (1996) found that of 2266 cancer patients referred to a cancer service, one-third had a single pain, one-third had two pains and one-third had three or more pains.

Ideally, a full physical examination should be included in the assessment to aid diagnosis and decisions about the most appropriate treatment. Further investigations may be required, for example radiography, scan and blood tests, so that a comprehensive evaluation of the pain problem is completed as a basis for pain management.

The physical dimensions of pain are well recognised and much of the progress gained in pain management in recent years is based on an understanding of pain pathways and pharmacological interventions. However, the sensory experience of pain is also affected by a multitude of psychological and social processes that can have a profound effect upon the way in which a person perceives pain and the way in which that pain is expressed to health professionals. This aspect of assessment should not be overlooked, as in many instances of complex pain it is only when the psychosocial and spiritual issues of pain are addressed that the pain can be brought under control.

FACTORS THAT MAY AFFECT THE EXPERIENCE OF PAIN

The effects of anxiety on pain are well documented and are perhaps most clearly seen in studies on postoperative pain, where a direct relationship between anxiety and pain has been clearly demonstrated (Nelson et al 1998). The meaning attached to the presence of pain when it is cancer-related is a strong reminder of the active nature of the malignancy and, therefore, the progression of the disease. One of the most distressing aspects of serious illness is the feeling of helplessness and loss of control that it engenders and this can strongly influence pain behaviours. Because of the nature of the disease, anxiety is likely to be a main feature of a cancer patient's existence. Twycross & Wilcock (2002) identify many factors as being influential, for example adjustment disorder, worries about family and finances, fear of treatments, thoughts about the past such as guilt and lost opportunities, fears for the future, physical and mental impairment and death. Depression is also strongly linked with chronic cancer pain and pioneering work by Bonica (1990) found that many patients feel hopeless and despairing and can find no meaning in their pain at all.

The experience of illness, according to Copp & Copp (1993), leads many to confront their own mortality and ultimate reality. They suggest that spiritual responses to illness include the need to find hope and meaning and purpose in life to make sense of the senselessness. Saunders, in the 1960s, was the first to develop the concept of 'total pain', which came to include the entire illness, i.e. physical symptoms, mental distress, social problems and spiritual needs. However, while palliative physicians and pain specialists acknowledge the importance of using a holistic approach in understanding the suffering of patients, this has not necessarily been linked to physical pain (Strang et al 2004). While psychological factors are judged to have an important role in the onset, severity, exacerbation or maintenance of pain (American Psychiatric Association 1994), the reverse is also true. A study by Strang (1997) demonstrated that symptom control also has an effect on existential issues, and when pain was well controlled patients had significantly fewer existential problems or fears for the future.

There is general consensus among palliative care specialists that both psychosocial and spiritual distress have a significant influence upon the experience of physical pain, and there are numerous anecdotes about the difficulties of controlling spiralling pain in patients who have unresolved fears, unexpressed anger and emotional conflict. Interestingly, despite the widespread acknowledgement of the impact of psychosocial issues on pain, there is little in the way of hard data about this phenomenon. The SIGN guidelines for pain (2000) observe that a patient's beliefs about cancer pain and their behaviours in response to it often lead to pain remaining unrelieved, yet the evidence available that investigates the effects of psychosocial interventions is negligible and mostly resides at levels 3 and 4, which are the weakest form of evidence. More research needs to be done to look at effective interventions to address this important area of palliative care, and the skills of the whole multiprofessional team should be employed to create a sense of calm and security and to address the spiritual dimensions of pain.

MANAGEMENT

The WHO reports that by using their guidelines pain can be completely relieved in 80–90% of patients and that acceptable relief is possible in most of the remainder (Grond et al 1996). Pain that is difficult to address using the WHO guidelines is considered as 'complex pain' and may need specialist palliative intervention. This section of the chapter will address pain management at two levels, that of *basic level palliative care* for uncomplicated pain, which is said to be 'a core skill that every health-care professional, in whatever setting should possess', and *specialist level palliative care*, which is 'led by clinicians with recognised, specialist palliative medicine training and deals with the more complex problems' (Scottish Cancer Co-ordinating and Advisory Committee 1996).

World Health Organization guidelines

The WHO programme for cancer pain relief in 1996 developed guidance for the pharmacological management of cancer pain and they recommended the following principles, which remain best practice:

- **By the mouth**: The oral route remains the least invasive and safest method of drug administration and provides a rapid onset of analgesia. The use of injections should be reserved for those patients who are unable to take medications orally or those who are unable to absorb drugs via the gastrointestinal route.

- **By the clock**: Pain is increasingly difficult to control if breakthrough is allowed to occur. Since most oral analgesics act only for 4 hours or less, oral analgesics should be prescribed 4-hourly in order to achieve therapeutic levels of analgesia rather than waiting for the pain to occur.

- **By the ladder**: The goal of palliative care symptom relief is for the patient to be pain-free with as few side effects of the medication as can be achieved. Following careful assessment, the analgesic dose must be titrated against the patient's pain until the maximum recommended dose is reached, the pain is relieved or the patient experiences serious side effects. The WHO programme for pain relief recommends three possible steps dependent upon the severity, type and cause of the pain. It is suggested that by using this treatment strategy up to 88% of patients will achieve pain relief (Ventafridda et al 1987, Zech et al 1995).

Step 1: Mild pain

Where the pain experienced by the patient is mild, step 1 of the ladder is appropriate. This involves the use of a non-opioid analgesic, e.g. paracetamol, or a non-steroidal anti-inflammatory analgesic (NSAID), e.g. diclofenac or ibuprofen.

Step 2: Mild to moderate pain

For moderate pain, step 2 analgesics should be used. This step includes weak opioids; most contain codeine, which should be in excess of 30 mg to be effective. Examples include dihydrocodeine and dextropropoxyphene. Some pains do not respond completely to opioids alone and this level of the analgesic ladder recommends the addition of a non-opioid such as paracetamol or an

NSAID to the prescription, as this has been found to be more effective than an opioid alone (McQuay & Moore 1997).

Step 3: Moderate to severe pain

The standard drug of choice for this level of pain is morphine plus step 1 non-opioids and adjuvants. The dose required to control each individual's pain will vary. Therefore the amount of analgesia should be carefully titrated against the response, while constant monitoring for adverse side effects and toxicity takes place. Normal-release preparations take about 20 minutes for onset and reach a peak at about 60 minutes. They are more suitable for initiating therapy for severe pain. A rescue dose of one-sixth of the total daily dose of morphine should also be prescribed (SIGN 2000) and this can be taken at any time for breakthrough pain. Breakthrough pain is described as an unexpected increase in pain to greater than moderate intensity, occurring on a baseline pain of moderate intensity or less (Foley 1998). Pain should be evaluated initially 30–40 minutes after giving the breakthrough dose.

If the pain is persistent then the breakthrough can be repeated but if pain is still troublesome after a further 60 minutes then full reassessment of the patient is required. Medication should normally be reviewed every 24 hours in relation to pain relief, side effects and toxicity. The total amount of morphine required, including breakthrough analgesia, is divided by six and prescribed 4-hourly, with the breakthrough dose altered accordingly. When pain is controlled and stable, controlled-release (prolonged action) morphine can be considered. The daily dose should be calculated and given as a once- or twice-daily preparation. An appropriate dose of normal-release morphine, e.g. Oramorph or Sevredol, should still be continued as breakthrough analgesia, which will be effective within 30 minutes and last for up to 4 hours.

Where pain is experienced on movement but not at rest (incident pain), caution should be exercised in increasing the overall daily dose as this may lead to opioid toxicity. This type of pain is better managed by providing anticipatory breakthrough analgesia and considering adjuvant analgesia and alternative treatments such as radiotherapy and stabilising surgery (SIGN 2000).

MONITORING PAIN

A significant role in pain management is played by the nurse who is best placed to monitor the patient's pain by virtue of their role in the administration of analgesia. It is helpful to establish:

- The site of the particular pain being experienced, using the body chart of the initial assessment, as the patient may have multiple pains and the pains can be labelled a, b, c, etc.
- Whether it is linked to movement or rest
- The level of pain, and this should be elicited from the patient.

Various pain tools are available for this purpose ranging from basic descriptors of the pain to visual analogue scores where a simple 100 mm line is presented without subdivisions. At one end of the line a descriptor such as 'No pain' is placed and at the other 'Worst possible pain'. Patients are invited to score where the pain is along this line. We have found it most useful, however, to use a numerical rating scale from 0–5, with 0 being 'No pain' and 5 being 'Worst possible imagined pain'. Described as 'simple, robust, sensitive and reproducible' (Skevington 1996), such tools enable the patient to describe the severity of the pain in such a way that it can be given a numerical rating. This can then be revisited for comparison following the administration of pain relief medication and, over a period of time, offers a clear indicator of the pattern of pain being experienced (Fig. 4.1). Farrer (2001) notes the importance of assessing treatment response and cautions that this is one of the most neglected aspects of pain assessment, leading to rapid escalation of the dose and resulting in patients experiencing toxicity.

KEY COMMUNICATION ISSUES

Surprisingly, some patients are reluctant to admit that they are experiencing pain, and this may be for a variety of reasons. Sontag (1991) implies that in our society's view a diagnosis of cancer carries with it a unique air of fear characterised by terms such as 'cancer victim' and the need to 'do battle'. Such analogies are influential and create a state of anxiety and fear. Patients may in some circumstances deny pain until it becomes intolerable, because to admit the pain would mean having to face their own impending death. The stoical stance that some cultures adopt may also encourage the patient to see the admission of pain as a sign of weakness and pain as something that should be endured without complaint (Bates et al 1993). This is particularly prevalent in British culture and it is often good practice to check with the patients regularly to see if they are in pain rather than relying on them to tell you spontaneously.

Twycross (1995) observes that a common misperception among patients is that if a cancer patient is prescribed morphine they are going to die soon.

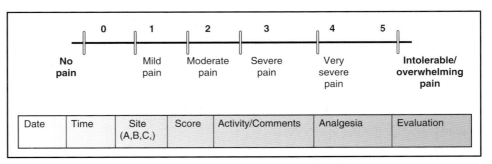

Figure 4.1 Highland Hospice pain monitoring chart

There are also a number of other beliefs about opioids that may influence acceptance of pain relief. An unpublished poll by the Napp pharmaceutical company among 1055 members of the public showed that 72% thought that morphine was addictive, 74% thought that it was dangerous, 40% thought that it impaired the ability to think clearly, 48% thought that it was associated with unpleasant side effects, 43% thought that it prevented normal life and 44% would be reluctant to take it (Smith 1995).

In reality, addiction is very rarely a problem because the pain acts as an antagonist to the opioid. More usually, when a patient is demanding injections every 2–3 hours it is because of inadequate pain relief and the behaviour ceases when the pain is properly managed with adequate dosage. Similarly, respiratory distress is rarely seen in patients with severe pain due to malignant disease provided the dose is titrated against the patient's pain. The correct use of morphine is likely to prolong life because pain will be relieved, there will be an increased appetite and ability to sleep and physical strength and activity will increase (Twycross 1995).

However, morphine does have some predictable side effects and the patient should be warned of what to expect. Initially, 30–60% of patients who are opioid-naive will develop nausea and/or vomiting (SIGN 2000). This usually settles within 5–10 days but an antiemetic such as metoclopramide or haloperidol in a low dose is generally effective in controlling this symptom. Drowsiness may occur in the first few days of regular opioids and subsequently if the dose is increased. This usually settles but the use of other drugs with a sedative side effect should be adjusted accordingly. The patient should be encouraged to persevere, in the knowledge that the problem will improve. Constipation commonly develops in most patients taking opioids and tolerance does not build up with long-term use, therefore, a prophylactic aperient should always be prescribed and a combination of stimulant and softening laxatives is recommended.

Other less common side effects that can occur include dry mouth, hypotension, confusion, poor concentration, gastroparesis, urinary retention and itch.

What could you do if you thought that a patient was concealing their pain? Suggestions:

- Establish reasons for reluctance to take opioids

- Try to dispel any misperceptions about opioids and give factual information

- Discuss realistically possible side effects and their duration to better prepare the patient and reduce anxiety and fear

- Articles and reading material could be provided as appropriate to the individual patient

- Give examples of patients with successful outcomes related to the use of opioids

- Offer to meet family members to minimise concerns

- Encourage questions at any time.

COMPLEX PAIN

When pain does not respond to the above strategies it is considered to be 'complex' pain and this requires specialist palliative care management. The pharmacological management of pain is predominantly the doctor's remit because complex pain states often have multiple facets, which are controlled by a variety of drugs, and there may be multiple pains. However, the nurse has the 24-hour custody of the patient and, consequently, has to make decisions about the administration of what is often a variety of prescribed drugs based on assessment of the patient's pain and knowledge of appropriate interventions. A sound knowledge of the pain pathways, influences and pharmacology is therefore essential in specialist palliative care.

OPIOID TOXICITY

Individuals will vary radically in their responses to opioids and this will depend upon whether the patient is opioid-naive, the degree to which the pain is responsive to opioids, the titration rate, renal and hepatic function and additional medication. Some types of pain are only partially opioid-responsive and the required escalating dosage can lead to side effects and toxicity. Part of the nurse's role is to watch for signs of opioid toxicity, which may include agitation, vivid dreams and nightmares, hallucinations, confusion and myoclonic jerks. Accompanying dehydration and alteration in renal function can compound the problem by accumulating toxins that would normally be excreted in the urine. If opioid toxicity is suspected then the dose should be reduced, adjuvant analgesics increased where possible, adequate hydration ensured and any confusion and agitation managed with haloperidol. In cases of toxicity or where there are severe side effects, morphine may be replaced by a different opioid. Alternative opioids have not been shown to have a superior clinical analgesic effect but they may have a different side effect profile, enabling the patient to be able to tolerate higher doses of the drug to control the pain (opioid switching). Examples include transdermal fentanyl, methadone, hydromorphone or oxycodone. Conversion to these opioids should be carefully monitored and controlled as they have different potencies from morphine.

NEUROPATHIC PAIN

Adjuvant analgesics that have been found to be effective in controlling neuropathic pain include tricyclic antidepressants such as amitriptyline, imipramine and clomipramine (McQuay & Moore 1997), and anticonvulsants such as carbamazepine, sodium valproate and gabapentin. The anti-inflammatory properties of steroids can also have a significant influence in pain management. Tumours often develop an area of inflammation with associated oedema that presses on neighbouring tissue and veins. Corticosteroids reduce the inflammation and therefore the total mass and associated pain. Therapeutic trials of high doses of steroids, e.g. dexamethasone, have been found to be effective in a variety of pain syndromes, including spinal cord compression and raised intercranial pressure. Steroids have the additional advantage of improving appetite, mood and general feeling of wellbeing, but have significant side effects. The dose and duration depend upon the clinical response to treatment. These adjuvants are usually used in conjunction with an opioid.

SENSITISATION AND 'WIND UP'

The use of the anaesthetic ketamine at subanaesthetic levels is gaining in popularity for the treatment of neuropathic pain states because of its ability to block the NMDA receptor at the dorsal horn. Side effects include transient hypertension, hallucinations, dysphoria and vivid dreams, so ketamine should only be used under specialist supervision.

ALTERNATIVE INTERVENTIONS

Although radiotherapy and chemotherapy are generally used as treatment modes, they can also be effective in the management of symptoms. Treatments are designed to create minimal disturbance to the lifestyle of the patient. Bone metastases with associated pain are generally very responsive to radiotherapy and treatment can make a significant improvement in the patient's pain. However, the duration of the response varies and there may be side effects because of the related underlying structures. Other pain problems that can be relieved include those resulting from brain metastases and spinal cord compression. Metastases in the long bones are prone to pathological fracture which will require internal fixation before pain will be improved. Bisphosphonates may also be beneficial for bone pain by reducing the production of proinflammatory cytokines (Crosby 1998).

Neurolytic and neurological procedures are much less common due to the drug advances in symptom control but spinal blocks, epidurals and intrathecal infusions are still crucial in a small number of patients where pain is resistant to drug therapy.

NON-DRUG INTERVENTIONS

When anxiety or spiritual distress are significant factors in the patient's pain, complementary therapies such as aromatherapy and massage, hypnosis and relaxation therapy can be effective in improving pain control in conjunction with spiritual care, good communication and counselling.

GASTROINTESTINAL PROBLEMS

INTRODUCTION

Nausea and vomiting in patients with advanced cancer are reported to have an overall incidence of 60% and 30% respectively (Mystakidou et al 1998), and patients with terminal cancer frequently experience nausea for extended periods, often more than 4 weeks (Bruera & Neumann 1998). These symptoms are particularly demoralising and demeaning and many patients find them equally as distressing as pain in terms of impact on quality of life (Dikken & Sitzia 1998, Dunlop 1989). The close and practical nature of nursing offers the opportunity for nurses to provide significant support and reassurance for patients at this distressing time. However, an understanding of the physiology of nausea and vomiting is crucial to effective nursing management, since antiemetics have differing effects and act by either blocking the neurotransmitters (Baines 1997) or by blocking the receptors on the physiological pathways to prevent activation by the transmitter (Hawthorn 1995).

PHYSIOLOGY

Vomiting is essentially a protective mechanism to rid the body of any ingested poison. Nausea is related to this process, being an unpleasant sensation that will stop further intake of the harmful substance. However the two events are not necessarily synonymous, since nausea does not always result in vomiting and in some circumstances vomiting can occur spontaneously without any precipitating nausea. When nausea occurs there is a disturbance in the normally constant contractions and relaxations of the stomach, which becomes flaccid in order to prevent further absorption of toxins. During vomiting the contents of the duodenum are reversed back into the stomach by a process of retroperistalsis (Lee et al 1985) and this culminates in a large contraction of the respiratory muscles and the muscles overlying the stomach, propelling the stomach contents out through the mouth (Hawthorn 1995).

When a toxic substance is ingested, or there are unusually high levels of normal body chemicals, specific detectors within the body identify the need to vomit and trigger the entire process. These main detectors are in the gastrointestinal tract, the labyrinthine apparatus in the ear and a specialised area of the brain called the chemoreceptor-trigger zone (CTZ), which is situated on the floor of the fourth ventricle. The CTZ is situated in an area outside the blood–brain barrier and can therefore access toxins circulating in the blood. It is also in contact with the cerebrospinal fluid and so in addition identifies toxic substances in this area. Following stimulation of these receptors, messages are relayed to the brain by the vagus nerve and communicated through neurotransmitters. Receptors are the recognition sites on the receiving cells that identify, bind to and are activated by the messenger molecule carrying the stimulus so that an emetic response is activated. Important receptors in the emetic pathway would appear to be dopamine receptors, which are present on the CTZ and vomiting centre (dopamine affects gastric motility), and 5-hydroxytryptamine-3 (5-HT$_3$) receptors, which are distributed in areas of the body involved in vomiting. There are also mechanoreceptors, which detect when the stomach or duodenum becomes overdistended or if changes occur in the pattern of gastric motility, and convey this information to the brain. The area of the brain that coordinates the whole vomiting process is situated in the brain stem close to the fourth ventricle and is called the vomit centre. The function of the vomit centre is to detect the need to vomit and then set in motion a complex sequence of events that includes nausea and retching and culminates in vomiting.

HIGHER CENTRES

The influence of psychological effects on nausea and vomiting should also not be underestimated. Anxiety-induced emesis is a common experience (Mannix 2004) and patients or their carers may be able to identify anxiety as the trigger for nausea. Anticipatory emesis is a classic example of the influence of the higher centres for patients who have suffered nausea and/or vomiting as a result of cytotoxic therapy. Any reminder of the experience can provoke a conditioned response.

EVALUATION

There are a number of causes of nausea and vomiting and these include chemical imbalances as a result of drugs such as opioids or because of metabolic disturbances caused by hypercalcaemia or hypernatraemia. Gastrointestinal problems of gastric stasis and constipation can be significant in emesis and may lead to outflow obstruction, while enlarged tumour bulk stretching the liver or abdomen or obscuring the gastric outlet will result in large-volume vomits. Cerebral tumours may lead to raised intercranial pressure, triggering nausea and vomiting, and anxiety can significantly exacerbate the situation. For the palliative care patient, causes can be multifactorial and good multiprofessional assessment is vital to accurate diagnosis and treatment. Assessment should include:

- A detailed history, including tumour histology and spread and previous treatment
- Onset of symptoms
- Physical examination
- Evaluation of biochemical status
- Factors that exacerbate or relieve symptoms
- Effects on activities of living
- Further investigations if necessary, e.g. radiological investigation.

MANAGEMENT

Pharmacological management principles are outlined in Table 4.1.

MONITORING

A key role is played by the nurse in the monitoring of the pattern and nature of the nausea and vomiting. The vomitus should be observed and its

TABLE 4.1
Pharmacological management of nausea and vomiting

Cause	Clinical features	Antiemetic management	Drug action	Side effects	Other interventions
Chemically induced nausea and vomiting; Drug-induced, e.g. opiates, cytotoxics, anticonvulsants; Metabolic-induced, e.g. uraemia, hypercalcaemia, liver failure	Constant nausea, other signs of toxicity, e.g. small pupils, drowsiness, confusion	Haloperidol Metoclopramide Domperidone / Cyclizine / Ondansetron	Dopamine antagonists – act on receptors in the CTZ and vomiting centre / Histamine antagonist – acts on the vomiting centre / 5-HT$_3$ antagonist – acts on receptors in CTZ	Extrapyramidal reactions, restlessness, agitation / Dry mouth, sedation / Headache, constipation, diarrhoea	Review drug regimen; check biochemistry; treat underlying cause of metabolic disturbance
Gastrointestinal causes: gastric stasis, outflow obstruction	Epigastric fullness and discomfort, acid regurgitation, early satiety	Metoclopramide	Increase rate of gastric and upper intestinal peristalsis and relax pylorus	Extrapyramidal reactions, colic and cramps in GI obstruction	Dietary advice; surgical intervention if appropriate; relieve constipation if appropriate
Enlarged liver – stretch, obstruction of gastric outlet, gastric stretch, tumour bulk in the abdomen – pressing	Large volume vomits which may contain undigested food, nausea relieved by vomiting, pain	Cyclizine	Acts on vomit centre	Dry mouth, sedation	Steroid therapy to reduce tumour mass. Temporary naso-gastric tube may be necessary

on gut or squashing stomach	and colic				
Constipation	Altered bowel habit	Cyclizine	Decreased gut peristalsis from stomach to large bowel. Slows gastric emptying, decreases volume of secretions	Dry mouth, sedation	Treat underlying cause. If subacute, relieve constipation with aperients/enemas
Bowel obstruction	Abdominal swelling, changes in bowel sounds, copious vomiting of fluid and faecal fluid as a late feature	Hyoscine hydrobromide Octreotide Haloperidol Levomepromazine	Acts on vomit centre and GI tract Reduces gastrointestinal motility and secretions Dopamine receptor antagonists	Dry mouth, ileus, urinary retention, blurred vision, occasionally agitation May potentiate hypoglycaemia Extrapyramidal reactions Restlessness, agitation Sedative effects	Surgical intervention if possible. Temporary nasogastric tube may be necessary
		Dexamethasone	Reduce tumour mass	Glucocorticoid effects, especially diabetes mellitus Mineralocorticoid effects. Cushing's syndrome	

Continued

TABLE 4.1

Pharmacological management of nausea and vomiting—Cont'd

Cause	Clinical features	Antiemetic management	Drug action	Side effects	Other interventions
Raised intracranial pressure: cerebral tumour; intracranial tumour; intracranial bleeding, infiltration of meninges by tumour; skull metastases, cerebral infection	Neurological signs: drowsiness, headache, dizziness, papilloedema, nausea and/or vomiting	Cyclizine	Histamine antagonist: acts on vomit centre and gastrointestinal tract	Dry mouth, ileus, urinary retention, blurred vision, occasionally agitation	
		Hyoscine hydrobromide Dexamethasone	Reduce cerebral oedema or tumour mass	Glucocorticoid effects, especially diabetes mellitus Mineralocorticoid effects. Cushing's syndrome	
Anxiety: anticipatory nausea and vomiting associated with chemotherapy	Waves of nausea and vomiting	Antihistamine or anticholinergics, if required Anxiolytic benzodiazepines	Act on vomit centre Agonists to GABA$_A$ receptors	Drowsiness Drowsiness, impaired psychomotor skills and hypotonia	Reassurance, relaxation, psychological techniques

Date	Time	Nausea	Vomiting	Comments	Medication	Time	Nausea	Vomiting	Comments	Medication
Evaluation:										
Date	Time	Nausea	Vomiting	Comments	Medication	Time	Nausea	Vomiting	Comments	Medication
Evaluation:										

Figure 4.2 Highland Hospice nausea and vomiting monitoring tool

characteristics recorded: amount, colour, odour, presence of blood, undi-
gested foodstuffs or faecal fluid; whether vomiting is associated with nausea
or occurs spontaneously and whether vomiting relieves nausea. In specialist
palliative care areas several drugs may be prescribed and the nurse will make
a decision on which is the most appropriate, based upon their assessment. The
outcome of the intervention should also be noted and recorded so that a clear
pattern emerges upon which management can be based (Fig. 4.2).

CASE STUDY 4.1
Management of vomiting

A 55-year-old woman is admitted to your area for the management of vomiting. She has
a diagnosis of ovarian cancer and, despite surgical de-bulking and chemotherapy, a recent
abdominal scan confirms an intraperitoneal mass. The oncologist has told her that her
prognosis is poor and that further chemotherapy is not an option.
History and presenting features include:

- No bowel movement for 5 days and she is not passing flatus
- Projectile vomiting in large amounts approximately twice daily and the vomitus is foul-
  smelling
- Intermittent colicky abdominal pain
- On examination, her abdomen is bloated and no bowel sounds are present
- Symptoms seem worse since commencing metoclopramide 2 days ago

Continued

●●●●●●

CASE STUDY **4.1**—CONT'D

Questions for consideration

1. What is the most likely cause for this lady's vomiting and why?

2. What investigations, if any, would be appropriate?

3. What antiemetics could be effective for this lady?

4. What surgical procedures may be necessary?

5. Given the poor prognosis, what psychological interventions may be of benefit?

Suggestions

1. On the basis of the clinical picture it is likely that this patient is suffering from severe constipation and subacute obstruction

2. It may be appropriate to order an abdominal X-ray to establish the likely cause of the obstruction

3. Discuss the meaning of the symptom to the patient and reassure that if initial interventions are not effective there are other options

4. If anxiety is a problem, treat as described on page 100

5. Prokinetic agents such as metoclopramide should be avoided, as they promote peristalsis and may exacerbate the symptoms of bowel obstruction

6. Dexamethasone may be used to reduce peritumour, oedema – benefits must be weighed against costs of steroid use.

7. Antiemetics:
   a. Octreotide – antisecretory: effective but costs may be prohibitive
   b. Hyoscine butylbromide – also antisecretory action and less expensive
   c. Cyclizine

8. Venting gastrostomy

9. Aromatherapy, hypnosis, relaxation therapy and acupuncture may be useful to interfere with stimuli that induce nausea

10. Sensitivity with food smells and oral hygiene

11. Individualised and holistic nursing care.

CONSTIPATION

INTRODUCTION

With between 40 and 57% of hospice patients requiring rectal intervention on a regular basis, constipation has to be a high priority for palliative nursing care, since nursing plays a key role in the management of this symptom. Palliative care patients are at particular risk of constipation and there are many influencing factors. For example, the tumour could be exerting external abdominal pressure or occluding the bowel wall, or there could be spinal cord damage or hypercalcaemia. The effects of the illness can also lead to dehydration, poor food and fibre intake, lack of exercise, weakness and confusion, which are all contributory features (Fallon & Welsh 1998). This is compounded by the constipating effect of many of the drugs used in palliative care and, in particular, the effects of opioids, which suppress forward peristalsis and raise sphincter tone (87–90% of patients taking strong opioids require laxatives (Bruera et al 1994, Sykes 1998)). Elderly patients are also likely to have other concurrent diseases predisposing to constipation.

If not addressed, the extended time that the contents remain in the gut results in increased water absorption, causing the faeces to become hard and eventually impacted. The faecal mass higher in the colon is then broken down by bacteria into a more liquid form, which can seep past the mass and may be mistaken for diarrhoea, thus confusing the diagnosis. Colicky, colonic pain frequently occurs as the colonic muscle contracts to expel the bowel contents. Nausea and vomiting are associated symptoms and urinary retention and cognitive impairment may also coexist. Complete absence of stool in the rectum may indicate colonic inertia.

EVALUATION

As with any palliative care symptom, a thorough assessment underpins sound management. It is important to elicit what the normal bowel pattern has been, if/when it changed, and the current pattern of defaecation. The appearance of the stool often gives an indication of the nature of the problem: small, hard stools may mean a slowing of the transit time through the bowel, while ribbon-like stools may point to stenosis. Blood in the stool could indicate tumour or haemorrhoids. Bowel habits vary across the population but, generally, if there has been no bowel evacuation for longer than 3 days this would raise concern.

Abdominal examination and rectal examination should be carried out if constipation is suspected. If it is unclear whether obstruction is present then an abdominal X-ray may help to distinguish between the two conditions. This is an important distinction to make, as interventions for constipation can cause severe pain in an obstructed patient.

MANAGEMENT

Any patient receiving morphine will require a laxative as a prophylactic measure. The choice of aperient for the constipated patient will be made on the basis of the action of the laxative and the consistency of the stool.

Modes of action of aperients

• Surface-wetting agents, such as docusate sodium and poloxamer, increase water penetration and therefore soften the stool but are seldom of adequate efficacy when used alone. More often they are used in combination with contact stimulants.

- Contact stimulant agents, e.g. bisacodyl, dantron, senna, sodium picosulfate, act on the large bowel to induce peristalsis.
- Bulk-forming drugs provide fibre and need to be taken with adequate water – they are seldom used in palliative care.
- Osmotic laxatives, e.g. lactulose, act primarily on the small bowel by exerting an osmotic influence, which retains water in the stool. If given alone in palliative care the amount used to be effective often causes bloating and colic.
- A combination of surface wetting agent and contact stimulant, e.g. co-danthrusate, co-danthramer, often produces a comfortable stool and is used in most UK hospices (Twycross & Wilcock 2002). Aperients should be taken on a regular basis and titrated to the required dose.

Some new developments and alternative approaches have been reported by Sykes (1999). There is interest in the use of cisapride and subcutaneous infusion of metoclopramide. The use of oral naloxone in opioid-induced constipation has also shown some success experimentally but opioid withdrawal can occur and more work needs to be done to clarify the role of such drugs in constipation management.

If constipation is severe or the patient is faecally impacted, it may be necessary to resort to rectal laxatives such as arachis oil if the stool is hard. Docusate sodium or sodium phosphate is more appropriate to stimulate peristalsis if the stool is soft. Highland Hospice has produced the protocol illustrated in Figure 4.3 for the management of constipation.

In some cases, as a last resort, it may be necessary to carry out a manual evacuation but this should always be under sedative cover such as midazolam or diazepam. It is easier to accomplish if the faeces are kept firm and are moved into the rectum by the administration of a contact laxative. Paraplegic patients may require regular rectal aperients and manual evacuation.

Non-pharmacological management

- Dignity and privacy in toileting
- Ensure adequate fluid intake
- Accurate daily recordings of stool consistency, ease of defaecation
- Encourage use of fruit cocktails and increase fibre intake, if possible
- Make sure food looks as attractive as possible
- Prophylaxis.

WORKING WITH THE FAMILY

When a family member is very ill their close relatives often operate on a heightened state of anxiety and fear. Loss of control can be an issue as trust must be placed entirely in the health-care professional's expertise and this can

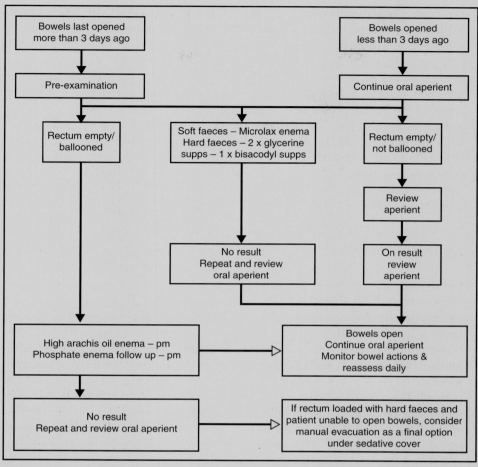

Figure 4.3 Highland Hospice – protocol for the assessment and management of constipation

leave people feeling very vulnerable. Problems can arise when family members do not understand why drugs are being prescribed or changed. They may also become angry with the staff when the disease progresses and it is not possible to prevent the deterioration of the patient. It is therefore essential to involve relatives in assessment of symptoms and discussions about rationales or changes in treatment and interventions. However, family members do have a tendency to overestimate the level of pain in their relatives (Clip & George 1992) and this can be misleading so the patient must always be the main assessor of the pain.

DEPRESSION

Depression coexists with other physical symptoms in palliative care patients (Radbruch et al 2003), and is one of the most frequently reported psychiatric symptoms in patients with advanced cancer (Block 2000). In 2004, Lloyd-Williams et al reported the findings from a prospective study that confirmed a close association between physical symptoms and depression in palliative care patients. One issue to be taken into account when discussing depression in the context of palliative care is the difficulty associated with distinguishing between sadness, appropriate at the end of life, and a true depressive illness. Another potential problem is screening for the symptom. Many specialist nurses report that they do not have the skills to assess for depression (Lloyd-Williams & Payne 2003). Although there are validated assessment tools available (Zigmond & Snaith 1983), the majority rely on patient participation, which is burdensome to patients who are not only dying but also have a depressive illness that may well further reduce their motivation and ability to contribute to the assessment process.

CONCLUSION

Symptoms are complex, demanding a multidimensional approach to their management. This should include non-pharmacological, pharmacological and multiprofessional components. No matter the specific symptom, a generic process should be adhered to, as discussed earlier in this chapter. This ensures that a methodical, scientific format is followed, which will facilitate a problem-solving approach and lead to satisfactory patient outcomes with the minimum time delay. No one health professional can facilitate all the needs of the patient. The skill of working in a successful interdisciplinary team is that each individual recognises their own professional and personal limitations. This enables individual practitioners to seek advice from, and respect the expertise of, their colleagues. This skill is perhaps the essence of the true professional and as such prioritises patient needs.

The US essayist and poet Ralph Waldo Emerson (1803–1882) reminds us that 'Shallow men believe in luck. Strong men believe in cause and effect' – good symptom control is not a matter of luck, rather knowledge and skill in applying a methodical process.

REFERENCES

Ahmedzai S, Davis C 1997 Nebulised drugs in palliative care. Thorax 52(Suppl 2):S75–S77

American Psychiatric Association 1994 Diagnostic and statistical manual of psychiatric disorders, 4th edn. American Psychiatric Association, Washington, DC

Andrewes T 2002 The management of breathlessness in palliative care. Nursing Standard 17(5):43–52, 54–55

Aranda S 2003 A framework for symptom assessment. In: O'Connor M, Aranda S (eds) Palliative care nursing. A guide to practice. Radcliffe Medical Press, Oxford, p 89–100

Armstrong E M 2001 Palliative care for all: the Scottish Executive's view. In: Palliative care for all. Responding to need not diagnosis. Scottish Partnership for Palliative Care, Edinburgh. Available on line at: www.scotland.gov.uk

Back I 2001 Palliative medicine handbook, 3rd edn. PM Books, Cardiff

Baines M J 1997 Nausea, vomiting and intestinal obstruction. British Medical Journal 315:1148–1150

Bates M S, Edwards W T, Anderson K O 1993 Ethnocultural influences on variation in chronic pain perception. Pain 52:101–112

Beck S, Schwartz A, Towsley G et al 2004 Psychometric evaluation of the Pittsburgh Sleep Quality Index in cancer patients. Journal of Pain and Symptom Management 27:140–148

Beckles M, Spiro S, Collice G, Rudd R 2003 Initial evaluation of the patient with lung cancer: symptoms, signs, laboratory tests and paraneoplastic syndromes. Chest 123:97–104

Birks C 1997 Pathophysiology and management of dyspnoea in palliative care and the evolving role of the nurse. International Journal of Palliative Nursing 3:264–274

Block S 2000 Assessing and managing depression in the terminally ill patient. Annals of Internal Medicine 32:209–218

Bonica J J (ed.) 1990 Cancer pain. In: The management of cancer pain. Lea & Febiger, Philadelphia, PA

Booth S 1998 Management of dyspnoea in advanced cancer. British Journal of Therapy and Rehabilitation 5:282–283

Booth S, Anderson H, Swannick M et al 2004 The use of oxygen in the palliation of breathlessness. A report of the expert working group of the Scientific Committee of the Association of Palliative Medicine. Respiratory Medicine 98:66–77

Bredin M, Corner J, Krishnasamy M et al 1999 Multicentre randomised controlled trial of nursing intervention for breathlessness in patients with lung cancer. British Medical Journal 381:901–904

Bruera E, Neumann C M 1998 Management of specific symptom complexes in patients receiving palliative care. Journal of the Canadian Medical Association 158:1717–1726

Bruera E, Portenoy R K 2001 Topics in palliative care. Oxford University Press, Oxford

Bruera E, Suarez-Almazor M, Velasco A et al 1994 The assessment of constipation in terminal cancer patients admitted to a palliative care unit: a retrospective review. Journal of Pain and Symptom Management 9:515–519

Bruera E, Schmitz B, Pither J, Neumann Hanson J 2000 The frequency and correlates of dyspnoea in patients with advanced cancer. Journal of Pain and Symptom Management 19:357–362

Chochinov H 2002 Dignity – conserving care – a new model for palliative care: helping the patient feel valued. Journal of the American Medical Association 287:2253–2260

Clinical Standards Board for Scotland 2002 Clinical standards for specialist palliative care. NHS Quality Improvement Scotland, Edinburgh

Clip E, George L 1992 Patients with cancer and their spouse caregivers: perceptions of the illness experience. Cancer 69:1074–1079

Cooley M, Short T, Moriarty H 2002 Patterns of symptom distress in adults receiving treatment for lung cancer. Journal of Palliative Care 18:150–159

Copp L A, Copp J D 1993 Illness and the human spirit. Quality of Life: A Nursing Challenge 2:50–55

Corner J, Plant H, Warner L 1995 Developing a nursing approach to managing dyspnoea in lung cancer. International Journal of Palliative Nursing 1:5–11

Crosby V 1998 A randomised controlled trial of intravenous clodronate. Journal of Pain and Symptom Management 15:266–268

Daut R L, Cleeland C S, Flannery R C 1983 Development of the Wisconsin Brief Pain Questionnaire to assess pain in cancer and other disease. Pain 17:197–210

Davis C 1997 ABC of palliative care: breathlessness, cough and other respiratory problems. British Medical Journal 315:931–934

Davis C L, Sheldon F 1999 Therapeutic innovations. In: Clark D, Hockley J, Ahmedzai S (eds) New themes in palliative care. Open University Press, Buckingham, p 223–238

De Conno F, Martini C 2001 Symptom assessment outcomes in home-based palliative care. In: Bruera E, Portenoy R K (eds) Topics in palliative care UK. Oxford University Press, Oxford, p 177–193

De Rond M, de Wit R, van Dam F et al 1999 Daily pain assessment: value for nurses and patients. Journal of Advanced Nursing 29:436–444

Dein S 2002 A place for psychostimulants in palliative care? Journal of Palliative Care 18:196–199

Dikken C, Sitzia J 1998 Patients' experiences of chemotherapy: side effects associated with 5 fluorouracil and folinic acid in the treatment of colorectal cancer. Journal of Clinical Nursing 7:371–379

Donnelly S, Walsh D, Rybicki L 1994 The symptoms of advanced cancer in 1,000 patients. Journal of Palliative Care 10:57

Doyle D, Hanks J, Cherny N, Calman K (eds) 2004 Oxford textbook of palliative medicine. Oxford University Press, Oxford

Dudgeon D 1994 Physician/nursing roles and perspectives in relationship to delivery of palliative care. Annals of the Academy of Medicine of Singapore 23:249–251

Dunlop G M 1989 A study of the relative frequency and importance of gastrointestinal symptoms, and weakness in patients with far advanced cancer. Palliative Medicine 4:37–43

Edmonds P, Higginson I, Altmann D et al 2000 Is the presence of dyspnoea a risk factor for morbidity in cancer patients? Journal of Pain and Symptom Management 19:15–22

Fallon M, Welsh J 1998 The management of gastrointestinal symptoms. In: Faull C, Carter Y, Woof R (eds) Handbook of palliative care. Blackwell Science, Oxford

Farrer K 2001 Pain control. In: Kinghorn S, Gamlin R (eds) Palliative nursing: bringing comfort and hope. Baillière Tindall/RCN, Edinburgh

Faull C, Woof R 2002 Oxford core texts: palliative care. Oxford University Press, Oxford

Field L 1996 Are nurses still underestimating patients pain post operatively? British Journal of Nursing 13:778–784

Fishman B, Pasternak S, Wallenstein S L et al 1987 The memorial pain assessment chart. A valid instrument for the assessment of cancer pain. Cancer 60:51–58

Fleming K 1997 The meaning of hope to palliative care patients. International Journal of Palliative Nursing 3:14–18

Foley K M 1998 Pain assessment and cancer pain syndromes. In: Doyle D, Hanks G W, Macdonald N (eds) The Oxford textbook of palliative medicine, 2nd edn. Oxford Medical Publications, Oxford, p 310–331

Friedrichsen M, Strang P, Carlsson M 2001 Receiving bad news: experiences of family members. Journal of Palliative Care 17:241–247

Grond S, Zech D, Diefenbach C et al 1996 Assessment of cancer pain: a prospective evaluation in 2266 cancer patients referred to a cancer service. Pain 64:107–114

Grossman S, Sheidler V, Swedeen K et al 1991 Correlation of patient and caregivers ratings of cancer pain. Journal of Pain and Symptom Management 6:53–57

Hately J, Scott A, Laurence V et al 2001 A palliative care approach for breathlessness in cancer: a clinical evaluation. Help the Hospices, London

Hawthorn J 1995 Understanding and management of nausea and vomiting. Blackwell Science, Oxford

Hawthorn J, Redmond K 2001 Pain: causes and management. Blackwell Science, Oxford

Hoban V 2003 Integrating complementary therapies. Nursing Times 99(30):20–23

Homsi J, Walsh D, Nelson K 2000 Psychostimulants in supportive care. Supportive Care in Cancer 8:385–397

Hotopf M, Chidgey J, Addington-Hall J, Lan Ny K 2002 Depression in advanced disease: a systematic review. Part 1. Prevalence and case finding. Palliative Medicine 16:81–97

Hough A 2001 Physiotherapy in respiratory care: an evidence-based approach to respiratory and cardiac management, 3rd edn. Nelson Thornes, Cheltenham

Hoyal C, Grant J, Chamberlain F et al 2002 Improving management of breathlessness using a clinical effectiveness programme. International Journal of Palliative Nursing 8:78–87

IASP 1994 Classification of chronic pain, 2nd edn. International Association for the Study of Pain, Seattle, WA

Ingham J, Coyle N 1999 Teamwork in end-of-life care: a nurse–physician perspective on introducing physicians to palliative care concepts. In: Clark D, Hockley J, Ahmedzai S (eds) New themes in palliative care. Open University Press, Buckingham, p 255–274

Jenkins V, Fallowfield L, Saul J 2001 Information needs of patients with cancer: results from a large study in UK cancer centres. British Journal of Cancer 84:48–51

Jennings A L, Davies A N, Higgins J P T, Broadly K 2004 Opioids for palliation of breathlessness in terminal illness (Cochrane Review). In: The Cochrane Library, issue 1. Update Software, Oxford

Kabel A, Roberts D 2003 Professionals' perceptions of maintaining personhood in hospice care. International Journal of Palliative Nursing 9:283–289

Kearney M 2000 A place of healing. Working with suffering in living and dying. Oxford University Press, Oxford

Keedwell P, Snaith R 1996 What do anxiety scales measure? Acta Psychiatrica Scandinavica 93:177–180

Kissane D W 2000 Psychospiritual and existential distress. The challenge for palliative care. Australian Family Physician 29:1022–1025

Klinkenberg M, Willems D L, van der Wal G, Deeg D J H 2004 Symptom burden in the last week of life. Journal of Pain and Symptom Management 27:5–13

Krishnasamy M, Corner J, Bredin M et al 2001 Cancer nursing practice development: understanding breathlessness. Journal of Clinical Nursing 10:103–108

Kutner J, Kassner C, Nowels D 2001 Symptom burden at the end of life: hospice providers' perceptions. Journal of Pain and Symptom Management 21:473–480

Kvale P 2003 Palliative care. Chest 123:284–311

Le Grande S, Walsh D 1999 Palliative management of dyspnoea in advanced cancer. Current Opinion in Oncology 11:250

Lee K Y, Park H J, Chey W Y 1985 Studies of mechanisms of retching and vomiting in dogs. Digestive Disease and Sciences 30:22–28

Lloyd-Williams M, Payne S 2003 A qualitative study of palliative care nurses' perceptions on depression. Palliative Medicine 17:334–339

Lloyd-Williams M, Dennis M, Taylor F 2004 A prospective study to determine the association between physical symptoms and depression in patients with advanced cancer. Palliative Medicine 18:558–563

Loftus L, Weston V 2001 The development of nurse-led clinics in cancer care. Journal of Clinical Nursing 10:215–220

Lothian Palliative Care Guidelines Group 2002 Breathlessness guidelines. Lothian Primary Care NHS Trust, Edinburgh

Macmillan Cancer Relief 2003 Professional resource catalogue. Macmillan Practice Development Unit, Southampton

Manning H 1995 Pathophysiology of dyspnoea. New England Journal of Medicine 333:1547–1553

Mannix K A 2004 Gastrointestinal symptoms: palliation of nausea and vomiting. In: Doyle D, Hanks J, Cherny N, Calman K (eds) Oxford textbook of palliative medicine. Oxford University Press, Oxford, p 459–467

McCaffery M, Beebe A, Latham J, Ball D 1997 Pain: clinical manual for nursing practice. CV Mosby, London, p 15

McMillan S, Brent J 2002 Symptom distress and quality of life in patients with cancer newly admitted to hospice home care. Oncology Nursing Forum 29:1421–1428

McMillan S, Moody L 2003 Hospice patient and caregiver congruence in reporting patients' symptom intensity. Cancer Nursing 26:113–118

McQuay H, Moore A 1997 Bibliography and systematic reviews in cancer pain: a report to the NHS National Cancer Research and Development Programme. NHS Publications, Oxford

Melzack R 1993 The McGill Pain Questionnaire. In: Melzack R (ed.) Pain measurement and assessment. Raven Press, New York, p 41–48

Minowa Y, Ide T, Nishino T 2002 Effects of inhaled furosemide on CO_2 ventilatory responsiveness in humans. Pulmonary Pharmacology and Therapeutics 15:363–368

Moore S, Corner J, Haviland J et al 2002 Nurse led follow up and conventional medical follow up in management of patients with lung cancer: randomised trial. British Medical Journal 325:1145–1155

Mystakidou K, Befon S, Liossi C, Vlachos L 1998 Comparison of the efficacy and safety of tropisetron, metoclopramide and chlorpromazine in the treatment of emesis associated with advanced cancer. Cancer 83:1214–1223

Nelson F V, Zimmerman L, Barnason R N et al 1998 The relationship and influence of anxiety on postoperative pain in the coronary artery bypass graft patient. Journal of Pain and Symptom Management 15:102–109

Nishino T, Ide T, Sudo T, Sato J 2000 Inhaled furosemide greatly alleviates the sensation of experimentally induced dyspnoea. American Journal of Respiratory and Critical Care Medicine 161:1963–1967

O'Brien T 2001 Neurodegenerative disease. In: Addington-Hall J, Higginson J (eds) Palliative care for non-cancer patients. Oxford University Press, Oxford, p 44–55

Paes P 2004 Breathless and fatigue in cardiac failure. European Journal of Palliative Care 11:9–11

Passik S, Donaghy K, Theobald D et al 2000 Oncology staff recognition of depressive symptoms on videotaped interviews of depressed cancer patients: implications for designing a training program. Journal of Pain and Symptom Management 19:329–338

Passik S, Kirsh K, Donaghy K et al 2002 Patient-related barriers to fatigue communication: initial validation of the Fatigue Management Barriers Questionnaire. Journal of Pain and Symptom Management 24:481–493

Payne R, Gonzales G R 1999 Management of pain. In: Doyle D, Hanks G W C, Macdonald N (eds) Oxford textbook of palliative medicine. Oxford University Press, Oxford, p 300

Radbruch L, Nauck F, Ostgathe C 2003 What are the problems in palliative care? Results from a representative survey. Support Care in Cancer 11:442–451

Ramfelt E, Severinsson E, Lutzen K 2002 Attempting to find meaning in illness to achieve emotional coherence: the experiences of patients with colorectal cancer. Cancer Nursing 25:141–149

Regnard C, Kindlen M 2002 Supportive and palliative care in cancer: an introduction. Radcliffe Medical, Oxford

Regnard C, Tempest S 1998 A guide to symptom relief in advanced disease, 4th edn. Hochland & Hochland, Hale

Royal Pharmaceutical Society 2004 British national formulary 47. British Medical Association and Royal Pharmaceutical Society of Great Britain, London

Scottish Cancer Co-ordinating and Advisory Committee 1996 Commissioning cancer services in Scotland. Report to the Chief Medical Officer. Scottish Cancer Co-ordinating and Advisory Committee, Edinburgh

Scottish Executive 2001 Cancer in Scotland: action for change. SEHB, Edinburgh

Serlin R, Mendoza T, Nakamura Y et al 1995 When is cancer pain mild, moderate or severe? Grading pain severity by its interference with function. Pain 61:277–284

SIGN 1998 Breast cancer in women. Publication no. 21. NHS Scotland, Edinburgh. Available on line from: www.sign.ac.uk

SIGN 2000 Control of pain in patients with cancer: a national guideline. Publication no. 44. NHS Scotland, Edinburgh. Available on line from: www.sign.ac.uk

SIGN 2004 Lung cancer review: a national guideline. NHS Scotland, Edinburgh. Available on line from: www.sign.ac.uk

Skevington S M 1996 Psychology of pain. John Wiley New York, p 39

Smith L 1995 The public's views of morphine. Unpublished research paper, Napp Pharmaceuticals Ltd, Cambridge

Sontag S 1991 Illness as a metaphor. Penguin Books, London

Steinhauser K, Christakis N, Clipp E et al 2000 Factors considered important at the end of life by patients, family, physicians and other care providers. Journal of the American Medical Association 284:2476–2482

Stone P 2002 The measurement, causes and effective management of cancer-related fatigue. International Journal of Palliative Nursing 8:120–128

Strang P 1997 Existential consequences of unrelieved cancer pain. Palliative Medicine 11:299–305

Strang P 1998 Cancer pain – a provoker of emotional, social and existential distress. Acta Oncologica 37:641–644

Strang P, Strang S, Hultborn R, Arner S 2004 Existential pain – an entity, a provocation, or a challenge. Journal of Pain and Symptom Management 27:241–250

Sutcliffe-Chidgey J, Holmes S 1996 Developing a symptom distress scale for terminal disease. International Journal of Palliative Nursing 2:192–198

Sykes N 1998 The relationship between opioid use and laxative use in terminally ill cancer patients. Palliative Medicine 12:375–382

Sykes N 1999 Constipation and diarrhoea. In: Doyle D, Hanks G, Macdonald N (eds) Oxford textbook of palliative medicine, 2nd edn. Oxford University Press, Oxford

Syrett E, Taylor J 2003 Non-pharmacological management of breathlessness: a collaborative nurse–physiotherapist approach. International Journal of Palliative Nursing 9:150–156

Tanaka K, Akechi T, Okuyama et al 2002 Impact of dyspnoea, pain and fatigue on daily life activities in ambulatory patients with advanced lung cancer. Journal of Pain and Symptom Management 23:417–423

Twycross R 1995 Pain relief in advanced cancer. Churchill Livingstone, Edinburgh

Twycross R, Wilcock A 2002 Symptom management in advanced cancer. Radcliffe Medical, Oxford

Twycross R, Wilcock A, Charlesworth S, Dickman A 2003 Palliative care formulary, 2nd edn. Radcliffe Medical, Oxford

Van der Molen B 1995 Dyspnoea: a study of measurement instruments for the assessment of dyspnoea and their application for patients with advanced cancer. Journal of Advanced Nursing 22:948–956

Ventafridda V, Tamburini M, Caraceni A et al 1987 A validation study of the WHO method for cancer pain relief. Cancer 59:850–856

Waller A, Caroline N L 1996 Handbook of palliative care in cancer. Butterworth-Heinemann, Newton, MA

Waller A, Caroline N 2000 Handbook of palliative care in cancer, 2nd edn. Butterworth-Heinemann, Newton, MA

Ward C 2002 The need for palliative care in the management of heart failure. Heart 87:294–298

Weitzner M A, Moody L N, McMillan S C 1997 Symptom management issues in hospice care. American Journal of Hospice and Palliative Care 14:190–195

Wilcock A 1997 Dyspnoea. In: Kaye P (ed) Tutorials in palliative medicine. ELP Publications, Northampton, p 227–249

Wilkinson S 1999 Communication: it makes the difference. Cancer Nursing 22:17–20

Woodruff R 1999 Palliative care, 3rd edn. Oxford University Press, Oxford

Woolf C J, Thompson S W N 1991 The induction and maintenance of central sensitisation is dependent on N-methyl-D-aspartic acid receptor activation: implications for the treatment of post-injury pain hypersensitivity states. Pain 44:293–299

World Health Organization 1996 Guidelines: cancer pain relief, 2nd edn. World Health Organization, Geneva

World Health Organization 2003 WHO definition of palliative care. Available on line at www.who.int/cancer/palliative/definition/en

Zech D F, Ground S, Lynch J et al 1995 Validation of World Health Organization guidelines for cancer pain relief: a 10 year prospective study. Pain 63:65–76

Zigmond A, Snaith R 1983 The Hospital Anxiety and Depression Scale. Acta Psychiatrica Scandinavica 67:361–370

FURTHER READING

Ashby M, Game P, Devitt D et al 1991 Percutaneous gastrostomy as a venting procedure in palliative care. Palliative Medicine 5:147–150

Campbell T, Hately J 2000 The management of nausea and vomiting in advanced cancer. International Journal of Palliative Nursing 6:18–25

Fainsinger R, Miller M, Bruera E et al 1991 Symptom control during the last week of life on a palliative care unit. Journal of Palliative Care 7:5–11

Grond S, Zech D, Diefenbach C, Bischoff A 1994 Prevalence and pattern of symptoms in patients with cancer pain: a prospective evaluation of 1635 cancer patients referred to a pain clinic. Journal of Pain and Symptom Management 9:372–382

Hardy J 2000 Medical management of bowel obstruction. British Journal of Surgery 87:1281–1283

Melzack R, Wall P D 1982 The challenge of pain. Penguin, Harmondsworth

Oberle K, Wry J, Paul P, Grace M 1990 Environment, anxiety and postoperative pain. Western Journal of Nursing Research 12:745–753

Puntillo K A 1994 Dimensions of procedural pain and its analgesic management in critical surgically ill patients. American Journal of Critical Care 3:116–122

Regnard C F B, Tempest S 1992 A guide to symptom relief in advanced cancer, 3rd edn. Haigh & Hochland, Manchester

Twycross R (ed.) 1997 Psychological symptoms. In: Symptom management in advanced cancer, 2nd edn. Radcliffe Medical, Oxford

Twycross R G, Fairfield S 1982 Pain in far advanced cancer. Pain 14:303–310

FIVE

Communication and support in palliative care

Jean Lugton, Doreen Frost, Susan Scavizzi

CONTENTS

Communication and support are among the most important aspects of palliative care. At the same time they are demanding of caregivers' own emotions and challenging in the skills they demand. The NHS Cancer Plan (Department of Health 2000) envisaged equality of access to resources and support for all people with cancer. This ideal is now beginning to be extended to include people with non-cancerous terminal conditions and people from minority ethnic groups, who were not accessing palliative care services to the same extent as the majority population. What are the implications of these changes for improving the support of terminally ill patients and their families?

AIMS OF THE CHAPTER

The purpose of this chapter is to unravel the meaning of the concept of support, a term in everyday use in nursing but often not clearly defined. This chapter will address the question: 'What do nurses (and other professionals) need to do to give support to patients who are receiving palliative care?' Various aspects of support will be explored, giving readers an opportunity to reflect both on the meaning of this important concept and on the implications for their practice. Illustrations of the meaning of support as perceived by women with breast cancer and their health visitors are taken from Lugton's (1994) research, which explored the links between support and identity/personhood. The importance of the concept of identity/personhood in nursing will also, therefore, be examined.

After you have read this chapter you should be able to:

- Recognise the ways in which personhood/identity in dying people and their relatives is threatened by terminal illness
- Support patients' own coping styles
- Identify effective aspects of support and communication (verbal, nonverbal, actions)
- Plan nursing interventions to maintain personhood in advanced illness
- Develop your communication practice.

THE DEVELOPMENT OF IDENTITY/PERSONHOOD

The greater part of identity or sense of self is developed and maintained through interaction with others. Everyday interactions among family members have profound effects upon the development of self. Social relationships and social support can be important factors in this adaptation and in the achievement of psychological wellbeing. Mead (1934) argued that the individual develops a self-concept through role taking. Hirsch (1981) maintained that people's social networks could both support and assist in redefinition of their identity. However, these social networks also reflect people's values and choices. The process of maintaining identities is thus interactive between people and their significant others.

CORE IDENTITIES

Of a number of social identities, a few can be considered as core identities because they form the basis of the individual's perceived self, being those self-perceptions that seem most important to the person. Examples of core identities for most people are their body image and sexuality. Nationality and culture are often very important. According to Armstrong & Fitzgerald (1996), each society has its own requirements for achieving and maintaining full adult personhood. For example, several key requirements for personhood in Western culture, including physical independence and control over bodily functions, are not universal (Armstrong & Fitzgerald 1996, Lawton 2000). Among Chinese populations, for instance, living independently is not a cultural expectation and it is the norm for elderly people to live with adult children (Ikels 1991).

People's significant others, such as their partners, parents, siblings and children, are likely to be included in their self-concepts. The attitudes and behaviour of people in these close relationships are important to the individual's self-esteem and security.

EFFECTS OF ADVANCED ILLNESS ON IDENTITIES

Research has shown that it is often difficult for people to maintain adequate concepts of self when undergoing changes caused by serious illness, which can spoil aspects of their established identities (Anderson 1986, Kelly 1991, 1992, Lugton 1994, Tait 1988). The degree to which an illness affects the individual's core identities varies from person to person. People who are terminally ill may face several identity crises, described here as threats. They have to move through these crises towards a more peaceful acceptance of their situation. Failure to do so means that identities remain under threat and the crises are unresolved. Some of these threats to personhood will now be considered (Fig. 5.1).

THE THREAT OF ILLNESS TO FUTURE LIFE AND PLANS

In health, most individuals can plan for the future with some confidence because they do not imagine that they will become ill and be unable to do the things they presently take for granted. Ideas about personal invulnerability and immortality begin in early childhood. Young children are often unable to understand the permanence of death, thinking that a relative who has died will return. Teenagers and young adults tend to see themselves as relatively indestructible, with an unlimited future. Apparently healthy, middle-aged people have an expectation of living to an old age. Often, people do not think about their deaths when they are in apparent good health. If they become aware that they have a potentially fatal disease, they are stopped in their tracks. It is a threat to the very core of self and can undermine their sense of security and ability to plan for the future.

Women with breast cancer had to cope with their fears of dying of the disease (Lugton 1994). Phyllis coped by perceiving herself as indispensable to her family.

You've got to die of something in the end. My mother died of lung cancer. She had secondaries before they discovered it had come from the breast. I'm not planning on doing that just now! I've got far too many responsibilities. I'm far too busy.

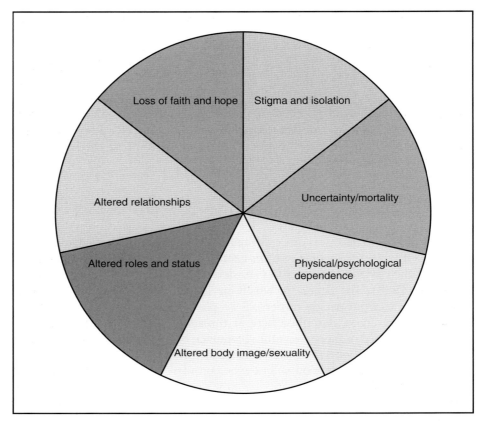

Figure 5.1 Identity crises facing the dying person.

Susan had been afraid of dying from cancer since her youth. She confronted her fears by remembering that she was only 46, strong enough to fight the disease.

> *I suppose when I was younger I thought 'What if I die of cancer?' That's everybody's fear, to die of cancer. I never thought at 46 that I would have cancer. Folk will say to you, 'You'll get on all right. You are strong enough. You're OK.'*

These examples show ways in which one group of women with breast cancer coped with the threat to their survival.

THE THREAT OF ILLNESS TO PHYSICAL AND PSYCHOSOCIAL INDEPENDENCE

In health most people regard themselves as competent and independent. Disease often makes them feel temporarily or permanently uncertain of their physical and psychological coping abilities. In a seminal paper, Maier & Seligman (1976) proposed a learned helplessness theory of depression, suggesting that a stressful situation could lead to depression if the individual believed that it was impossible to control the situation.

Erikson (1965) maintained that gaining autonomy is an important part of development of the self. Loss of independence can be shattering to self-esteem. Johnson (1991) found that the process of gaining control after a heart attack involved three dimensions: an ability to predict outcomes, to make informed decisions and to act on decisions. Heart attack victims had a sense of uncertainty, which diminished predictability. They also lacked understanding of their bodies, undermining their sense of power and control. No longer being able to trust their abilities and relying on others' support undermined their independence.

THE THREAT TO BODY IMAGE AND SEXUALITY

Support of the sexual identities of patients with advanced disease is discussed in depth in Chapter 7 and is only briefly mentioned here. The threat to life posed by the illness does not always override anxieties about sexual identity, which is so much a part of personhood. For example, in Lugton's (1994) research, Carol, who had advanced breast cancer, disliked her appearance because she had a fungating tumour. She always took a foam bath to avoid looking at herself, saying that she felt dirty because of her cancer. Even patients with long-standing and apparently good relationships were anxious about the possible effects of cancer on their sexual relationships. Retaining her femininity despite a double mastectomy and hair loss was important to Margaret.

It's very important to have a good wig. To be caught without it can be really shattering. You think, 'I can't look so terribly different with no hair,' but oh my goodness you do. Your head looks so wee. It's as if half your personality had been whipped off as well. But wanting to wear a wig and having to are two different things. It's nice to have your own hair. It's part of being feminine isn't it?

Edith, whose cancer had caused her to lose a lot of weight, often felt depressed about her physical appearance. Her husband was supportive.

Then I lost an awful lot of weight. Then I swelled up in the tummy. I looked like one of those poor little mites you see on TV with the thin arms and thin legs and pot tummy. I don't have a light on to go to bed. My husband and I had our first little barney for a long time. It sparked off over a dress he wanted me to get. I said, 'Oh what's the point? I've got that much in my wardrobe that I can't wear because I'm going up and down in size.' I've always put on this brave face. Just now and again, you can't. It's only you and your husband that has to accept it and mine never showed any repugnance.

THE THREAT TO SOCIAL ROLES AND STATUS

With progression of disease, people are likely to feel less confident in their roles as partners, friends and workers. Some roles may have to be given up. Lynam's (1990) research into the support of young adults with lymphoma and sarcoma emphasised the importance to identity, of their ability to fulfil social roles. All her respondents defined themselves in terms of their social roles and relationships and the feelings derived from them. Women with breast cancer also worried about their competence to carry out their normal work and social roles (Lugton 1997a). Many found themselves temporarily unable to do so and a few were permanently unable to cope.

Serious illness and its treatment impose physical limitations. These are often temporary and are cast aside on the road to recovery. However, in advanced disease, physical dependence often increases as the disease progresses. Maintaining their employment was important to many patients with breast cancer (Lugton 1994). Carol, who had advanced breast cancer, had prided herself on taking little sick leave from work, until she had to take time off for hospital treatment. Her disease and treatment made her feel tired. However, her work was important to her identity. She wanted to continue full-time for as long as possible.

Before all this happened I was never off, you know. I find that if I'm working I feel that much better. I think it gives you a purpose. It takes your mind off the problems. I do feel I need to work.

Anna, who had advanced cancer, wanted to work but was unsure of her ability to cope. She later had a course of chemotherapy but this made her feel tired and old. Her illness and its treatment had undermined her self-esteem.

There are so many things I want to do and I just can't do them. You just can't help doubting yourself.

THE THREAT TO RELATIONSHIPS

In health many people feel secure in their important relationships. Close relationships form a part of a person's identity and give feelings of security and competence. As the seriousness of their illness becomes manifest, people often go through a period of feeling less confidant in their relationships. Indeed, they may experience negative reactions from some relatives and friends whose own security is threatened by the illness. Lugton's (1994) research among 35 women with breast cancer revealed that, for 14 of them, social networks were predominantly supportive. Relatives and friends seemed able to cope with the patient's illness without perceiving it as in any way threatening to themselves. However, 20 networks offered women with breast cancer a mixture of support and strain. There were long-standing relationship difficulties between some women in this group and their network members.

In a number of instances, a relative was ill or unable to cope with the woman's illness, regarding it as in some way threatening to them. One woman had a predominantly stressful network owing to dysfunctional relationships within the family and a lack of friends.

Sometimes relatives and friends do not want to recognise the seriousness of an illness because the patient's inability to fulfil their normal roles threatens their own accepted roles and identities. For example, Janice was very depressed after breast surgery and felt that her husband and children made light of her illness, not acknowledging her feelings.

It was quite hard because it wasn't until I was really quite down that they sort of acknowledged that I was feeling low. I had to shout quite loudly about it. In fact Ben [her husband] has always been very busy and he was rushing about. He was perhaps the last one to notice.

However, illness also offers opportunities for increased richness in relationships because of increased awareness of how much others care. Margaret had advanced cancer. Her husband, who was a doctor, decided to spend more time with her.

He decided he would retire early. He decided last year when I was getting chemotherapy and he was getting home late. It meant I had to wait sometimes the whole day till he was finished. We thought, 'This is silly. We should be spending more time together, not muddling on trying to get this one to pick me up and him having the stress of not being able to do this.'

The strain existing in some social networks illustrates the potential for professional staff both to provide the missing support themselves and to facilitate improved relationships between patients and their significant others (Lugton 1997a). Glaser & Strauss's (1965) research showed that communication within families could become closed when one member was seriously ill and others became anxious. Family members were aware of the situation but were unable to discuss their concerns. This is an area where nurses can be helpful in trying to open up communication.

THE THREAT OF STIGMA AND ISOLATION

In health, most people regard themselves as 'normal', integrated into their families and communities. Serious illness can make them feel powerless and unsure of their status, especially if they are subjected to others' negative expectations and labelling. For example, anyone with cancer has to face society's fatalistic attitudes to malignant disease. The sufferer is often reduced in people's minds from being a whole and normal person to being a tainted, discounted one, a stigmatising experience shared by families of patients with cancer. Anna found her advanced breast cancer embarrassing because it was incurable and some people avoided her.

It's an embarrassing disease. At times I feel as if I've got this big sign up say-ing 'Beware cancer'. There are a lot of people who'll not go near you if they know you've got something like that. You feel as if you should be ringing a bell, saying 'Unclean' or something. You tend to keep it to yourself. Other people, you feel, are watching you, just waiting on you popping off.

A disease like cancer is a mystery to many people, as its causes are unknown, adding to its aura of fatality.

THE THREAT TO FAITH AND HOPE

A life-threatening illness may cause a person to grow spiritually or fall into doubt and despair. In Lugton's (1997a) research patients sometimes spoke of the need for spiritual support. For example, Sheila valued the spiritual sup-port offered by her church friends.

There's a lot of prayers being said by a lot of people. I'm in their thoughts. You don't think it's doing anything but it does. It brings you through.

A person's spirituality is much broader than their religious beliefs or lack of them. It is an important part of identity. McIllmurray et al (2001) conducted a questionnaire survey of the psychosocial needs of adult cancer patients who were at various stages in the cancer journey. They found that needs relating to spiri-tual issues were less commonly expressed but strongly felt. 'Support from a spir-itual adviser' was a significantly higher level of need for patients at recurrence and at the move to palliative care than for patients at other moments. Chapter 6 explores ways in which spiritual distress can manifest itself during terminal ill-ness and ways in which nurses can care for clients who have spiritual problems.

(((●)))

REFLECTION POINT 5.1

Threats to personhood

Think of a patient you have nursed. What were the ways in which their person-hood/identity was threatened by the terminal illness? What were their core identi-ties (self-perceptions that seemed most important to them)?

SUPPORTING PERSONHOOD IN ADVANCED ILLNESS

An individualised approach to patients with a terminal illness involves recog-nising each person's identity and the reactions to illness that are characteristic of that individual and of their family. Lugton's 1994 research into the experiences of women with breast cancer indicated that the underlying 'essence' of support (both professional and informal) to these women was the way it maintained their identities, their sense of self. In some circumstances, support also helped them to make necessary changes in their self-concepts, by adapting their self-perceptions to their changed circumstances. Patients received from doctors, nurses and health visitors information and psychological support that enabled them to appraise the nature and seriousness of the threat of breast cancer to their wellbeing. Their uncertainty and anxiety was reduced by the availability of health-care workers to support them. In particular, health visitors were perceived to be accessible and approachable and able to provide them with personalised support.

In a qualitative study, Kabel & Roberts (2003) examined the attempts made by staff to maintain the personhood of patients in two hospices in north-west England. The questions for hospice staff were whether they acted to restore a damaged personhood or to maintain a threatened one, or whether terminal illness inevitably leads to loss of personhood. Themes emerged from their study showing that hospice staff supporting personhood by:

- Normalising the distressing symptoms, making an effort to maintain eye contact with patients experiencing distressing or embarrassing symptoms
- Acknowledging the delicate balance between providing total care for patients and promoting their independence, and respecting their decisions about personal and medical care
- Helping patients to have control over their personal appearance and environment (patients were allowed to decorate their bedsides with photos and items from home to personalise their space)
- Caring for the unconscious patient – nurses talked to and touched patients and encouraged the family to do the same as they might still be able to hear.

Copp (1999) identified that, as death became imminent, nurses appeared to separate the person's body from the personal self. She suggested that people construct this separation as part of the process of ensuring a sense of continuity and meaning after death, with an absence of separation constituting the total annihilation of the person, body and self. However, Lawton (2000) was critical of the claims made by the hospice movement to maintain personhood and found that dying patients were often reduced to the status of a body.

REFLECTION POINT 5.2
Supporting personhood in terminal care

Does terminal illness inevitably lead to a loss of personhood? Think of a patient you have recently cared for. How did you support the personhood of the patient? What were the successes? What were the difficulties?

ENHANCING INFORMAL SUPPORT

Lugton's (1997a) research into supporting personhood showed the importance of informal support enhancement. The main types of informal support the women received from family and friends were opportunities for confiding, support from fellow patients undergoing a similar experience, practical help, companionship, emotional support and affirmation of their value. As nurses we should assess the patient's informal support needs, preserve existing support by minimising disruption and encourage missing aspects of support through, for example, support groups. Peer support groups and day centres for people undergoing treatment for advanced diseases can help to relieve social isolation.

It is important for nurses to be aware of family dynamics and to practise family-focused care. Nurses working with people with advanced illness have an important role in relation to enhancement of supportive relationships. It is essential to understand the dynamics of the social network otherwise we may undermine one of the strongest potential resources people have in coping with the disease, the social relationship. Encouraging patients and their families to make meaningful connections between events in the course of the illness is important in maintaining identities (Flanagan & Holmes 2000).

WHEN TO BEGIN SUPPORT?

To be effective, support should begin early in the disease process. Dixon et al (1996) noted the importance of including patients' fears of recurrence as an integral part of the nursing assessment of cancer patients. He reported that patients worried about how their families would cope if they should die. They wondered how they would be treated, whether they would be allowed to stay at home, whether medical staff would say that there was nothing more that could be done, leading to a sense of abandonment, how they would die and if they would experience severe symptoms.

SUPPORTING PATIENTS' OWN COPING STYLES

Nurses can play a vital role in helping people to assess their situations, what support is available to them and the adequacy of their coping resources. Coping involves mobilisation of personal resources (psychological and tangible). In a critique of Kubler Ross's five-stage model of the dying process, Buckman (1999) proposed, in its place, a three-stage model that is more closely tied to personhood than to stages in the disease process. He noted that people facing death demonstrate a mixture of reactions that are characteristic of the patient, not of the diagnosis or stage of the disease.

Progress through the dying process is marked not by a change in the type or nature of emotions but by resolution of the resolvable elements of those emotions (Buckman 1999, p. 52).

Buckman claimed that the three-stage system helps professionals to understand what they are hearing from the patient, to respond with greater sensitivity and to predict what is likely to occur next. The initial stage, 'facing the threat', starts when the person first faces the possibility of dying from the disease. People may show a variety of emotions, representing their usual coping strategies and reactions in a crisis, for example anger or denial. The 'chronic stage', being ill, follows as the person resolves those elements in their initial response that are resolvable and shows a diminution of intensity of emotion. The third stage is defined by the person's 'acceptance of death'. However, a few patients die without ever overtly acknowledging the imminence of their death (Lugton 1994). Margaret had lived with her recurrent breast cancer for 18 years and demonstrated a fighting spirit. Now she seemed to be on a downward path.

I find the time between remissions seems to be shorter and shorter. I think that makes you very frightened. I found the last time I came to the clinic, I didn't take it in. Normally, I would ask questions and ask for something to be explained to me and then I've got it. But I didn't. I was in a daze. I couldn't even remember what the doctor said to me.

Nurses can restore patients' ability to cope by helping them to clarify problems and deal with negative emotions. They can also provide practical help. Nurses can encourage patients to explore and express their feelings, discuss problems, make plans and develop coping strategies. The ability to make decisions is an important aspect of autonomy and patients should be involved in discussions about all aspects of their care.

Nurses can also assess whether patients are in an anxiety state or clinically depressed. Learning new skills develops a positive self-image. Patients may have to cope with, for example, a new body image, wearing a prosthesis or stoma bag. Those receiving chemotherapy have to cope temporarily with caring for a wig. They need support from nurses to acquire these skills. Support needs to be balanced against people's need to perceive themselves as coping. Sometimes, patients' family and friends can be overprotective towards them. This can affect their self-esteem and identity as independent people, capable of giving as well as receiving support (Lugton 1994).

REFLECTION POINT 5.3

Coping styles

With a colleague discuss ways in which you each coped with a problem. Did you have similar or different coping styles? What help were you wanting from friends or relatives to help you to cope?

DEVELOPING THERAPEUTIC RELATIONSHIPS IN PALLIATIVE CARE

Nursing is about relationships and interactions. It is not, as some nursing models imply, about what the nurse does to the patient. It is about continuity of relationships to maintain growth. Proctor (1996) notes that nurse–patient relationships are, to an extent, invisible and therapeutic relationships may not be so highly valued by health-care organisations as more obvious measures of effective nursing care. Indeed, much of the information required by management as an indication of the effectiveness of nursing services seems to be quantitative. Morse et al (1992) claimed that the heart of effective nursing support was the nurse's ability to identify with the patient's experiences:

> The caregiver must be emotionally involved or able to identify with the sufferer. The caregiver must be willing and able to experience or share with the other's suffering and to respond meaningfully and appropriately to the sufferer. The essence of the nurse–patient relationship is the engagement, the identification of the nurse with the patient.
>
> Morse et al 1992, p. 811

Luker et al (2000) noted that emotionally supportive relationships appear to depend on nurses familiarising themselves with patients' experiences, in order to get to know them and to be able to work with them. In a North American study, Davies & Oberle (1990) conducted in-depth interviews with one supportive care nurse and showed how the nurse connected with patients, establishing rapport and developing a bond. Maintaining this bond involved spending time with patients and giving of the self. In an ethnographic study, Bottorf et al (1995) found that nurses communicated emotional support in a variety of ways, verbally (affirming statements, reassurance, empathy, encouragement, sympathy) and non-verbally (touch and proximity). These comforting strategies acknowledged patients' concerns and created an atmosphere of acceptance.

Emotional involvement with patients can leave aspects of nurses' identities exposed and vulnerable. Morse et al (1992) recognised that it was not desirable for caregivers to be constantly engaged in relationships. Other responses were often appropriate to protect the caregiver or were needed by the patient. Health visitors sometimes found their involvement with patients with breast cancer stressful (Lugton 1994). Anna had advanced breast cancer and her health visitor had this experience.

> It's quite involving. You tend to think about it as you come away as well. The visits can take quite some time. In fact Anna has almost gone through a grief-type reaction. I can see a big need there. Mind you, it would be very draining.

There are compensations for making an emotional commitment to the patient. The caregiver often receives reciprocal support. However it is important that professionals support each other in these situations. Nurses working in the community can be particularly vulnerable if there are fewer opportunities for sharing their feelings with colleagues. Professional relationships with patients can often be supportive to patients because they are not embedded in any past or future roles and do not carry expectations of reciprocity, as do relationships with kin and friends. During illness many patients feel obliged to protect their family and friends by hiding their true feelings. Women with breast cancer commented on the supportiveness of confiding in someone 'outside' their social circles (Lugton 1994). For example, Carol reported that her family was unwilling to talk about her illness because they could not cope. Being separated from her husband, she wanted to share her worries about herself and her sons' future. She was unable to do this. She felt that she could confide in her health visitor.

It's nice to have someone who knows what I'm talking about but is sort of an outsider. It helps because I'm beginning to see it from her point of view as well as my own. The family is hopeless about this.

We should be aware that patients' protective attitudes can sometimes extend to professional helpers as well (Lugton 1994). Patients may protect their doctors from their anxieties, putting up with discomforts without complaint, presenting a bright face. A health visitor attending the hospital outpatient breast cancer clinic noted:

The thing that struck me about those clinic sessions was what a false impression the doctors might get about the patients. The patients on the whole were quite bright and positive with the doctors and joked with them. At some of the clinics, the patients would stay in the rooms and get undressed. I would stay with the patients and they would say, 'This is a nightmare', or something totally opposite to how it sounded to the doctor.

Patients' coping ability is increased by the availability of nurses who are perceived as accessible and approachable and able to provide personalised support. This support can be in the background, available if needed. In this respect nurses can be like attachment figures described by Bowlby:

Presence of an attachment figure is to be understood as implying ready accessibility rather than actual or immediate presence and absence implies inaccessibility. Not only must the attachment figure be accessible but he/she must be willing to respond in an appropriate way to someone who is afraid.

Bowlby 1975, p. 234

Several patients with breast cancer described this attachment to health visitors (Lugton 1994). Anna commented on her relationship with her health visitor:

She's my lifeline. I know she's there. I suppose it's a bit like a kid with a night light. You know it's there if you want it. She's really made a tremendous difference.

We have to convey to patients verbally and non-verbally that we can both understand and cope with their distress. Power plays a more obvious role in professional than in informal relationships. Professionals who control their relationships with patients by dominating interactions and controlling accessibility are seen as unsupportive. By contrast, those who are openly available to see patients and discuss anxieties are seen as very supportive. Adverse effects of power on effective support are evident when professional agendas dominate their interactions with clients. Thus, professionals can use their expertise to exercise power over patients or to empower them. For example, Ina, who had been receiving treatment for breast cancer, was worried about a lumpy breast following radiotherapy. She unsuccessfully sought professional reassurance (Lugton 1994).

The radiotherapists don't notice. It's just their own wee bit they are interested in. Then the doctor says, 'Take your things off'. Then he just goes, 'Oh yes'. I mean, it's ridiculous. Why do we bother, because they don't look at the thing? I never felt he asked me anything. I thought, 'I'm going away'. I just can't get out quickly enough.

Wallace (2001) maintained that, in order for communication with patients to be therapeutic, nurses providing palliative care should be conversant with communication theories and models.

Peplau (1988) maintained that in terminal illness the discovery of meanings can often be the most important work carried out in the nurse–patient relationship. Mathieson & Stam (1995) noted that encouragement of self-expression helps to reinforce patients' identities as individuals. Person-centred counselling theories which emphasise the individual's concepts of self, can also assist nurses in developing empathic relationships with patients (Egan 1990, Rogers 1967). In a small qualitative study, Richardson (2002) found that patients having palliative care identified two types of therapeutic interaction with nurses. While recognising the nurse's role in the relief of physical symptoms, the patient's perception of feeling better was generally focused on psychological wellbeing. The patients felt valued and of individual importance. The focus on the patient as a person affirmed them as an individual.

Heron's (1990) theoretical model is helpful in developing the communication skills necessary for supporting patients and their families. He suggested six possible categories of helpful intervention.

Authoritative interventions

Authoritative interventions are practitioner-led. The nurse takes responsibility for the client, guiding their behaviour. Authoritative strategies are described as prescriptive, informative and confronting.

- **Prescriptive**: the helper seeks to direct the behaviour of the client
- **Informative**: the helper gives the client information
- **Confronting**: the helper tries to raise the client's consciousness about an attitude or behaviour.

Facilitative interventions

Facilitative strategies aim to help patients be more autonomous through emotional release, self-knowledge and learning, and affirmation of their value and being. These are cathartic, catalytic and supportive interventions.

- **Cathartic**: the helper encourages the client to release painful emotions such as fear
- **Catalytic**: the helper elicits self-discovery and problem solving in the client
- **Supportive**: the helper affirms the worth of the client's attitudes, qualities and actions.

((((●))))

REFLECTION POINT 5.4
Authoritative and facilitative interventions

Think about your own communication style in a recent interaction with a patient or relative. How much of the conversation was authoritative, how much was facilitative? Do you think you gave the patient the support they wanted?

COMMUNICATION AND SUPPORT

Many patients with cancer suffer from psychological distress (Greer et al 1992, Hopwood et al 1991) but several studies have demonstrated that health professionals trained in communication skills can ameliorate patients' psychological distress. Wilkinson (1999) noted that good communication consists of the ability to assess the patient's communication needs and tailor communication to these needs while maintaining realistic hope. Koopmeiners et al (1997) investigated behaviours of health professionals that influence patients' hope. They found that taking time to talk, giving information, demonstrating caring behaviours and being friendly, respectful and honest were all areas of communication that promoted hope.

In a pilot study, Bailey & Wilkinson (1998) asked patients to describe their idea of a good communicator. Most patients mentioned the importance of being a good listener or being available to listen to their particular concerns, asking simple questions and using open, not leading questions.

COMMUNICATION CHALLENGES IN PALLIATIVE CARE

We communicate our support to others both verbally and non-verbally, and there must be consistency between these two forms of communication if we are to be perceived as genuine. We should therefore try to relate to dying people on a personal as well as a professional level. Benjamin (1981) emphasised the necessity of congruence between verbal and non-verbal communication in effective counselling.

NON-VERBAL COMMUNICATION

It is important to increase our awareness of non-verbal communications. Speaking about the insights gained through the use of video during counselling training sessions, Benjamin noted that: 'We can judge for ourselves the extent to which our words match our actions – We can see ourselves as the interviewee may see us – Most of all, do we only sound genuine or do we look genuine as well?' (Benjamin 1981, p. 67)

In a video programme (video interactive guidance) used to improve communication skills in children and families, non-verbal communication such as joint gaze and the use of gesture have been found important in the construction of meaning (Biemans 1990). Forsyth & Kennedy (1998–1999) stated that non-verbal communication and turn-taking must be in place before verbal communication becomes effective. It has been estimated that non-verbal communication carries four times the weight of verbal communication (Henley 1973). For example, three major themes emerged from Perry's (1996) study of exemplary oncology nurses. Two of these concerned the importance of non-verbal communication, i.e. dialogue in silence and mutual touch, in providing support. Silence emerged repeatedly from the study as an approach that was used by exemplary nurses in the study. Most of these silences were rich in non-verbal communication. Messages that were difficult or even impossible to speak were sent from nurse to patient and patient to nurse in silence.

Silence was important for listening and hearing the message and Perry recommends listening with openness. Sometimes silent messages were 'encoded in actions' of the nurses. Small details, like folding the patient's pyjamas or warming their milk if they like it that way, seemed trivial but transmitted powerful messages to patients. The second non-verbal theme identified by Perry was mutual touch. Sometimes this was non-physical, as when nurses were skilled at encircling a patient by having an arm just behind the patient's back or around the patient's shoulders. Sometimes eye contact was combined with touch to provide a potent communication medium.

Perry's third theme encompassing non-verbal and verbal behaviour was the use of humour. This was described as a light-hearted attitude, common among the skilled nurses in the study. These nurses deliberately chose most of the time to see the positive, humorous side of situations for the benefit of both themselves and their patients. Benjamin (1981) also advocates the use of humour as a means of support. He is careful to point out that he does not mean sarcasm, ridicule or cynicism but a light touch of humour that stems from empathic listening and reflects a positive outlook on life.

It may well consist of no more than a raised eyebrow, a smile, a gesture. When it breaks through though, it brings two partners in the interviewing process closer together by establishing an additional bond. For want of a better term, I can only call this bond, genuine caring for each other and confidence of the helping nature of human rapport.

Benjamin 1981, p. 159

PROMOTING HOPE

One of the most important messages to convey to a person with advanced illness is one of hope. This can be difficult, especially at times of relapse or deterioration. Most patients' main anxiety will be uncertainty about the future. Nurses can help patients cope with these anxieties, not with false reassurance but by encouraging them to talk about their fears and by providing appropriate medical information. It is important that, in the earlier stages of advanced disease, patients are able to put their illness into perspective, so that they can participate in other aspects of life. Nurses can help patients to think positively about the things that they are still able to do. For example, many people with advanced illness struggle to remain involved with family and community life. Some will want to continue working for as long as possible. Work is a way of leading a normal life despite having advanced disease. In a small phenomenological study of the meaning of hope to patients with cancer receiving palliative care, Flemming (1997) found that the greatest threat to loss of hope was the loss of control over significant present circumstances, which threatened the existence of a future. Maintenance of the individual's perception of control over loss was essential to preserving hope. In a study of what dignity means to those who are terminally ill, McClement et al (2004) identified factors that support and undermine dignity in these patients. One aspect of the patient's dignity-conserving repertoire is 'the continuity of self', i.e. the patient's belief that the essence of self is intact despite advanced illness. The implication for staff is that they should view patients apart from their disease and communicate and affirm those aspects of their personhood not affected by illness.

HELPING PEOPLE WITH COMMUNICATION DIFFICULTIES

People with verbal communication difficulties can experience emotional distress caused by loneliness, lack of self-esteem or depression. Communication problems may result in the person feeling socially excluded. These people may include those who have had a stroke or who suffer from learning difficulties. Kopp (2000a) noted that language impairments or problems with hearing could often occur in settings where elderly people were nursed.

Burgess (2004) reported that the palliative care needs of people with dementia had received little attention to date. She maintained that a palliative care approach from diagnosis is beneficial because it addresses people's emotional needs as well as those of their families and carers. Ham (1999) suggested that, if people with dementia are not aware of their condition at an early stage, they cannot make choices about their future care. Time to come to terms with the diagnosis may enable them to make any financial, spiritual and medical decisions while they are still able to do so. Viewing dementia as a disability rather than a disease allows us to view the person with dementia as actively coping with their impairment and entitled to adequate quality of life (Downs 2002). There is a growing body of evidence to show that people are adapting to living with dementia (Sabat 2002). One of the important management issues in the care of the person with dementia is pain management. Indicators of pain are often non-specific and may included changes in sleep, mood, eating and mobility. There are various 'discomfort scales' available that assess pain by non-verbal expressions, for example, noisy breathing and/or frightened expressions and tense body language (Hurley et al 1992).

COMMUNICATION WITH CHILDREN

Staff often depend on families to communicate with children when a family member is seriously ill. However, sometimes families would like help with this. Sheldon (1994) found that parents may underestimate their children's needs, partly in the belief that they are protecting them and partly because they themselves are exhausted and distressed by preparing to say goodbye to a partner. Also, the family's ability to support children will depend on pre-existing communication and coping styles (Pfeffer et al 2000). The Clinical Standards Board for Scotland (2002; as of 2003, now known as NHS Quality Improvement Scotland) outlined the need for children to be given information to help them understand the likely outcome of the patient's illness. Sheldon (1997) noted that greater emphasis is now being placed on including children in open discussion about the situation and their own emotional responses.

The adoption of a preventative approach is increasing in the UK (Rolls & Payne 2003). Macpherson & Cooke (2003) introduced a workbook for families of hospice patients to help parents better understand their children's knowledge of the patient's illness and to begin to explore their children's thoughts and feelings. Offering the workbook to seven families with children under 12 was intended to show that staff were open and prepared for discussion. The children used the workbook in different ways, some completing it immediately, others doing so gradually. Some chose to draw and write, some only to write, and some to use drawings or photographs only. All the children enjoyed having the workbook. It provided opportunities to interact and build relationships with the staff. However, the authors noted that it was important to fully inform parents about the workbook as it raised issues about death and dying that might be unacceptable to some parents who needed to come to terms with the situation themselves before being able to support their children.

DEVELOPING COMMUNICATION PRACTICE

Both patients and nurses have styles of communication that are part of their personality. Kopp (2000b) noted that a person's style of communication is linked to personal history and can be difficult to change. However, good communicators can modify their styles, for example, become more assertive if they are not getting what they want or less forceful if other people are getting upset.

A habit of reflecting on our communication and support with each patient and family will help us to improve our support. Johns (1996) noted that the advent of the reflective practitioner shifts reliance on prescriptive models of nursing towards reflective practice, which is grounded in reflective cues that tune the practitioner in to the human encounter. Reflective practice involves a process of grasping and interpreting the moment (assessment) in the light of past experience (evaluation) and responding with appropriate intervention in light of envisaged outcomes (planning).

This reflection on experience develops the quality of interventions. Nurses can try to understand their own feelings and the ways in which these may unconsciously play a part in their interactions. Porritt (1990) identified three ways in which we can become more self-aware: awareness of the outside world, awareness of the inner world and awareness of each moment of experience.

REFLECTION POINT 5.5
Becoming more self-aware

Kopp (2000b) suggested that a good way of increasing self-awareness is to carry out a SWOT (strengths, weaknesses, opportunities, threats) analysis of our communication skills. We can then see where our strengths and weaknesses in communicating with clients lie and identify opportunities and threats that can aid or obstruct effective communication. A colleague might be able to help us do this.

As stated earlier, an important aspect of effective communication is turn-taking. Giving and taking turns in conversation is one of the key contact principles in video interactive guidance. Simpson (1999) noted that effective communication in children or adults is characterised by initiative and reception, where turns are even and short. Using the same video programme, Lugton & Sneddon (2001) found that, after training, health visitors' feedback to parents encouraged parents to be 'active partners' in finding solutions to achieving satisfying communication with their children. Health visitors did this by taking short turns when conversing with parents and checking for shared understanding. After training there were clear improvements in health visitors' feedback to clients. Notably, shared turns between parents and health visitors increased from 10 to 25%. Client turns, where the client did most of the talking, increased from 15 to 27%. This shows the importance of professionals listening to people and 'activating' them by encouraging them to express their feelings and views. Thus the communication becomes patient centred rather than dominated by the professional person's agenda.

((((●))))

REFLECTION POINT 5.6
Turn-taking in communication with patients

When talking to patients and relatives, how much do you 'activate' them by turn taking during the conversation?

Wilkinson et al (1999) noted that patients and their families are often dissatisfied with their interactions with health professionals and that such communication difficulties also cause stress to health professionals. Heaven & Maguire (1997) found that, although a 3–5-day communication course improved nurses' skills, it failed to noticeably develop their ability to identify their patients' concerns. Wilkinson (Wilkinson et al 1999, Wilkinson 2002) advocated communication training that developed the skills necessary for effective dialogue. The content included attitudes to cancer, communication with patients, relations and colleagues, non-verbal and verbal communication skills, assessing psychological distress, facilitating skills, techniques for handling difficult questions and raising self-awareness. Teaching was by use of observation, constructive audiotape feedback, demonstration videos and role play discussions. The communication programme was integrated into 6-month postbasic courses in cancer and palliative care. On completion of a communication skills training programme, there was a significant improvement in nurses' skills. These were evaluated according to nine key areas of communication. All nine individual areas of the assessment showed statistically significant improvements post-intervention. The areas that showed most improvement were those with high emotional content.

Wilkinson et al (1999) evaluated the effects of the programme 2.5 years after the nurses had completed the course. There was no significant deterioration or further improvement in eight of the nine areas of assessment skills evaluated. However, in the area of psychological assessment there was a significant improvement. The researchers noted that these results suggested that nurses became more confident in the emotional areas of care as a result of training. The psychological assessment performance was measured in terms of the nurse's ability to pick up cues and explore in depth how the patient's illness had affected their life and psychological wellbeing. Wilkinson et al (1999) noted that the programme's unique feature was that it did not just focus on communication skills but also on knowledge of cancer, death and dying, and raised nurses' awareness of how they communicated.

The integrated approach of 26–30 hours was more costly in terms of lecturers' and students' time than a 3–5 day course.

COMMUNICATION AND SUPPORT IN THE COMMUNITY

SUPPORTING CHOICE ABOUT PREFERRED PLACE OF CARE

Palliative care providers have always aimed to enable people to choose where they want to die. However, in recent years, more efforts have been made to identify their wishes and support them in their choice, whether through hospices, hospital palliative care teams, day centres, support in the community or crisis intervention services. In a national telephone survey of the preferred place of care in terminal illness, Higginson (2003) found that results were similar to those found in a systematic review of 18 earlier studies. Preferences for home death among patients, families, professionals and the general public ranged between 49 and 100%. What was new in the latest study (Higginson 2003) was the finding of a higher preference for hospice care (24%) than in previous studies.

The desire to die at home was often frustrated (Higginson 2003), although most people with a terminal illness spend time at home after their diagnosis. Pemberton et al (2003) introduced a Preferred Place of Care document (PPC) to monitor the number of deaths at home for all terminally ill patients in Lancashire and South Cumbria. The aim of completing the document was to enable patients and their main carers' wishes about their preferred place of care to be identified and discussed. The use of the document highlighted the importance of opening up discussion about difficult issues of care that might not otherwise be addressed. Sources of support available to carers and patients requiring palliative care in the community setting can be identified. The importance of holistic individual assessment is highlighted by examples of diverse patient case histories and outcomes. Pemberton (2004) concluded that patients were finding use of the PPC empowering and that relatives were finding comfort in carrying out the patient's wishes.

TEAM CARE IN THE COMMUNITY

In palliative care, the team approach is vital to effective support. Clear lines of communication between hospital and community staff are essential. In a study of link health visitors' support for patients with breast cancer in the community, the health visitors expressed satisfaction with the information they received from the breast unit on discharge sheets and all of them felt comfortable phoning the hospital ward if they encountered problems or required information. The link health visitors acted as resources for their colleagues in the community so that they in turn could provide better support to these patients (Lugton 1997b). In a study exploring nursing outcomes for patients with advanced cancer following intervention by Macmillan specialist palliative care nurses, Corner et al (2003) found that Macmillan nurses functioning within a multiprofessional team were able to achieve positive outcomes for their patients. They were particularly effective when they acted as an intermediary between the medical team and the patient. Where positive outcomes were observed in complex situations, this was due to: 'Macmillan nurses orchestrating the involvement of multiple services or agencies, as well as working to reduce family conflict' (Corner et al 2003, p. 574).

Comparing team assessments of end-of-life communication with patients with advanced cancer in three European countries (UK, Ireland, Italy), Higginson & Costantini (2002) noted the importance of communication between the different professionals involved in care of these patients to avoid contradictory or redundant information and ambiguity. Multiprofessional palliative care teams cared for all patients in the study. Longer time in the care of the team was associated with fewer communication problems, indicating that the teams had improved communication. Effective communication was especially important where there were spiritual problems, need for care planning and poorer patient insight and family insight. Higginson & Costantini (2002) concluded that a multiprofessional approach to care is needed, with staff able to offer support in all these wider aspects.

AN EXAMPLE OF MAXIMUM AGENCY INVOLVEMENT

Corner et al (2003) found that negative outcomes could result from too many health professionals being involved, so that the patient was unable to differentiate the particular contributions of individuals. District nurses try to promote independence. Packages of care can sometimes take it away. The following example illustrates how provision of services by multidisciplinary professionals at too early a stage was detrimental to the patient and family because their potential coping strategies were compromised.

CASE STUDY **5.1**
Ben

Ben was a 70-year-old married man living with his wife in sheltered accommodation. He had a diagnosis of Barrett's oesophagus progressing to a malignancy. This was identified when his oesophagus ruptured during a routine admission for oesophageal stretch. Following insertion of a stent to facilitate swallowing and to ensure adequate nutrition, he was transferred from the local hospital to a hospice for convalescence. Prior to this event he had led an active life. He was heavily involved in arranging social activities for the residents in his housing complex as well as enjoying playing bowls with his wife at the local green. Prognosis was uncertain but a reasonable quality of life was expected, with a return to some of his previous interests.

On his discharge home, hospital staff informed Ben's wife that her husband's care would be provided on a daily basis by the community nursing service. This information was given without consultation or prior discussion with the district nursing service, which already knew Ben through regular contact with the residents in the housing development. Therefore, the family's expectations of care were that there would be maximum input by various agencies to achieve what they perceived as optimum care. Teamwork has been identified by Torrington et al (1989) as essential but, in this case, although the teams were well established and familiar, the lack of communication between key workers contributed to the subsequent difficulties.

On discharge, the district nurse's assessment was that Ben would be capable of self-care with minimal support to encourage a degree of independence for as long as possible. Regular reviews and support were planned. Inappropriate information supplied to the family by hospice staff compromised this assessment and resulted in it becoming necessary to provide maximum nursing input at too early a stage in Ben's illness. As anticipated, this resulted in Ben adopting the mantle of the sick role and his wife becoming very anxious and dependent. Ben did not return to any of his previous interests or hobbies and spent increasing amounts of time in his flat. Concurrently, his wife made life changes, in that she also curtailed her social activities.

Although maximum agency support for patients requiring palliative care would seem to provide optimum care for both the patient and family, in this situation, poor communication between secondary and primary care resulted in inappropriate nursing input at too early a stage in the patient's disease. Ben survived for a further 18 months but required frequent hospice respite admissions because of his wife's and family's anxiety. Their anxiety was heightened because, initially, Ben was not encouraged by his family to retain his independence, resulting in minor events being perceived as critical and requiring a medical solution. This was compounded by the fact that hospice provision was situated outwith the area, some distance from Ben's home. This made visiting difficult.

Following Ben's death, his wife continued to perceive the need for extended visits from both nursing and GP services, as a result of her dependence over the long period of her husband's illness. She required ongoing support for many months before she was able to accept her loss and grief. Poor communication and nursing intervention at an inappropriate stage resulted in the family's potential coping strategies being curtailed.

On reflection, when Ben's case was presented through a joint seminar with the hospice, Macmillan nurses, GP and district nurses, it was recognised that mistakes had been made and that the best interests of the patient and family had not been served. All professionals had tried to provide the best possible care but their responses had been reactive, dependent on the patient and family's anxiety, rather than carefully considered options. The professionals should have tried to gain insight into the root of this anxiety. Use of a patient care pathway might have facilitated the expected course of the patient's journey and enabled professionals to forward plan care and to avoid unnecessary admissions (Doyle 1998).

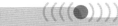

AN EXAMPLE OF HOLISTIC CARE IN THE COMMUNITY

Integrated care pathways for the dying patient have been developed to transfer the hospice model of care into other care settings and to promote multiprofessional team working by requiring roles to be clearly defined. One such care pathway has been described by Ellershaw et al (1997). The pathway provides guidance on different aspects of care, including psychological and spiritual care and family support. In a study of hospital nurses' perceptions of the pathway, nurses reported finding that it had a positive impact on patients, their families, nurses and doctors (Jack et al 2003). The pathway helped to foster effective communication with families. This included care of relatives after the patient's death. It also resulted in a reduction in documentation. However, sounding a note of caution on care pathways, Daniels (2004) pointed out that within palliative care it is difficult to define an expected course of care: if the framework is too rigid then it might 'blinker' professionals to the variable needs of the individual patient. In standardising palliative care, we risk losing the individualised approach, a key element of nursing and palliative care practice. However, Daniels noted that standards and frameworks should not limit the scope of practice, rather they should ensure that the key elements are provided, at the same time enabling the provision of individualised care, the premise of palliative care.

Wenrich et al (2003) cited the need to consider the patient and carers as unique individuals with consideration of their social situation and personal preferences. Attention should be centred on holistic care rather than focusing only on the disease process. In contrast to the first case study, where there was maximum multiagency involvement, Case study 5.2 demonstrates minimal professional support, which was nevertheless in accordance with the patient's wishes.

CASE STUDY 5.2

Yvonne

Yvonne was a middle-aged professional woman living in private accommodation with her husband. Their two adult children were both university students, studying abroad. Yvonne and her husband were both in full-time employment, leading active working and social

CHAPTER FIVE   COMMUNICATION AND SUPPORT IN PALLIATIVE CARE   157

lives, prior to Yvonne's illness. While on a skiing holiday abroad, Yvonne had an accident requiring a hospital admission for a treatment of a fracture. On return home Yvonne contacted her GP because she believed recent rectal bleeding and constipation were due to the effects of prescribed analgesia. On investigation her GP was concerned that there could be an underlying malignancy and referral was made to her local district general hospital. Yvonne was not unduly anxious as she had always enjoyed good health and, until her accident, had had minimal contact with health professionals. However a diagnosis of rectal carcinoma was made, resulting in extensive abdominal surgery with the formation of a stoma.

On discharge from hospital Yvonne was referred to the District Nursing Service for an assessment of her nursing needs – Beaver et al (2000) identified district nurses as the main professional carers for patients dying at home. Information on discharge was sent to the GP practice. It indicated advanced disease, with a poor prognosis, which had been discussed with Yvonne and her husband. Prior to the initial district nursing assessment visit, the available information suggested that the nursing need would be for palliative care and support.

On visiting the couple, it became apparent that Yvonne did not perceive herself as being terminally ill and would only accept help on her own terms. Throughout her illness, she remained in control of the boundaries of what would be tolerated. Although her attitude addressed the need for patient participation, the nursing staff viewed her management, at times, to be chaotic. Non-verbal cues and Yvonne's body language left no doubt of her wishes to continue to function as a strong, highly intelligent individual who tolerated nursing visits as a necessary evil. Yvonne's husband appeared to benefit from the support of the district nurse in that he was more receptive to practical advice and any suggestions offered. Yvonne refused to consider the involvement of other agencies. This left her husband without optimum support, although visitors had never previously been encouraged. District nursing visits continued over the next 3 months, as Yvonne's illness progressed, until she died at home, in the presence of her family.

On reflection, the district nursing team recognised that Yvonne's symptom control and particularly her pain management had not been optimal but that the care given was tailored to what was acceptable to the patient. Although they felt that the support they had given was inadequate, this was not the perception of the family. A bereavement visit to the family was pre-empted by Yvonne's husband coming to the Health Centre to thank the staff involved for allowing Yvonne to remain in control of her life during her illness.

REFLECTION POINT 5.8
Patients who want minimal intervention

Have you cared for a patient like Yvonne? As a professional, how did you feel about the patient setting the boundaries of acceptable care?

CARE OF PATIENTS FROM ETHNIC MINORITIES – OVERCOMING LANGUAGE BARRIERS

Communication has an important role in delivering effective palliative care services to ethnic minority groups. O'Neill (1994) indicated that, among the reasons for low uptake of palliative care services by ethnic minority groups, were professionals who were uninformed about the customs of ethnic minority patients, the Christian image of hospices and language barriers. In a major study, Hill & Penso (1995) noted that communication difficulties were a major concern to health professionals and source of distress to patients whose first language was not English, and that there was an inappropriate use of other hospital staff as interpreters and a lack of available interpreters. Many care teams relied on family members to help them translate. This created problems, as family members might be selective in their translation so as not to distress patients (Spruyt 1999). The conclusions of a small study by Randhawa et al (2003) were that interpreters should be trained to work in palliative care and that guidelines should be developed for use of family members as interpreters. In Bradford, a Macmillan ethnic minorities liaison officer works across primary and secondary care services. Much of the work is done directly with patients during visits with health professionals (Jack et al 2001).

The uptake of palliative care services offered by the district nursing service to ethnic minority groups in our own area in Scotland is low. The following case study illustrates the difficulties in caring for a patient with limited knowledge of English, despite help received from a translating service.

CASE STUDY 5.3
Mrs Chang

Mrs Chang is a 50-year-old married woman living in private accommodation with a large extended family. She is part of the local Chinese community, originating from Hong Kong. Although resident in the UK for many years and having raised a family here, her command of the English language is limited. Her adult sons act as her interpreters. In 1997, accompanied by her son, Mrs Chang presented to her GP with a 2-year history of a mucoid cough with occasional haemoptysis. Hospital investigations confirmed an inoperable lung tumour, which was treated with chemotherapy and radiotherapy. A hospital lung cancer support nurse provided support at this time. In May 2003, liver and bone metastases were confirmed by scan.

Mrs Chang was referred by her GP to the District Nursing Service in October 2003, when she was complaining of general fatigue and lumbar pain radiating to her leg. Liaison between district nurses and the Macmillan service resulted in a plan for district nursing input to establish a relationship with the family, with Macmillan involvement if required. The focus of the first visit centred on medication management, bowel management and the supply of pressure-relieving and other nursing equipment.

Language difficulties as well as cultural perceptions compromised communication from the onset. On the initial visit to Mrs Chang, her son acted as interpreter. Her body language indicated that she was in great pain and discomfort, resulting in agitation and an inability to sit. The assessment necessitated asking questions of a personal nature, which embarrassed her son, and her irritation was apparent. The nurse felt inadequate in a situation in which she would normally have full control.

Following a discussion with the GP, a decision was made that, in order to provide quality care, a female interpreter with good command of both languages and knowledge of ethnic customs and attitudes would be required. This decision was reached because of the potential barriers to effective ongoing communication and support that were evident at the initial visit. Although Mrs Chang's son's English was fluent, there were concerns that, having been raised in this country, his understanding of Chinese was uncertain, particularly in relation to medical terminology. Also under consideration were the mother–son relationship and their preferences. While there were other female relatives in the house, including Mrs Chang's mother, it appeared that they were unable or unwilling to offer practical assistance. Research into Chinese family culture revealed that it would be perceived as demeaning for a mother or older female relative to assist with personal care.

Contact was made with a Chinese development worker who met all the requirements. She was able to accompany Mrs Chang to all hospital appointments, acting as her advocate, and fed back relevant information to the district nurse. She assisted in home visits with the nurse as necessary.

With strategies in place, visits continued in the belief that information translated was fully understood and accepted. Although physical symptoms were controlled, with subsequent improvement in Mrs Chang's wellbeing and the removal of many of the barriers to effective communication, it became apparent at a hospital appointment to discuss chemotherapy that Mrs Chang did not appreciate the concept of palliative care and her limited prognosis. Prior to the involvement of the support worker, Mrs C's son had provided all translations at hospital visits. Although information on disease progression had been factual and honest, it became obvious that this had not been relayed to or understood by Mrs Chang. A breakdown in communication due to language barriers appeared to have played a part in her lack of understanding of this issue.

This has been identified in other groups when being faced with bad news. Robinson (1999) recognised denial as a common and effective coping response when dealing with an unwanted diagnosis in the initial stages. Perhaps it is the only means by which a patient can survive the ordeal and preserve their status in the family.

The issue was addressed by providing an extended hospital appointment with the palliative support nurse to discuss progression of the disease and symptom control. This resulted in Mrs Chang telling the district nurse that she felt very sad and asking for an indication of her life expectancy.

Mrs Chang's care is ongoing to date and, although strategies are in place to facilitate improved communication, problems continue as a result of cultural differences in the perception of disease and Mrs Chang's ability and desire to tolerate pain. Mrs Chang is aware of her medicine regime as it has been translated into Chinese but continues to self-medicate according to her own wishes. It is proving difficult to plan terminal care because of the reluctance of the support worker to be involved in assisting the district nurse to discuss preferences with Mrs Chang and her family.

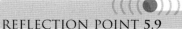

Ethnic minority patients

In your work situation, how well do you care for terminally ill patients from ethnic minorities? Is the standard of care on a par with that of other patients? If not, how could it be improved?

SUPPORT FOR SUFFERERS OF NON-MALIGNANT DISEASE

While there is an extensive literature and research on communicating with people with advanced cancer, people suffering from non-cancerous diseases also need sensitive support. A postal survey carried out for the Multiple Sclerosis Society in 1999 concluded that the diagnosis of the disease was poorly managed, little information was given and little ongoing support was offered. Box et al (2003) reported on a survey of the information needs of people with multiple sclerosis in the UK throughout the course of the disease and found a great discrepancy between information required and received. In a study of 20 patients with lung cancer and 20 with advanced heart failure, Murray et al (2002) found that patients with cardiac failure had less information about and poorer understanding of their condition and were less involved in decision-making than patients with lung cancer. They rarely recalled being given any written information, prognosis was rarely discussed and there was little acknowledgement that end-stage cardiac failure is a terminal illness. They suffered social isolation, progressive losses and the stress of monitoring a complex medication regime. Cardiac patients received less health, social and palliative care services and their care was often poorly coordinated. Their primary care contacts were mainly with the general practitioners. Murray et al (2002, p. 936) conclude that:

> *Unclear prognostic indicators and a desire to protect patients from potentially distressing information are barriers to effective communication between patients and professionals. The lessons learned from caring for cancer patients – an individualised approach to information giving, promotion of their coping strategies, appropriate training for professionals – should be applied to those with other life threatening illnesses.*

From local community nursing audits and personal experience in supporting patients with progressive, non-cancerous disease, we have found that active nursing management appears to be equitable between patients with cancer and non-cancerous disease. However we have found that the dearth of respite provision, overnight support, specialist medical and nursing backup and voluntary input has direct implications on the quality of support we can give. Charitable organisations are responsible for funding many of the palliative care services available to cancer sufferers, while other people with chronic, non-malignant diseases do not receive the same level of media interest and celebrity support, with consequent disadvantage (Table 5.1). Compounding the inherent difficulties in planning and discussing palliative care for non-cancer sufferers is the difficulty in recognising end-stage disease, due to the chronic disease process combined with acute exacerbations. There is now a consensus that palliative care provision for chronic disease sufferers and their families needs to be improved. Murray et al (2002) cited the World Health Organization (1999) palliative care approach model as a standard to achieve.

DAY CARE

Palliative day care has expanded rapidly but the types of care offered are variable. The small amount of research on palliative day care is mainly descriptive. People attend palliative day care for peer support as well as for nursing care and respite for themselves and their carers (Corr & Corr 1992). McDaid

TABLE 5.1

Palliative care support systems for cancer sufferers and patients with non-malignant conditions

Services Primary health-care team	Specialist services	Hospital
GP	Macmillan nurse	Dietetics
District nurses	Oncologist	Physiotherapist
Health visitors	Macmillan day care	Hospital day care
Podiatrist	Complementary therapy	Social work
Physiotherapist		Occupational therapy
Pharmacist		
Resources Local authority	Voluntary groups	Health
Social work services		Day centre
Finance/benefits		Respite/hospice care
Housing		Marie Curie home care
Equipment provision		Spiritual
Care agencies		

Services and resources more generally available to cancer sufferers are in italic type

(1995) noted that palliative day care is suitable for patients who are not actively dying but who have diminished ability to fulfil their family and societal roles.

Higginson et al (2000) conducted a survey of day care in the North and South Thames Regions in England. Most day care units had doctors, nurses, chaplains, managers, aromatherapists and hairdressers but the presence of chiropodists, occupational therapists, social workers, dietitians and music and art therapists was much more variable. The most common activities were review of patients' symptoms or needs, bathing, wound care, physiotherapy, hairdressing and aromatherapy. Most patients (90%) had cancer. Other diseases were HIV/AIDS, motor neurone disease and stroke. In a small ethnographic investigation of communication among patients attending palliative day care, Alison Langley-Evans (1997) found that, in the day care environment, patients talked readily about cancer, illness and death. She considered that provision of a social environment for patients with a terminal disease may be as important as one-to-one counselling by a professional. The majority of the patients talked openly about their illness and their awareness of and preparation for death. Langley-Evans noted: 'the light hearted and humorous nature of the patients' 'death talk' serves an important psychological function in allowing themselves to distance themselves from their own deaths while simultaneously permitting and acknowledgement of their terminal condition' (Langley-Evans 1997, p. 1101).

In an audit of palliative day care in a West Lothian hospital, patients were asked how they had benefited from attending the centre (Grafen 2000). The benefits most mentioned were contact with other people (78%), emotional support (56%), boost to self-esteem (39%) and help with symptom control (39%).

In our opinion, day care is useful for many patients but not for everyone. It can help socially isolated people. However, some people, while they like the facilities, do not want to talk about the process of dying. It is important that we are aware of and respect these differences.

SUPPORTING STAFF

Caring for patients with a terminal illness and supporting their relatives is known to be a source of occupational stress (Llewellyn & Payne 1995). Warshaw (1989) found that occupational stress is associated with anxiety, depression, job dissatisfaction and reduced quality of life. The closeness of the nurse–patient relationship in palliative care means that nurses can get involved with patients and their families, sharing in their emotions. How do staff then express their own feelings? Benica et al (1992) found that repeated exposure to the death of patients was an important factor in professional burnout. However, Field (1998) presented evidence that district nurses find palliative care rewarding despite restrictions on care delivery.

In an Australian study, Wilkes & Beale (2001) found that nurses from both urban and rural settings were stressed when caring for palliative care patients at home. Both groups found family relationships and role conflict to be major stressors in their workplace. Nurses found it difficult to be a friend, a nurse and a counsellor at the same time. Isolation in rural areas exacerbated stress for rural nurses. Support was often informal debriefing with their peers or family.

Usually, nurses giving palliative care get their support informally from within the multiprofessional team. The benefits of this type of support are well-recognised (NCHSPCS 1995). However, in our opinion, nurses need respite sometimes, because they can get burnt out easily. This is sometimes not acknowledged in small teams. In a small comparative study of death anxiety in hospice and emergency nurses, Payne et al (1998) found that hospice nurses had lower death anxiety and were more likely to recall both good and difficult experiences related to patient care. Unlike hospice nurses, Accident & Emergency nurses reported that they were unable to discuss problems with colleagues.

Clinical supervision can help nurses to cope with work-related stress. Dunne (2003) noted that it allows nurses to discuss and reflect on issues in a non-threatening environment, with possible therapeutic effects. However, Dunne also noted that clinical supervision is not well implemented in NHS trusts despite being advocated as good practice (UKCC 1996).

Kushnir et al (1997) set up Balint-type groups in an Israeli paediatric oncology ward. Michael and Enid Balint first set up these groups in London as research/training seminars on psychological problems in general practice (Balint 1957). Group members discuss any clients about whom they feel concerned and aspects of their work they find troubling. Kushnir et al (1997) found that the issue of death and dying was the main subject discussed. The most stressful experience for paediatric oncology nurses was the death of patients with whom they had established close relationships, as well as the feeling of helplessness when they experienced suffering, relapse and sudden death. Other subjects discussed were the professional image of the oncology nurse, perceived isolation from medical staff and emotional overinvolvement with patients. Kushnir et al concluded that more sharing and discussion of issues related to the deaths of young patients in the presence of an experienced group leader would have been beneficial to staff.

((((●))))

REFLECTION POINT 5.10
Burnout in palliative care

In palliative care, nurses can get 'burnt out' very easily. Do you agree with this statement? What kind of formal and informal support is available to you? Can you think of more ways in which you could be supported in your work?

SUMMARY

As nurses, we should examine our own motives for feeling less attracted to supporting people with some conditions than others. It may be that these conditions and situations threaten aspects of our personal or professional identities. Support for patients with terminal illness can be emotionally draining and nurses need support from colleagues and managers. They need to develop teamwork and learn to receive as well as give support. They need to have some insight into their feelings and to be able to acknowledge when they are upset. They need to be aware of distancing strategies they can use in communication to protect themselves from pain. Personal experiences can influence our attitudes to work with dying people. Self-awareness is one of the qualities Egan (1990) considered necessary in effective counselling. Other qualities were empathy, genuineness and unconditional acceptance of others. A climate of trust is created not only by what is said but also by the understanding shown in facial expression, tone of voice and gestures. Recognition and support come not only from colleagues but, perhaps surprisingly, also from dying people and their relatives. By developing their understanding of the role of support in enabling terminally ill people and their relatives to pass through critical phases of their illness and bereavement to self-acceptance, nurses have a major role to play, both in providing sensitive, professional support and in promoting patients' and relatives' informal support networks.

REFERENCES

Anderson M J 1986 The nursing contribution to the aftercare of mastectomy. Report prepared for the Scottish Home and Health Department. University of Edinburgh, Edinburgh

Armstrong M J, Fitzgerald M H 1996 Culture and disability studies: an anthropological perspective. Rehabilitation Education 10:247–304

Bailey K, Wilkinson SM 1998 Cancer patient perceptions of nurses' communication skills. International Journal of Palliative Nursing 4:300–305

Balint M 1957 The doctor, his patient and the illness. Pitman, London

Beaver K, Luker A, Woods S 2000 Primary care services received during terminal illness. International Journal of Palliative Care Nursing 6:220–227

Benica S W, Longo C B, Barnsteiner J H 1992 Perceptions and significance of patient death for paediatric critical care nursing. Critical Care Nursing 12:72–75

Benjamin A 1981 The helping interview, 3rd edn. Houghton Miffin, Boston, MA

Biemans H 1990 Video home training: theory, method and organisation of SPIN. In: Kool J (ed.) International Seminar for Innovative Institutions, Ryswijk, Netherlands. Ministry of Welfare, Health and Culture, The Hague

Bottorf J L, Gogag M, Engelberg-Lotzkar M 1995 Comforting: exploring the work of cancer nurses. Journal of Advanced Nursing 22:1077–1084

Bowlby J 1975 Attachment and loss separation (anxiety and anger). Pelican Books, Middlesex

Box V, Hepworth M, Harrison J 2003 Identifying information needs of people with multiple sclerosis. Nursing Times 99(49):32–36

Buckman R 1999 Communication in palliative care: a practical guide. In: Doyle D, Hanke G, Macdonald N (eds) Oxford textbook of palliative medicine, 2nd edn. Oxford University Press, Oxford

Burgess L 2004 Addressing the palliative care needs of people with dementia. Nursing Times 100(19):36–39

Clinical Standards Board for Scotland 2002 Standards for specialist palliative care. NHS Quality Improvement Scotland, Edinburgh

Copp G 1999 Facing impending death: experiences of patients and their nurses. EMAP Healthcare, London

Corner J, Halliday D, Haviland J et al 2003 Exploring nursing outcomes for patients with advanced cancer following intervention by Macmillan specialist palliative care nurses. Journal of Advanced Nursing 41:561–574

Corr C A, Corr D M 1992 Adult hospice day care. Death Studies 16:155–171

Daniels L 2004 Standardise or individualise: finding a balance. International Journal of Palliative Nursing 10:108

Davies B, Oberle K 1990 dimensions of the supportive role of the nurse in palliative care. Oncology Nursing Forum 17:87–94

Department of Health 2000 The NHS cancer plan. A plan for investment. A plan for reform. DH, London

Dixon R, Lee-Jones C, Humphris G 1996 Psychological reactions to cancer recurrence. International Journal of Palliative Nursing 2:19–21

Downs M 2002 Dementia as a disability: implications for practice. In: Benson S (ed.) Dementia topics for the millennium and beyond. Hawker Publications, London

Doyle D 1998 Domiciliary palliative care. In: Doyle D, Hanks G, MacDonald N (eds) Oxford textbook of palliative care, 2nd edn. Oxford University Press, Oxford, p 962–993

Dunne K 2003 The personal cost of caring (Guest editorial). International Journal of Palliative Nursing 9:232

Egan G 1990 The skilled helper: a systematic approach to effective helping. Brooks/Cole, Pacific Grove, CA

Ellershaw J, Foster A, Murphy D et al 1997 Developing an integrated care pathway for the dying patient. European Journal of Palliative Care 4:203–207

Erikson E H 1965 Childhood and society. Penguin, Harmondsworth

Field D 1998 Special, not different: general practitioners' account of their care of dying people. Social Science and Medicine 46:111–120

Flanagan J, Holmes S 2000 Social perceptions of cancer and their impacts: implications for nursing practice arising from the literature. Journal of Advanced Nursing 32:740–749

Flemming K 1997 The meaning of hope to palliative care cancer patients. International Journal of Palliative Nursing 3:113–118

Forsyth P, Kennedy H 1998–1999 Trainee guider's handbook. SPIN VIP: Scottish Project in Viewing Interaction Positively. Dundee University, Dundee

Glaser B G, Strauss A L 1965 Awareness of dying. Aldine, Chicago, IL

Grafen M 2000 Perceptions of palliative day care: an audit, April 1998–March 1999. West Lothian Healthcare NHS Trust/St John's Macmillan Centre, Livingston, West Lothian

Greer S Moorey S, Baruch J D R, Watson M 1992 Adjuvant psychological therapy for patients with cancer: a prospective randomised trial. British Medical Journal 304:675–680

Ham R J 1999 Evolving standards in patient and caregiver support. Alzheimer's Disease and Associated Disorders 13:527–535

Heaven C, Maguire P 1997 Disclosure of concerns by hospice patients and their identification by nurses. Palliative Medicine 11:283–290

Henley N 1973 Power, sex and non verbal communication. Newbury House, Rowely, MA

Heron J 1990 Helping the client: a creative, practical guide. Sage, London

Higginson I J 2003 Priorities and preferences for end of life care in England, Wales and Scotland. National Council for Hospice and Specialist Palliative Care Services, London

Higginson I J, Costantini M 2002 Communication in end of life cancer care: a comparison of team assessments in three European countries. Journal of Clinical Oncology 20:3674–3680

Higginson I J, Hearn J, Myers K, Naysmith A 2000 Palliative day care: what do services do? Palliative Medicine 14:277–286

Hill D, Penso D 1995 Opening doors: improving access to hospice and specialist palliative care services by members of the black and ethnic minority communities. Occasional Paper 7. National Council for Hospice and Specialist Palliative Care Services, London

Hirsch B J 1981 Social networks and the coping process. In: Gottleib B H (ed.) Social networks and social support. Sage, Beverly Hills, CA, p 149–171

Hopwood A, Howell A, Maguire P 1991 Psychiatric morbidity in patients with advanced cancer of the breast: prevalence measured by two self-rating questionnaires. British Journal of Cancer 64:349–352

Hurley A, Volicer B J, Hanrahan P A et al 1992 Assessment of discomfort in advanced Alzheimer's patients. Research in Nursing and Health 15:369–377

Ikels C 1991 Ageing and disability in China: cultural issues in measurement and interpretation. Social Science and Medicine 32:649–665

Jack B, Gambles M, Murphy D, Ellershaw J E 2003 Nurses' perceptions of the Liverpool Care Pathway for the dying patient in the acute hospital setting. International Journal of Palliative Nursing 9:375–381

Jack C M, Penny E, Nazar W 2001 Effective palliative care for minority ethnic groups: the role of a liaison worker. International Journal of Palliative Nursing 7:375–380

Johns C 1996 Developing reflective models of nursing. Lothian College of Health Studies, 1st Biennial Nursing and Midwifery Conference, Heriot Watt University, Edinburgh

Johnson J L 1991 Learning to live again: the process of adjustment following a heart attack. In: Morse J M, Johnson JL (eds) The illness experience. Sage, London

Kabel A, Roberts D 2003 Professionals' perceptions of maintaining personhood in hospice care. International Journal of Palliative Nursing 9:283–289

Kelly M P 1991 Coping with an ileostomy. Social Science and Medicine 33:115–125

Kelly M P 1992 Self, identity and radical surgery. Sociology of Health and Illness 14:390–415

Koopmeiners L, Post-White J, Gutnecht S et al 1997 How healthcare professionals contribute to hope in patients with cancer. Oncology Nursing Forum 24:1507–1513

Kopp P 2000a Communicating with patients. Nursing Times 96(27):45–47

Kopp P 2000b Enhancing communication skills. Nursing Times 96(29):45–47

Kushnir T, Rabin S, Azulai S 1997 A descriptive study of stress management in a group of paediatric oncology nurses. Cancer Nursing 20:414–442

Langley-Evans A 1997 Light-hearted death talk in a palliative day care context. Journal of Advanced Nursing 26:1091–1109

Lawton J 2000 The dying patient's experiences of palliative care. Routledge, London

Llewellyn S, Payne S 1995 Caring: the costs to nurses and families. In: Broome A, Llewellyn S (eds) Health psychology: processes and application, 2nd edn. Chapman & Hall, London, p 109–122

Lugton J 1994 The meaning of social support: a descriptive study of informal networks and of health visitors' formal role in supporting the identity of women with breast cancer. Unpublished PhD thesis, University of Edinburgh, Edinburgh

Lugton J 1997a The nature of social support as experienced by women with breast cancer. Journal of Advanced Nursing 25:1184–1191

Lugton J 1997b Health visitor support for patients with breast cancer: 1. Nursing Standard 11(33):33–37

Lugton J, Sneddon E 2001 Health visitors' application of video technology as an intervention in child and family focussed programmes of care. Report for the Queen's Nursing Institute, Scotland

Luker K A, Austin L, Caress A, Hallett C E 2000 The importance of knowing the patient: community nurses' constructions of quality in providing palliative care. Journal of Advanced Nursing 31:775–782

Lynam M J 1990 Examining support in context: a redefinition from the cancer patient's perspective. Sociology of Health and Illness 12:169–194

McClement S E, Chochinov H M, Hack T F et al 2004 Dignity conserving care: application of research findings to practice. International Journal of Palliative Nursing 10:173–179

McDaid P 1995 Day care. In: Penson J, Fisher R (eds) Palliative care for people with cancer. Edward Arnold, London, p 150–157

McIllmurray M B, Thomas C, Francis B et al 2001 The psychosocial needs of cancer patients: findings from an observational study. European Journal of Cancer Care 10:261–269

Macpherson C, Cooke C 2003 Pilot of a workbook for children visiting a loved one in a hospital. International Journal of Palliative Nursing 9:397–403

Maier S, Seligman M E P 1976 Learned helplessness, theory and evidence. Journal of Experimental Psychology 105:13–46

Mathieson C M, Stam H J 1995 Renegotiating identity, the cancer narratives. Sociology of Health and Illness 17:283–306

Mead G 1934 Mind, self and society. University of Chicago Press, Chicago, IL

Morse J M, Bottorff J, Anderson G et al 1992 Beyond empathy: expanding expressions of caring. Journal of Advanced Nursing 17:809–821

Multiple Sclerosis Society 1999 Are we being served? Health care experiences of people with MS of the health services. Mori, London

Murray S, Boyd K, Kendall M et al 2002 Dying of lung cancer or cardiac failure: prospective qualitative interview study of patients and their carers in the community. British Medical Journal 325:929–940

NCHSPCS 1995 Working Party on Clinical Guidelines on Palliative Care: information for purchasers. National Council for Hospice and Specialist Palliative Care Services, London

O'Neill B 1994 Ethnic minorities – neglected by palliative care providers? Journal of Cancer Care 3:215–220

Payne S A, Dean S J, Kalus C 1998 A comparative study of death anxiety in hospice and emergency nurses. Journal of Advanced Nursing 28:700–706

Pemberton C 2004 Understanding the preferred place of care document: its place in practice. Contact, Spring. RCN Palliative Nursing Group, London

Pemberton C, Storey L, Howard A 2003 The preferred place of care: an opportunity for communication. International Journal of Palliative Nursing 9:439–441

Peplau H E 1988 Interpersonal relations in nursing. Macmillan, London

Perry B 1996 Influence of nurse gender on the use of silence, touch and humour. International Journal of Palliative Nursing 2:7–14

Pfeffer C R, Karus D, Siegal K, Jiang H 2000 Child survivors of parental death from cancer or suicide: depressive and behavioural outcomes. Psycho-Oncology 9:1–10

Porritt L 1990 Interaction strategies. An introduction for health care professionals. Churchill Livingstone, Edinburgh

Proctor S 1996 Fuzzy boundaries: multi-professional working and visibility in nursing practic. Paper for the Royal College of Nursing of the United Kingdom Research Society, Annual Nursing Research Conference, Newcastle upon Tyne

Randhawa G, Owens A, Fitches R, Khan Z 2003 Communication in the development of culturally competent palliative care services in the UK: a case study. International Journal of Palliative Nursing 9:24–31

Richardson J 2002 Health promotion in palliative care: the patient's perception of therapeutic interaction with the palliative care nurse in a primary care setting. Journal of Advanced Nursing 40:432–440

Robinson A W 1999 Getting to the heart of denial. American Journal of Nursing 99:43–53

Rogers C R 1967 On becoming a person. Constable, London

Rolls L, Payne S 2003 Childhood bereavement services: a survey of UK provision. Palliative Medicine 17:423–432

Sabat S 2002 Surviving manifestations of selfhood in Alzheimer's disease dementia. International Journal of Social Research and Practice 1:7–10

Sheldon F 1994 Children and bereavement – what are the issues? European Journal of Palliative Care 1:42–44

Sheldon F 1997 Psychosocial palliative care: good practice in care of the dying and bereaved. Stanley Thornes, Cheltenham

Simpson J 1999 The theory of secondary intersubjectivity and its relationship to video interaction guidance. Paper delivered at the SPIN USA International Working Conference, Westford, MA, May

Spruyt O 1999 Community based palliative care for Bangladeshi patients in East London. Accounts of bereaved carers. Palliative Medicine 13:119–130

Tait A 1988 Whole or partial breast loss: the threat to womanhood. In: Salter M (ed.) Altered body image: the nurse's role. John Wiley, Chichester, p 167–177

Torrington D, Weigtman J, Johns K 1989 Effective management, people and organisations. Prentice-Hall, Hemel Hempstead

UKCC 1996 Guidelines for professional practice. United Kingdom Central Council for Nursing, Midwifery and Health Visiting, London

Wallace P R 2001 Improving palliative care through effective communication. International Journal of Palliative Nursing 7:86–90

Warshaw L J 1989 Stress, anxiety and depression in the workplace. Report of the NYBGH/Gallup Survey. Conference on Stress, Anxiety and Depression in the Workplace, New York

Wenrich M D, Curtis R, Ambrozy D A et al 2003 Dying patients' need for emotional support and personalised care from physicians. Journal of Pain and Symptom Management 25:236–246

Wilkes L M, Beale B 2001 Palliative care at home: stress for nurses in urban and rural New South Wales, Australia. International Journal of Nursing Practice 7:306–313

Wilkinson S 1999 Schering Plough Clinical Lecture. Communication: it makes a difference. Cancer Nursing 22:17–27

Wilkinson S 2002 The essence of cancer care: the impact of training on nurses' ability to communicate effectively. Journal of Advanced Nursing 40:731–738

Wilkinson S, Bailey K, Aldridge J, Roberts A 1999 A longitudinal evaluation of a communication skills programme. Palliative Medicine 13:341–348

World Health Organization 1999 Cancer pain relief and palliative care. Technical Report, Series 804. WHO, Geneva

CHAPTER SIX

Spirituality in palliative care

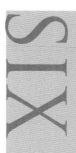

Jacquelyn Chaplin, David Mitchell

CONTENTS

INTRODUCTION

Spirituality is a term that is widely used and included as an integral feature of health care in general and palliative care in particular. It is one of four clearly recognised areas of holistic palliative care: physical, psychological, social and spiritual. Despite its ready recognition, it is a concept that has proved difficult to define, and most writing on spiritual care begins with the author's definition and understanding. This chapter seeks to explore spirituality and spiritual care as it relates to palliative nursing practice. In particular, it will examine spirituality in the context of having a sense of meaning and purpose in living and the factors that contribute to an individual's sense of meaning: hope, being there, and peace. It also questions whether the much sought after definition of spiritual care is actually needed – or is it more helpful to be open to a broad concept?

Within palliative care, issues of spirituality come into sharp focus, especially in practice. How health-care professionals can respond to people struggling with the difficult 'why' questions, or a sense of hopelessness, will be discussed.

The experience of spiritual pain will also be explored. Is pain the best word or is it better to speak of distress? In palliative care, spiritual care includes the patient's family/carers; if one is distressed that affects the other, so the nurse's role in supporting the family will be discussed.

A crucial element of spiritual care is self-awareness and, before we set out to care for others, we need to think through what we ourselves understand and believe about life, death, illness and relationships. Further discussion will examine how nurses can use that understanding in a non-judgemental way to journey with others to where they are and what they believe in.

We also need to be aware that we are part of a care team and be open to using the skills of the team, as multiprofessional teamwork is a core element of palliative care. The need for greater understanding of each other's role in spiritual care and the skills that each professional brings are also important. Not least is an understanding of the contribution that can be made by the profession with specialist expertise in spiritual care – chaplaincy, a profession that is about much more than religion.

Having explored the concept of spiritual care and the impact on patients, family carers and ourselves both as individuals and part of a team, we are naturally led to think about how we put it into practice. One aspect that will be considered is whether spirituality lends itself to the use of an assessment tool and, if so, how it should be used. Considering competence in spiritual care, would a competency framework offer a different approach to assessment?

The chapter concludes with a discussion of some current and future challenges, which include the changing demographics of society, the challenge of caring for people with non-cancerous conditions, developing spiritual care practice, spirituality within research, and the ultimate challenge of understanding our own mortality.

AIMS OF THE CHAPTER

- To broaden readers' understanding of the concept of spirituality and its relevance to palliative care
- To examine issues and challenges faced by health-care professionals in assessing and addressing the spiritual needs of patients and family/carers
- To challenge readers to reflect on their own spirituality and how that may influence the care they provide

Personal reflection features throughout the chapter. There are activities that will encourage you to reflect and work through your personal understanding and awareness of spirituality. In addition, a case study is offered to help you focus your thinking on your personal experience, your own understanding of what you believe and, importantly, how you put that into practice in palliative care.

CAPTURING THE CONCEPT

Spirituality is a difficult concept to define, discuss and audit (Hunt et al 2003). It is unique and individual to each person and the descriptive language used in spiritual care is often subjective and diverse and does not lend itself to clear expression. It follows, therefore, that in terms of identifying, assessing and addressing spiritual needs, accepted methods of assessing and planning care are unlikely to be useful. However, such individuality and variety of expression may in fact be a strength; not only does it enable health-care professionals to deepen their understanding of the people they care for but the experience may also positively influence a broader and more holistic approach to be used in the care of patients and their families/carers.

The first and most important distinction in spirituality is to distinguish *spiritual* and *religious* (Cobb 2001). Spirituality is often mistakenly equated with religion: religion can be an important factor in a person's spirituality, but how important will depend on the individual. Spirituality is much broader than religion and would draw together everything in a person's life that gives them a sense of meaning.

Spirituality is about people, and all people are different! Do we therefore *need* a definition of spirituality, or is there another, more open approach? If we conclude that spirituality involves an individual sense of meaning and is influenced by human relationships, it is inevitable that it will be different for everyone. Taking into consideration the difficulty of language and expression, the subjective and diverse ways in which it can be expressed, it may be that the real strength and understanding of the concept of spirituality will come from an openness and willingness to engage in its diversity of expression and experience (Mitchell & Sneddon 1999).

The NHS in Scotland has issued guidelines that offer a helpful definition for spiritual and religious care (Scottish Executive 2002):

- **Religious care** is given in the context of the shared religious beliefs, values, liturgies and lifestyle of a faith community
- **Spiritual care** is usually given in a one-to-one relationship, is completely person-centred and makes no assumptions about personal conviction or life orientation.

The essence of spirituality is its person-centredness and its understanding of the way in which the key elements of our humanity link together. When asked to describe their spirit, many people will take their fingers and put them towards their heart and describe it as the bit inside that makes you who you are, that makes you individual and different. As Byrne (2002) notes, there is no defined language of spirituality and often it is a word used to describe all that is 'left over' or can't be explained in body or mind.

The traditional model of body, mind and soul has grown into a model where the soul becomes the spirit and also includes the impact that others have on our lives (World Health Organization 1990). In Figure 6.1 we see an example of how we might think of ourselves as human beings. The spirit is the essence of who we are as people and within that person we have a body, a mind, and relationships with people who are important to us. What the diagram also helpfully makes clear is the interrelatedness of each of the elements: whenever one area of our person is affected by an event, there is a natural impact on the other areas.

A SENSE OF MEANING

To help grasp the interrelatedness of spirituality as part of being human, we need to be aware of a personal sense of meaning. Ask yourself the question: What is most important to me in my life – what gives me my meaning? Try and identify three or four key elements.

You are probably thinking about family, friends, health and work. Often, other interests like music, reading or football are also there and perhaps religion or faith too. These are elements of meaning common to us all as people, and they come into sharp focus in illness and when we feel our remaining life may be limited.

The following three sections are offered as a framework to understanding meaning as it relates to us as people and to give a background for considering the key elements of spiritual care.

HOPE

Hope is a universal concept that we all share. Our tradition at each New Year is to reflect on the past year but, regardless of whether we deem it a

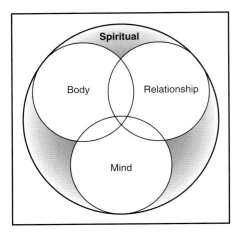

Figure 6.1 The body, mind and relationships model of spirituality (adapted from Twycross 1999).

good or bad experience, we look forward to a good New Year. Hope is very much our way of coping with life's variety of experiences, especially the difficult and uncertain times. Hope is also a fluid and changing concept that is influenced by current and past life experiences. It changes throughout the life journey and the changes come into sharp focus when illness occurs. At a time of diagnosis or recurrence of a disease, hope will often be focused on an available treatment and that it will be successful. Move forward to end of life care and our hope shifts to a pain-free and peaceful death, and often away from ourselves entirely – 'I hope my family will be OK'.

BEING THERE

An important part of being human are the relationships that matter to us in life, as seen in Figure 6.1, and the question of what gives us meaning in life. For people with cancer, the second and most common fear of the disease, after pain, is of being alone. This fear can be focused on being isolated from family, being apart from God or from health-care professionals. As disease progresses, patients can fade from the vision of family, friends, work, society, and fewer visits are needed from fewer professionals, all of which can contribute to a sense of abandonment (Stanley 2002). 'Being there' can counter feelings of abandonment but it can also be challenging. To *be there* without *doing* is not easy and demands time and experience. Experience also suggests that there is a paradox in the need in patients for someone to be there: why do so many patients die when the family who have been sitting by the bedside for hours or days leave the room to go to the toilet or to make tea?

PEACE

Pain and symptom control are crucial in achieving a sense of peace; however, the concept is much broader than physical needs. Often you need to control the pain and symptoms to allow the patient to think about the wider issues; however, it is common in palliative care for the spiritual issues to be a significant factor in controlling pain and symptoms. If relationships are important to us as human beings, if our sense of meaning is focused on family and our hope is that our family will be OK, it is hardly surprising that all will impact on our sense of peace. Add to that personal questions of How will I know when I am dying? How is it likely to happen? How long have I got? and it's clear that there are a host of factors that can influence a sense of peace in patients and their families/carers. The key elements in achieving peace are information, honesty and a recognition that sometimes the answer has to be 'I don't know'. It also requires an honest recognition that sometimes we can't resolve all a patient's needs but it may be that we can help them cope with their needs and find peace.

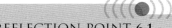

REFLECTION POINT 6.1

Fostering a sense of meaning

Think of someone you have known and/or cared for and reflect on that person:

- What were their hopes?

- What were their feelings and fears?

- What were the pain and symptom issues, including the broader spiritual issues?

- What were your feelings as a carer?

- How could you foster hope, being there, and peace to enhance your care?

SPIRITUAL ISSUES IN PALLIATIVE CARE

Receiving a diagnosis of serious illness is often accompanied by feelings of fear, uncertainty about the unknown future and a need to examine personal values and priorities (Halldorsdottir & Hamrin 1996). Treatment brings with it many uncertainties and physical, social and practical demands as people negotiate their own unique treatment calendar (Schou & Hewison 1999). When faced with the reality of recurrence or advanced disease, individuals often find that this can be even harder to come to terms with (Barraclough 1999).

Entering the terminal phase of illness also challenges spirituality because it brings issues of mortality sharply into focus. When we are healthy and life is going on as normal, few of us think about and deal with issues related to our own mortality. Having a life-threatening illness often results in people questioning the value of life and the meaning of death at a personal level.

Speck (1998) suggests that death for most people brings together the past, present and the future as they explore their spiritual identity. Frequently, a key part of this spiritual examination is a review of their life, including both the challenges they have faced and their achievements. This life review can contain many positive elements, often in relation to close relationships, but it is important to recognise that it can also evoke feelings of guilt or regret over past actions or inactions. Personal belief systems may also be challenged and re-examined, especially in relation to individual beliefs about the cause of illness and, for some, their faith and religious beliefs.

At the same time, people can experience feelings of anger that may be focused on professionals, at life in general or at a higher being who has 'let them down'. This anger often demonstrates a need in patients to understand their present situation and what their illness means for them in the future. In particular, palliative care patients may have real concerns as to the way in which they will live until they die, how they will die and the impact that their dying and death will have on their family.

In essence, facing death is often characterised by feelings of uncertainty, loss of control and fear and, as a result, individuals often embark on a process of self-examination and questioning.

THE 'WHY?' QUESTIONS

In the context of palliative care, searching for meaning and purpose in life often results in individuals asking a range of difficult and searching questions. These questions can be wide and varied but some of the most commonly asked are:

- Why did I get cancer?
- Why me?
- What have I done to deserve this?
- Why has this happened now when I am ready to enjoy my children . . . retirement . . . grandchildren?
- Why does God allow this to happen?
- Why does my family have to suffer watching me like this?
- Why am I dying? I'm only 30 . . . 40 . . . 50 . . . and older people are still alive!

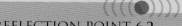

REFLECTION POINT 6.2
Difficult questions

Reflect on your professional experience of caring for people who are dying. Select one person who you have cared for where you had to deal with a difficult question of a spiritual nature. This may be the same patient that you selected in Reflection point 6.1 or a different individual.

- What form did the question take?

- How did you respond to the question?

- What were your feelings at that time?

Dealing with these types of question can be one of the most challenging aspects of palliative care practice and it is important to recognise that they may be asked of any professional involved in palliative care, not just nurses. However, nurses have prolonged and intimate contact with people, as do health-care assistants, and often have to respond to such questions. Responding in such a situation requires effective communication skills, a degree of personal and professional confidence and a mature sense of spiritual self-awareness. Box 6.1 outlines six steps that provide a framework for dealing with such questions.

Box **6.1**

Six step framework for responding to spiritual distress

1. **Do not rush in with an answer.** Recognise that many people are not looking for an answer to their question but rather the opportunity to air their thoughts, in order to give vent to their feelings and clarify their own thinking. Indeed, there is often no answer, and saying 'I don't know' is both appropriate and honest.

2. **Listen actively.** Listen to what is being said and to what is unsaid – there may be deeper issues that the patient wants to discuss and they are 'testing the water'. Observe non-verbal and verbal communication and use silence in order to give the patient the opportunity to reflect on what they are saying. Spiritual care in this context requires our full attention, to do anything less gives the impression to the patient that these issues are not important.

3. **Explore what has prompted this question.** Use facilitative communication skills to explore what has prompted this person to ask this question at this time. An openness to allow the discussion to be led by the patient may threaten our sense of control but ensures that we are exploring what is important to that individual at this point in time. It is important that we do not presume that we know what the issues are – each person is unique, with a unique combination of experiences and issues.

4. **Respond to the patient's feelings.** Exploration of spiritual issues in the context of palliative care often evokes strong emotions such as anger and may result in the individual becoming emotionally distressed. Acknowledging these emotions in a non-judgemental way is important, as it validates the individual's right to feel the way that they do. In addition, experiencing these intense emotions can be frightening and people often highly value the presence of another person. Therefore 'being there' for people at this time in their life is an important contribution to their care.

5. **Be aware of your own feelings.** Dealing with questions of a spiritual nature is demanding and we need to be aware of our own feelings and how they influence what we say, think and do. Pay particular attention to whether your feelings and responses are encouraging the patient to examine their feelings, or whether they are blocking the patient's responses. Be aware that there may be times when you are particularly fragile or vulnerable. Trust your own feelings and instincts.

6. **Refer to other professionals when appropriate.** It is important to recognise that other professionals may be better qualified than you to deal with some issues. Referral to a chaplain who has particular skills in dealing with spiritual distress may be appropriate. Alternatively, referral to psychological services may be appropriate if someone demonstrates evidence of psychological disorders such as anxiety and depression.

It is appropriate to express a word of caution at this point. The framework identified may be helpful but should not be seen as being prescriptive. It is important that we respond to individuals as ourselves, in our own way. So while a framework may act as a guide, the most important element of any response that we can make in this situation is to focus on the person and we can best do so by being ourselves. There are no 'magic words'!

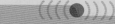

REFLECTION POINT 6.3
Responding to spiritual distress

Now reconsider the situation that you reviewed in Reflection point 2 and assess your level of skill in relation to the six steps outlined above, using a scale of 0–10 with 10 being the highest level of skill achievable. Try to be as honest as possible. It is likely that you assessed your skill as being higher for some aspects of this framework than for others. It may also be the case that there is room for some improvement.
Now consider two things:

- How might you achieve such an improvement?

- How might you respond if faced with a similar situation tomorrow?

HOPELESSNESS

Some people who face the prospect of dying appear to be so overwhelmed that they can no longer sustain a sense of hope in the future. Many of us have had the experience of caring for individuals who appear to have given up hope and we know that this can be very challenging. As has been identified already, a sense of hope is important to spiritual wellbeing, yet the relationship between hope and spirituality is not entirely clear. A lack of hope or hopelessness is characterised by a lack of interest and involvement in everyday life and a withdrawal from the company of others. Recognising individuals who have a sense of hopelessness is relatively easy. They are often socially withdrawn, lack interest in everyday living, appear to care little about their physical state and, if asked, may say that they don't care or don't see the point in going on.

There is general consensus that a sense of hope is essential to life (Chaplin & McIntyre 2001, Dufault & Martocchio 1985, Farran et al 1995). Nurses, with other health-care professionals, have the potential to hinder or foster hope in palliative care patients (Herth & Cutliffe 2002). In the context of palliative care, it has been identified that the hope that can be fostered is linked to two different elements of hope; living in hope and hoping for better days or moments (Benzein et al 2001). McIntyre & Chaplin (2001) suggest a simple framework for fostering hope in palliative care patients that focuses on promoting comfort, maintaining attachments with important people and affirming the sense of self-worth of the individual. This is consistent with the framework for spiritual care outlined in this chapter whereby being there for people is the key to providing support in order that people find a sense of hope and peace.

One challenge for those working in palliative care is to ensure that hoped for goals are realistic. This is particularly difficult, as it may not always be clear, especially in relation to survival, because accuracy in estimates of survival is poor. A second challenge is to identify those individuals whose sense of hopelessness is part of a state of clinical depression. The diagnosis of depression is particularly problematic in palliative care, in part because the physical symptoms of loss of appetite, sleep disturbances and fatigue are also characteristic of advanced malignant disease (Hotopf et al 2002). As a result, a sense of hopelessness is often used as an important indicator of clinical depression. However, it is unclear whether the implementation of hope-fostering strategies throughout the patient's illness might prevent a sense of hopelessness occurring.

SPIRITUAL DISTRESS

A number of people who receive palliative care may have spiritual pain or distress. Spiritual distress is when a person experiences feelings of despair in relation to their intrinsic personal beliefs and values. Spiritual distress is linked to the concept of total pain, which recognises that pain can have not only a physical component but also an emotional, a social and a spiritual component (Saunders 1984). Spiritual distress is also closely linked to suffering. Cassell (1991, p. 33) describes suffering as 'the state of severe distress associated with events which threaten the intactness of the person'. It has also been identified that suffering is linked to feelings of a lack of control and an overwhelming sense of fear of what the future holds.

Spiritual distress can be overlooked, as there seem to be no readily visible signs or answers. However, it is possible to assess spiritual distress and appropriate action can be taken to lessen the distress experienced if nurses and other professionals are aware of the indicators of spiritual distress and the strategies that professionals can use to offer support.

CASE STUDY 6.1
Jim

Jim is admitted to the hospice for symptom control. His pain goes up and down for no apparent reason; he has difficulty sleeping and he is agitated. Following admission, his medication is steadily increased but there is little effect. Jim has bouts of pain and agitation, requiring regular breakthrough medication. Jim also finds it difficult to sleep at night and asks for something to help him sleep.

Jim's son Robert visits regularly and spends most afternoons with his dad. Robert discloses to staff that he has been getting help from a clinical psychiatric nurse for 5 years but feels he is coping well with his dad's illness, realising that it is serious and he maybe doesn't have long to live. Jim's wife and stepdaughter never visit and don't phone to ask how he is. When Jim needs clothes from home, the occupational therapist visits and combines the visit with a home assessment.

The medical team feels that Jim has something on his mind but he is reluctant to talk. The team refers Jim to the chaplain to 'drop by' and visit.

The chaplain meets Jim, and Jim's first question is: 'Do you do funerals, son?' quickly followed by 'Would you see me all right when the time comes?'

- What are pointers to spiritual pain/distress?
- What could be the causes of Jim's distress and how could you deal with them?
- What could be done to ease Jim's distress?

Assessing spiritual distress often involves recognising and interpreting the 'ordinary' aspects of people's lives: family and social relationships, their sense of meaning and purpose, their religious beliefs and financial and practical concerns. Indicators of spiritual distress can be considered under three main categories: non-verbal behaviour, verbal responses and the patient's environment. The main indicators, adapted from Twycross (1999), are set out in Box 6.2.

Treating spiritual distress requires us to foster hope and a sense of meaning in life and living. It also requires us to give of ourselves and be a companion to the person in distress as well as a professional. In some circumstances, for example where family relationships are the primary source of the distress, it may also be appropriate to facilitate reconciliation, where this is possible. Practical and financial issues also need to be addressed as they can add to the level of distress, and this is where other members of the multiprofessional team, for instance the social worker, can also play a key role.

Box 6.2

Indicators of spiritual distress

Non-verbal behaviour

- Loneliness

- Depression

- Anger

- Agitation

- Stoicism

- Prays/uses religious material

- Sleep disturbances

- Unusually high levels of analgesics required

- Distressed reaction to visitors

Continued

BOX 6.2—CONT'D

Verbal responses

- Repeatedly asks the 'Why' questions

- Puts on a brave face – 'I can't let my family/church down'

- Expressions of intense suffering

- Vocalises feelings of helplessness – 'I'd be better off dead'

- Talks about God/religion without gaining comfort

Patient's environment

- Religious books and medals are around

- Religious music used

When spiritual distress has a religious focus it may be appropriate to refer the patient to a member of the clergy who can help them to explore the main issues that are important to them. It is important that strategies that are being implemented are understood by the whole team, so that a concerted approach to care is achieved.

CASE STUDY 6.1—CONT'D

The indicators of Jim's spiritual pain/distress included:

- Poor pain control
- Agitation
- Trouble sleeping
- Family concerns
- Questioning what would happen when he died.

Outcome

The chaplain used the question about whether he could conduct Jim's funeral as a way of talking through his family concerns. By going behind the question and asking who will be organising the funeral, he encouraged Jim to open up and explain that, although he lived with his wife, he didn't like her. He was concerned for his son and how he would cope. On discussing his wishes for a funeral and how much it would cost, it became clear that money was an issue and that he didn't trust his wife with money; his house was in joint names with his wife, but he had his own bank account. The talk focused on how important it was for Jim to make a will because, as it stood, his son would have the death certificate as his next of kin and could therefore arrange Jim's funeral, but it would be his wife who would have access to the money to pay for it.

That day Jim saw a lawyer and made a will. The next day, Jim and the chaplain met with Jim's son, Robert, and discussed Jim's concerns, which were shared by Robert. Robert was also concerned he wouldn't be thinking straight when his dad died and, following discussions, went to the funeral directors and took out a funeral plan (a prepaid and arranged funeral), paying for the funeral with his dad's money.

Following the interventions by the chaplain, the multidisciplinary team met to discuss Jim. His pain was controlled, his medication was reduced and stabilised, he was not agitated and he had a normal sleep pattern. Jim never discussed his funeral service and died a week later, with Robert by his side. Robert coped well, his clinical psychiatric nurse, stepdaughter and two friends attending the funeral.

FAMILY DISTRESS

The case study discussed above highlights clearly that for many people who face death, as in life, their family is of great importance. While families are often of paramount concern to the patient, it is important to recognise that the family can also be a source of stress and distress to the patient. Caring for the family can also be a source of stress and distress to nurses and other professionals.

Every family is composed of a unique set of people, each with their own beliefs, views and philosophy of life and death. As each patient is unique and different, so each family is unique and different. It is essential, therefore, if we are to provide holistic palliative care, that we take time to determine the structure and relationships of each of our patients' families. Liossi et al (1997) advocate the use of a genogram, a simple family tree, to document the structure of the family, and suggest that simple notes and symbols can be included in this pictorial representation of the family in order to describe relationships within the family. The importance of including details about the nature of relationships within families is highlighted in the previous case study. Although he was married, Jim's relationship with his wife was not supportive in the time leading up to his death. It shows that there are real practical benefits from a systematic approach to documenting information about the family. Each member of the multiprofessional team does not need to ask similar questions, all members of the team can use the information, and bereavement issues may be highlighted for specific family members.

As already stated, each family member has their own unique perspective on life, death and religion. This can lead to assumptions being made within the family about the patient's beliefs and wishes. It can also mean that the patient does not feel comfortable talking about issues of a spiritual nature with members of their family, as they do not want to 'upset them'. This is particularly the case when it comes to talking about death and what to do after the death. For many patients, planning their funeral and dealing with practical issues like finance and inheritance can be a positive experience. Yet how often have you heard relatives saying, 'Don't talk like that, you've got to be positive', or listened as they changed the subject? One reason why relatives act in this way is because they are trying to 'protect' the patient. Another reason is that a dual process of adaptation is going on within the family at this time.

Coming to terms with dying is a process, not an event, and as such takes time (Copp 1999, Kubler-Ross 1969). Coming to terms with the fact that someone you love is dying is also a process, which has been linked to anticipating the grief that is to come (Costello 1999). In many families, these two processes are going on together, yet they are often not synchronised. Indeed, in many circumstances, different family members deal with their anticipated loss in different ways. Recognising when there are differences of this nature in the family is an important aspect of palliative nursing care. Discussing with the patient and the family their views, wishes and concerns and acting as a bridge between patient and family can contribute to the patient's sense of meaning and purpose in living and can help both the patient and the family to plan for the future.

In large families, many issues can occur as the stresses and strains of looking after the patient are felt. While this experience can draw families more closely together, it can also be the case that difficulties that previously existed in family relationships may emerge under the strain of watching someone they love die. This can cause some difficulty for both the patient and the family and can also present difficulties for professionals, who may feel that they are being cast in the role of referee. Additionally, in some circumstances, patients may seek reconciliations with estranged family members that are not always supported by the whole family. In this type of situation, our key role, as professionals providing care, is to listen to the concerns and wishes of the patient and the different family members while at the same time remembering that the patient's quality of life is paramount. Regular good communication with the family, using agreed pathways of communication, can be helpful in this situation. Nevertheless, the complexities of modern families, with divorce and remarriage being common, makes this a particularly challenging aspect of palliative care.

SPIRITUAL SELF-AWARENESS

Providing spiritual care in the context of palliative care often involves establishing relationships where highly personal information and feelings may be shared (Kelly 2002). In order to recognise the need for spiritual care and to provide this care for others, it is necessary that we, as professionals and individuals, know ourselves. Like all other human beings we need to make sense of and find meaning in what we do, both in our personal and our professional lives. In palliative care, there are a number of reasons why this awareness of self at a spiritual level is so important.

Firstly, in order to appreciate the spirituality of others we need to be able to appreciate our own essence of self. Secondly, unless we are aware of our own feelings and spirituality, we run the risk of dealing with issues that are ours rather than dealing with issues raised by the patient or the family for whom we are providing care. Furthermore, as someone providing care, we need to be aware of both our professional and personal limitations. There may be other members of the team who are more able to deal with spiritual issues than we are ourselves and there may be issues that we feel we cannot deal with because our personal lives are such that we are more vulnerable at that time. Spiritual self-awareness also involves asking ourselves whether at any point in time we have any particular areas of stress and distress that might influence our ability to provide care for people. It is important that we all recognise that we have our own special needs and that these are not static: they change from moment to moment, from day to day, from year to year, in the light of our experiences at a personal and a professional level. Finally, many people who face the reality of imminent death examine their own views on the meaning of life, death and religion. In order to support people who are doing this, we as professionals need to understand our own views on these important aspects of life. Speck (1998) suggests that this aspect of palliative care can be partic- ularly challenging, as the questions asked by people who are dying may echo questions in our own minds.

In essence, in order to understand others and in particular to understand their spiritual needs, it is important that we know ourselves. Part of this process is clarifying our own values and beliefs. It takes a degree of personal maturity to feel comfortable with who you are, to know where you have come from and to identify those aspects of your life that you value most highly.

You have already been asked to think about what gives your life meaning and purpose. Let us explore this further by considering the following questions:

- What is your philosophical outlook on life?
- What are your own personal views on death, suffering, religion and the possibility of life after death? How comfortable do you feel about discussing these personal values and beliefs with others?

As well as reflecting on our own values and beliefs, we must also consider our intrinsic response to the beliefs of others, particularly those that we may not share. An openness to others and their beliefs is founded upon the ethical principle of respect for persons (Beauchamp & Childress 1994). The health- care principle of respect for persons supports each individual's right to make decisions and to have views that are fundamentally theirs. Respect and caring are vital elements in the role of health-care professionals in all settings, includ- ing palliative care. We demonstrate a respect for others by valuing them as people and by recognising each person's right to make decisions about in which they live and the way in which they wish to die.

Part of this respect is an openness and an awareness of other beliefs and faith systems. We live within a multicultural and multifaith society and this pres- ents a number of challenges. How much do you know about the individual spiritual beliefs of the patients for whom you care, and how willing are you to find out about them? It has already been identified that the explanation of spirituality and spiritual need is limited by the language we use. How comfortable do you feel about discussing their spiritual beliefs with others? It has been identified that some nurses avoid such discussions, as they can be too emotionally and personally challenging or they do not have the communication skills to do so (Ross 1997).

Providing spiritual care for people, particularly at the end of life, is a process whereby we learn as much about ourselves as we do about the patients and families for whom we provide care. How open are you to being challenged and to being changed? Kelly (2002) argues that spiritual care begins with the health-care professional who seeks to offer such care and goes on to stress that the heart of spiritual care is the personhood and the spirituality of the care giver. If we accept this, then we have to recognise that part of giving spiritual care is the way that we may be changed as a person by providing that care.

Being challenged, being changed and growing as an individual can be exciting on the one hand but on the other may be frightening, and we also have to consider how we support our colleagues and ourselves during this process. For some time in nursing, reflection has been recognised as a strategy whereby nurses can critically examine and learn from the 'messy reality' of practice (Schon 1983). Wright (1998) asserts that using reflection effectively can often result in nurses embarking on a spiritual journey as they explore practice situations that are personally relevant.

One such mechanism that allows the use of reflection within a formal framework is clinical supervision. Clinical supervision is a way in which we can deal with some of the challenges that providing spiritual care presents to professionals. It provides a forum where in-depth critical analysis of clinical situations can be undertaken. A fundamental element of this critical analysis is analysis of one's actions, beliefs and feelings. Reflective practice, therefore, is supportive not only of continuous professional development but also the ethos of personal lifelong learning. Furthermore, Cobb (2001) asserts that the application of reflective practice to spiritual care can help professionals to develop their knowledge of spirituality into the 'art' of spiritual care practice.

The skills of reflection also provide us with a mechanism to identify our own spiritual needs and to evaluate how we meet those needs. As people we must develop and regularly implement strategies to ensure that our spiritual wellbeing is maintained. What gives you spiritual nourishment? How do you take care of the spiritual element of you as a person? Self-awareness is the key to spiritual wellbeing.

SPIRITUAL ASSESSMENT AND CARE

THE MULTIPROFESSIONAL TEAM

Teamwork is readily acknowledged as an essential element of providing palliative care. While the more complex aspects of spiritual care demand specialist expertise, it is widely acknowledged that spiritual care can be and often is provided by all members of the multiprofessional team (Association of Hospice & Palliative Care Chaplains 2003).

WHO MAKES UP THE TEAM?

The National Health Service Plan gives a commitment to breaking down barriers between staff and ending hierarchical ways of working (Department of Health 2000). In their place will be flexible team working between different professionals and flexibility across traditional boundaries. This approach is further supported by recent NHS plans for cancer care that acknowledge the crucial importance of specialist multidisciplinary teamwork in palliative care and give a commitment to multidisciplinary education to support and develop the effectiveness of such teams (Department of Health 2000, Scottish Executive Health Department 2001).

The composition of a multiprofessional team will depend on the care setting:

- **In the community** it could include the general practitioner (GP), district nurse, clinical nurse specialist and others as required
- **In a nursing home** it could be the GP(s), nursing staff, district and clinical nurse specialists and others.

In hospitals and hospices it is easier to be prescriptive and standards for specialist palliative care in Scotland have been issued stating clearly the composition of the core team in different settings (Clinical Standards Board for Scotland 2002; as of 2003, now known as NHS Quality Improvement Scotland):

- **In hospices** the core team comprises chaplain, doctors, nurses, occupational therapist, pharmacist, physiotherapist and social worker. The core team should also have ready access to a named list of other professionals
- **In hospitals** the core team consists of doctors and nurses, with ready access to a list of other named professionals.

SKILLS AND BOUNDARIES

In any team the use of complementary skills gives a comprehensive perspective to the quality of care, and particularly so in a palliative approach to care (Cobb 2001). A team will be enhanced and comprehensive care enabled if members are aware of each other's skills and expertise and are not threatened by the inevitable occasions when professional boundaries need to blur. This is particularly true of spiritual care, with its individual and diverse nature. The skills necessary for effective spiritual care are human skills that transcend the professions and include communication skills, levels of awareness, insight and discernment. Confidence in the complementary abilities of the team can be enabled and encouraged through staff induction programmes, regular team meetings and multiprofessional education and training.

Regardless of how well a team communicates and how comfortable the members are with each other's skills and boundaries, it is the patient who will choose to whom they will talk, and where and when. Privacy is often preferred and this perhaps explains why so many deep and spiritual conversations take place with nursing staff in the intimate setting of a bath or in the quiet of the early hours of the morning.

CHAPLAINCY

The chaplain or director of pastoral/spiritual care is the professional regarded as having specialist expertise in spiritual care. Chaplaincy often has its roots in religion; however, there is a clear distinction between the role of the religious representative and chaplain. While the religious representative seeks to support and encourage people in faith, the chaplain is there to respond to the needs of the other person, regardless of their faith, background or life stance. Chaplaincy provides generic spiritual care. However, a personal faith provides the chaplain with a base from where they can journey with people of different religious traditions and those who hold another life stance (humanist, pagan, etc.). A measure of the growing expertise and professionalism of chaplaincy has been the development of the Association of Hospice and Palliative Care Chaplains and the publication of *Standards for Hospice and Palliative Care Chaplaincy*, which acknowledge the importance of multiprofessional teamwork and the potential for all health-care professionals to assess spiritual needs and provide spiritual care (Association of Hospice & Palliative Care Chaplains 2003).

ASSESSING SPIRITUAL NEEDS

The language of assessment and developing care plans to meet particular needs are well established in nursing and health care, but is it the right approach to ensure spiritual care?

The concept of spiritual care has been questioned, in part because it is not clearly defined (Draper & McSherry 2002). Nevertheless, spirituality is very much part of the language of health care at a personal and political level. However, rhetoric alone cannot justify the significance of spirituality, and spiritual assessment must reflect the needs of individuals and recognise the inevitable overlap with other concepts of need, including the social, psychological and religious (Kellehear 2000, Swinton & Narayanasamy 2002).

If we agree that spiritual assessment is an important element of holistic care planning, then we must consider what tools should be used. A small number of tools are available, although, as they are often based around a standard for spiritual care and focused on a patient questionnaire, the tools are designed more for audit of a service than for an exploration and assessment of an individual's spiritual need. However, even when based on a service audit, there is a recognition that, rather than seeking to view spiritual care from a problem-solving perspective, it is more appropriate to think of supporting a patient on a journey (Catteral et al 1998).

To think of a spiritual journey is helpful, for a journey allows a change of pace and direction. This raises the question as to whether a spiritual assessment tool can be workable, since an assessment made at any given point in the journey could be out of date as soon as it has been made. Moreover, how often should this assessment be carried out: weekly, daily, hourly, every time someone is with the patient?

A more helpful approach can be based around guidelines that encourage staff to be more person-centred in their approach. One such model suggests the Five Rs of spirituality: **R**eason, **R**eflection, **R**eligion, **R**elationships and **R**estoration. Using the Five R approach, there are suggested questions within each section that would elicit needs and allow them to be recorded (Govier 2000). However, even with helpful guidelines there are other factors that need to be taken into consideration in spiritual assessment. There is the issue of timing. When is spiritual assessment carried out? Is there enough time if it needs a longer conversation? Is the ability of the person carrying out the assessment adequate? Does the person have the necessary skills to complete the assessment, such as communication skills, awareness, discernment, insight, experience? What form should the documentation of the assessment take?

Perhaps these questions point us in the direction of assessment that is not so dependent on a tool but rather is enabled by the skills and competence of all members of the multiprofessional team.

ASSESSING RELIGIOUS NEEDS

For those patients who have a religious element to their spirituality, it is important that it too is assessed and addressed. Although we are reputed to live in a secular society, there are many people who believe in a God, although they don't follow a particular faith or practice. We are also living in a multicultural and multifaith society where many communities find they have a broad ethnic mix that encompasses a wide variety of religious beliefs and practices.

If you consider Christianity as a religion, we know that there are many different branches of the religion and it matters to patients and their family/carers that, in seeking to meet their religious needs, we understand the denomination or Church they belong to. Each Church has different beliefs and practices and, while there is a core belief in God and in Jesus, his son, across all denominations, within Christianity the differences in practice can be significant, and especially so to patients who are devout in their faith. It is important to understand that all the world faiths, including Hinduism, Islam (Moslems), Judaism and Sikhism are also diverse and, although Buddhism is a philosophy of living rather than a religion, it also has many different schools of thought and practice.

Within palliative care there is a particular need to be aware of specific religious traditions around illness and dying. Many people will find comfort and meaning in their faith and associated sacraments and rites at such a time. For others, it may cause immense distress. Faith can also impact on symptom control; for example, a Buddhist patient may want to tolerate pain as death approaches in order to be as fully aware as possible when the time comes (Neuberger 1999).

It is important too that, in caring for a person's body after death, religious needs are taken into consideration. Some faiths have particular requirements concerning the sex of the person handling the body, the way the body should be prepared and placed, the removal of tubes and needles, and views on post-mortems. Most hospices and hospitals have guidelines for the care of deceased patients of different faiths and cultures. However, the best guide is to be prepared and to ask the patient or their family in advance. Remember, all religions have diversity in practice and the only way to be sure you get it right and do not cause offence is to ask the patient and their family.

There are various ways of meeting religious needs and often referral to the chaplain is the most straightforward. Although chaplains may have their own personal faith background, they are appointed for the spiritual and religious care of all patients, visitors and staff. A chaplain will have particular skills and expertise in matters of faith and will know the relevant questions to ask and, if not able to meet the religious need themselves, will know who to contact. Many chaplains prepare a list of local faith leaders that staff can refer to. However, such local directories need to be updated regularly, and for particular faith groups that are less well known, it is more useful to use faith group websites or national directories of religions for the UK (Weller 2001) to access up to date information on the local faith leader.

Included in patient notes there is often a space for noting the religion of a patient. We need to be aware of the assumptions we make on that information and think before we action any referral for religious support. Not all patients will want to see their faith leader, therefore it is important to ask before referring. The clearest guidance and advice to follow in all assessment and addressing of religious needs is to *ask the patient and family*.

We have already stressed the importance of self-awareness in spiritual care. A question often asked by health-care professionals who are religious themselves and are aware of religious needs in their patients is: Should I share my own faith with patients and families? As a guide, it is OK to share what you believe if asked to respond to a search for meaning in a patient or family/carer. However, it is important that the beliefs you share will contribute positively to patient care. To say that you are concerned that a patient is 'destined for hell and eternal damnation' because they don't share your faith, even if that is what you believe, is abuse (Gordon 2000). As in all spiritual care, our aim should be to support patients and their family/carers. If this is an issue for you, it may be helpful to discuss it with your chaplain or your own faith leader.

COMPETENCE IN SPIRITUAL CARE

The Department of Health has issued a working draft of the NHS knowledge and skills framework and development review guidance (Department of

Health 2003). This document aims to identify the knowledge and skills that individuals need to apply in their post, guide their development and provide a framework for staff review and development. It sets out a framework of up to five levels of experience/grade relating to different dimensions of care. Spiritual care is an activity that all staff will be expected to meet at level 2. By level 3, spiritual care is an intervention expected of the individual staff member, and at levels 4 and 5 it is a recognised element of care and intervention involving different professional groups and agencies.

The competency-based approach to spiritual care is becoming increasingly adopted. Alongside national initiatives, various professional organisations are producing competency-based documents. The Royal College of Nursing is developing competencies for many areas of nursing. One example states that nurses should be able to provide care that takes into account the spiritual beliefs of the patient and be able to support others in developing these skills regardless of care setting (Royal College of Nursing 2003). The accompanying performance criteria give examples of how evidence might be achieved: observation of practice, evidence describing requirements of specific patient groups, awareness and case studies.

Both the NHS and RCN documents demonstrate the ready acceptance and inclusion of spiritual care. What they lack, however, is the detail: what is competence in spiritual care and how can you audit it? This aspect has been taken forward by Marie Curie Cancer Care in its publication of spiritual and religious care competencies for specialist palliative care (Marie Curie Cancer Care 2003). Although primarily developed for hospice care, the competencies are relevant to more general palliative care.

These competencies acknowledge the difficulties of definition, language, evidence and the individuality of spiritual care. They are set out in a familiar three-column competence format, working from Knowledge through to Skills and on to Actions. There are four levels of competence relating to different aspects of patient and family/carer contact:

1. Staff and volunteers with casual contact with patient/family

2. Staff and volunteers whose duties require personal contact with patients/families

3. Staff and volunteers who are members of the multiprofessional team

4. Staff and volunteers whose primary responsibility is the spiritual and religious care of patients, visitors and staff.

Each level sets the competence that each member of staff and volunteer should be expected to demonstrate. They include:

• Appropriate understanding of the concept of spirituality at that level

• Awareness of their own personal spirituality

• Recognition of personal limitations

• Recognition of when to refer on

• Documentation of perceived needs and referral options.

At level 3, which relates to members of the multiprofessional team, assessment, interventions and outcomes should be documented. Confidentiality and the recording of sensitive and personal patient information are also introduced at this level. However, a number of questions arise. What will be recorded in the patient's notes? Is the patient aware that it will be recorded? What personal information can be disclosed to others?

Level 4 gives a competency framework for the expertise required of the chaplain or director of spiritual care, which includes being a resource, offering staff support, providing education and training, and influencing the development of national initiatives.

One weakness in all competency frameworks is in measurement, and it is particularly difficult in areas that, by nature, don't lend themselves to clear definition and may be difficult to observe. The Marie Curie Cancer Care competencies offer suggestions for audit of spiritual care that include a review of documentation to demonstrate competence, and have published assessment tools that can be linked to the personal performance review and development process for staff (Marie Curie Cancer Care 2004).

LIMITATIONS OF ASSESSMENT TOOLS AND COMPETENCY FRAMEWORKS

Clearly, spiritual care does not easily conform to recognised methods of assessment and care planning. By nature, the focus of care needs to be individual to each patient and family, with care being provided by the multiprofessional team. The concept of spiritual care does, however, lend itself to the recognition of a patient journey, where the needs of the patient change frequently and are particular to the moment. Spiritual care cannot be addressed by using a tick box assessment on admission or shortly after. It benefits considerably from a process of continuous assessment. The key to such a form of assessment is the knowledge, skills and actions of the multiprofessional team. By encouraging an awareness and development of competence in spiritual care, continuous assessment of spiritual needs is not only practical, it will greatly enhance the quality of care offered to all patients and their families, and develop and enhance the skills of individual health professionals, the multiprofessional team and the unit.

PERSONAL CHALLENGES

As already explored above, self-awareness in health-care professionals is a crucial factor in providing spiritual care. Reflecting on your personal practice and on the case study above may have raised personal issues and challenges. Linked to that will be issues that arise in different health-care settings such as:

- The range and expertise of professionals available within the multiprofessional team

- The availability of members of the team
- The staff/patient ratio and time available to spend with patients and family/carers
- Access to specialist spiritual support (chaplaincy).

The resources available within a hospice will be different from a hospital, where staffing levels may be lower. There may be less time for individual patients, and the chaplain may not have dedicated time allocated to the palliative care team. This also applies to nursing homes and the community, where the professionals on the team might not meet regularly and chaplaincy is often provided by faith leaders rather than dedicated chaplains.

However, regardless of challenges of the different health-care settings, you may find it helpful to reflect on the reality of your situation and consider what areas of spiritual care you are comfortable with and able to meet personally. More importantly, you might also reflect on what areas of spiritual care you are uncomfortable with and use the following questions to develop a strategy to help you respond appropriately and in a way that will benefit patients and their family/carers:

- How can I enhance my skills to enable me to provide a greater level of spiritual care?
- Who can I refer on to when I assess that the issues are more complex and need different skills or specialist expertise?

CURRENT AND FUTURE CHALLENGES

It is important to recognise that providing spiritual care occurs within the context of current developments in modern-day society, developments in palliative care and developments in our own life. A number of challenges will be discussed here: the impact of changes in the demography of our society, the broader application of palliative care for people without cancer, the need to have an evidence base for spiritual care practice and facing our own mortality.

DEMOGRAPHIC CHANGES IN SOCIETY

Cancer is a disease primarily of the elderly, with an estimated 65% of people with cancer being over 65 years of age (Cancer Research Campaign 2001). In addition, in the UK we are living in a society where people are living longer and, as a result, the number of elderly people is growing year on year (Department of Health 2000). These two changes in our society mean that there is a growing demand for palliative care services for elderly people.

It is worth highlighting the fact that elderly patients with cancer often have other coexisting conditions such as cardiac disease and dementia. Providing spiritual care for a person who has dementia presents its own unique challenges. It has already been highlighted that the essence of spirituality is that which gives a person meaning and purpose in living. Fundamental to assessing spiritual need and providing spiritual care is being able to discuss with each person the unique focus of the meaning of their life and what gives their life a purpose. How we achieve this when we are caring for people with dementia, who may be unable to express their thoughts and views, is less clear. In this situation, it is important that we do ask the patient their views, wishes and concerns, as we cannot assume that they are unable to express these coherently. However, in practice, if this is unsuccessful, we often have to rely on their carers for information about the patient's beliefs and values. In addition, getting to know the person in this way can be supplemented by paying attention to their behaviour and their non-verbal expressions of their personality and beliefs. For those professionals who have responsibility for caring for the individual with dementia earlier in their illness, it is important to anticipate future decline in cognitive ability by discussing their wishes for the future with the patient and documenting this information. This may take the form of an advance directive or may be a less formal document.

CARING FOR PEOPLE WITH NON-MALIGNANT CONDITIONS

The origins of palliative care in the UK are firmly based in cancer care. However, as discussed in Chapter 5, the need to extend palliative care to people who have non-cancerous conditions is being responded to by palliative care providers in hospices, in primary care, in hospitals and in nursing homes. It is worth considering the challenges that providing spiritual care to people with diseases such as motor neurone disease, multiple sclerosis and cardiac disease presents to practitioners.

One of the ways in which providing care for people with non-cancerous illnesses is challenging is that often these illnesses have a much less predictable course than many types of cancer and it can be difficult to determine when the terminal phase of the illness is entered. For example, epidemiological data demonstrate that most lung cancer patients will be dead within a year of diagnosis but multiple sclerosis is characterised by different patterns of relapsing and remitting deterioration that may last for 20 or 30 years. At first consideration, these differences can seem to have a profound effect on the context and practice of providing spiritual care, especially in terms of discussing people's views and wishes about how and where they will die and what they wish to do in preparation for that event.

However, if we reflect on the model of spiritual care offered earlier in this chapter and assess its relevance, being there for people to help them find a personal balance between hope and peace is clearly an appropriate approach regardless of the medical diagnosis. We need to adopt a person-centred approach that recognises that people will explore spiritual issues when it is important to them that they do so. Furthermore, as long as we are able to 'pick up on their cues' and respond to the patient's and family's need in an individual way, then the provision of spiritual care is not linked to medical diagnosis but rather to the uniqueness of people as people. The fact that as palliative care professionals we find this area of practice a challenge is perhaps due to our relative inexperience in this area and our feelings of lack of awareness of the particular features of these non-cancerous illnesses. Both these issues can be addressed by personal reflection, education and collaborative working with appropriate expert practitioners in the field of nursing, for example clinical nurses specialists in motor neurone disease or multiple sclerosis.

DEVELOPING PRACTICE IN EVALUATING SPIRITUAL CARE

In order to ensure that resources are being used effectively and efficiently and that patient need is being met, spiritual care requires to be evaluated (NCHSPCS 1997). Evaluation of spiritual care provision should help to identify those interventions that are most effective. Furthermore, publication and dissemination of the evaluation results will contribute to an evidence base for practice and help to share good practice. However, like many other aspects of palliative care, evaluation of spiritual care presents major challenges. Those with a responsibility for audit may have to be creative in identifying suitable approaches, which take account of the complexities and difficulties not only of providing spiritual care but of determining appropriate outcome measures.

While the importance of spiritual care is recognised in the literature, it has, to a significant degree, been left off the research agenda (McGrath 1997). In part, this is because of the complexities inherent in researching such a 'soft' subject, which does not lend itself to objective measurement. This is an epistemological challenge that those involved in researching palliative care practice need to meet. In addition, those involved in providing spiritual care also have to learn the skills of conducting research with palliative care patients. It could be argued that the nature of spiritual care naturally lends itself to a qualitative approach to research, which has been identified as having the potential to make a significant contribution to understanding of the patient's experience and practice (Froggatt et al 2003). Therefore, those involved in conducting research, approving research and funding research need to develop their knowledge and understanding of the philosophical, theoretical and practical frameworks on which qualitative research is based.

FACING OUR OWN MORTALITY

It has been identified already that dealing with spiritual issues challenges us because it brings our own mortality sharply in to focus. This is never more so than when we care for someone who is similar to us in terms of age, family structure or lifestyle. The feeling that 'this could be me' is something that many nurses and other professionals experience at some time in their career, whether it relates to a young adult with leukaemia, a mother with breast cancer or an older adult looking forward to retirement. The uniqueness of people and our own humanity mean that at times we may have a particularly strong and personally significant relationship with some of our patients and their families. As a result, responding to the spiritual needs of these patients and families can evoke a spiritual need in ourselves to face the reality that we will all die and that for some of us it will be sooner rather than later.

While there is growing interest in the spiritual coping strategies that patients employ when dealing with life-threatening illness, there is limited research exploring how professionals deal with these spiritual issues. How do you deal with the stress that caring for such patients can engender? One way of dealing with stress is to acknowledge that such situations are personally stressful and to try to prepare ourselves for such situations in the future.

REFLECTION POINT 6.4
Facing up to our own mortality

Reflect on and try to answer the following questions:

- How comfortable do you feel thinking about your own death?

- How prepared are you for the fact that you will die? (For example have you made a will, have you discussed funeral plans with others, have you made plans for the ongoing care and support of the people who mean a lot to you?)

- What are the most important things that you want to achieve before you die?

- What have you managed to achieve thus far/what are you doing about trying to achieve them?

- What do you believe will happen to you after you die?

You may find it difficult to answer these questions immediately and some may benefit from considerable reflection. However, these questions do challenge us to consider our own spirituality and in particular our beliefs and values and our own mortality. As professionals who care for others who are themselves asking these questions, it may be helpful for us to consider them. Taking time to reflect on these questions may help to prepare us for providing care for others in the future. As well as knowing our spiritual selves it is important that we care for and value ourselves.

CONCLUSION

Spirituality is the unique essence of the person, the core of their existence, characterised by a personal sense of meaning and purpose in life. An individual's spirituality is linked to their personal beliefs, values and 'life stance'. These are unique and may or may not be related to religion. So spirituality can be experienced in different ways, by different people and, as a result, is expressed in different ways.

Understanding the spiritual dimension of people is essential to the provision of person-centred holistic palliative care. Part of that understanding is being open to the diverse ways in which spirituality can be experienced and expressed. In the context of palliative care, spiritual care can be provided using a framework whereby being there for people and sharing their experience can support people as they seek to achieve a balance between hope and peace. All members of the multiprofessional team can make a contribution to spiritual care.

A number of spiritual issues frequently arise in palliative care regardless of whether that care is provided in acute hospitals, in hospices, in people's own homes or in nursing homes. In facing their own mortality, patients question their past life, their beliefs, their priorities in living and what will happen after they die. This self-searching can be a painful experience, which can be supported by professionals by using a simple framework when faced with these difficult questions. Recognising spiritual distress and exploring the origins and focus of that distress may require the skills of the whole team, with the chaplain having particular skills and expertise in this area.

In order to provide spiritual care, professionals require a degree of spiritual self-awareness. Spiritual self-awareness is a never-ending process that can be enhanced by the use of reflective skills in a way that allows practitioners to explore their own spirituality as well as analysing their contribution to spiritual care. It requires a degree of examination at both a personal and a professional level.

It is important to acknowledge that spirituality and spiritual care do not occur in isolation but are affected by, and in turn affect, developments in society, developments in palliative care and the ability of professionals to face their own mortality. In this chapter, a number of current and future challenges have been identified and briefly discussed. These included the implications of an increasingly elderly population, providing spiritual care for people with non-cancerous illnesses, developing an evidence base for spiritual care practice and facing our own mortality. It is anticipated that facing these challenges will generate considerable debate in the future.

REFERENCES

Association of Hospice & Palliative Care Chaplains 2003 Standards for hospice and palliative care chaplaincy. Association of Hospice & Palliative Care Chaplains, Help the Hospices, London

Barraclough J 1999 Cancer and emotion. John Wiley, New York

Beauchamp T, Childress J 1994 Principles of biomedical ethics. Oxford University Press, Oxford

Benzein E, Norberg A, Saveman B 2001 The meaning of the lived experience of hope in patients with cancer in palliative home care. Palliative Medicine 15:117–126

Byrne M 2002 Spirituality in palliative care: what language do we need? International Journal of Palliative Nursing 8:67–74

Cancer Research Campaign 2001 The challenge we face. Cancer Research Campaign, London

Cassell E 1991 The nature of suffering and the goals of medicine. Oxford University Press, Oxford

Catteral R A, Cox M, Greet B et al 1998 The assessment and audit of spiritual care. International Journal of Palliative Nursing 4:162–168

Chaplin J, McIntyre R 2001 Hope: an exploration of selected literature. In: Kinghorn S, Gamlin R (eds) Palliative nursing: bringing comfort and hope. Baillière Tindall, Edinburgh

Clinical Standards Board for Scotland 2002 Clinical standards for NHS Quality Improvement Scotland, specialist palliative care. Edinburgh

Cobb M 2001 The dying soul: spiritual care at the end of life. Open University Press, Buckingham

Copp G 1999 Facing impending death: experiences of patients and their nurses. NT Books, London

Costello J 1999 Anticipatory grief: coping with the impending death of a partner. International Journal of Palliative Nursing 5:223–231

Department of Health 2000 The cancer plan. Department of Health, London

Department of Health 2003 The NHS knowledge and skills framework and development review guidance: draft. DH, London

Draper P, McSherry W 2002 A critical review of spirituality and spiritual assessment. Journal of Advanced Nursing 39:1–2

Dufault K, Martocchio B 1985 Hope: its spheres and dimensions. Nursing Clinics of North America 20:379–391

Farran C J, Herth K, Popovitch J M 1995 Hope and hopelessness: critical clinical constructs. Sage, Thousand Oaks, CA

Froggatt K A, Field D, Bailey C, Krishnaswamy M 2003 Qualitative research in palliative care 1990–1999: a descriptive review. International Journal of Palliative Nursing 9:98–104

Gordon T 2000 Reflections on religious dogmatism in the care of the dying and bereaved people. Scottish Journal of Healthcare Chaplaincy 3:18–22

Govier I 2000 Spiritual care in nursing: a systematic approach. Nursing Standard 14:32–36

Halldorsdottir S, Hamrin E 1996 Experiencing existential changes: the lived experience of having cancer. Cancer Nursing 19:29–36

Herth K A, Cutliffe J R 2002 The concept of hope in nursing 3: hope and palliative care nursing. British Journal of Nursing 11:977–983

Hotopf M, Chidgey J, Addington-Hall J, Lan Ly K 2002 Depression in advanced disease: a systematic review: Part1. Prevalence and case finding. Palliative Medicine 16:81–97

Hunt J, Cobb M, Keeley V L, Ahmedzai S 2003 The quality of spiritual care – developing a standard. International Journal of Palliative Nursing 9:208–215

Kellehear A 2000 Spirituality and palliative care: a model of needs. Palliative Medicine 14:149–155

Kelly E 2002 Preparation for providing spiritual care. Scottish Journal of Healthcare Chaplaincy 5: 11–16

Kubler-Ross E 1969 On death and dying. Macmillan, New York

Liossi C, Hatira P, Mystakidou K 1997 The use of the genogram in palliative care. Palliative Medicine 11:455–461

McGrath P 1997 Putting spirituality on the agenda: hospice research findings on the 'ignored' dimension. Hospice Journal 12:1–14

McIntyre R, Chaplin J 2001 Hope: the heart of palliative care. In: Kinghorn S, Gamlin R (eds) Palliative nursing: bringing comfort and hope. Baillière Tindall, Edinburgh, p 129–145

Marie Curie Cancer Care 2003 Spiritual and religious care competencies for specialist palliative care. Marie Curie Cancer Care, London

Marie Curie Cancer Care 2004 Assessment tools: spiritual and religious care competencies for specialist palliative care. Marie Curie Cancer Care, London

Mitchell D, Sneddon M 1999 Spiritual care and chaplaincy. Scottish Journal of Healthcare Chaplaincy 5:2–6

NCHSPCS 1997 Making palliative care better: quality improvement, multiprofessional audit and standards. National Council for Hospice and Specialist Palliative Care Services, London

Neuberger J 1999 Dying well. Hochland & Hochland, Hale

Ross L 1997 The nurse's role in assessing and responding to patients' spiritual needs. International Journal of Palliative Nursing 3:37–42

Royal College of Nursing 2003 Emergency nursing care competencies. Royal College of Nursing, London

Saunders C 1984 The management of terminal illness. Edward Arnold, London

Schon D A 1983 The reflective practitioner. Temple Smith, London

Schou K C, Hewison J 1999 Experiencing cancer. Open University Press, Buckingham

Scottish Executive 2002 Spiritual care in the NHS Scotland. National Health Service Health Department Letter 76. Scottish Executive, Edinburgh

Scottish Executive Health Department 2001 Cancer in Scotland: action for change. Scottish Executive Health Department, Edinburgh

Speck P 1998 Spiritual issues in palliative care. In: Doyle D, Hanks G W C, McDonald N (eds) Oxford textbook of palliative medicine. Oxford University Press, Oxford

Stanley K 2002 The healing power of presence: respite from the fear of abandonment. Oncology Nursing Forum 29:935–940

Swinton J, Narayanasamy A 2002 Response to 'A critical review of spirituality and spiritual assessment'. Journal of Advanced Nursing 40:158–160

Twycross R 1999 Introducing palliative care. Radcliffe Medical, Abingdon

Weller P (ed.) 2001 Religions in the UK: directory 2001–2003. Multi-Faith Centre of the University of Derby and the Inter Faith Network for the UK, Derby

World Health Organization 1990 Cancer pain relief and palliative care. World Health Organization, Geneva

Wright S 1998 The reflective journey begins a spiritual journey. In: Johns C, Freshwater D (eds) Transforming nursing through reflective practice. Blackwell Science, Oxford

Sexuality and palliative care

Richard Gamlin

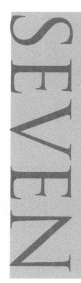

We had been together for 25 years and always enjoyed the beauty of love making, the tenderness, and the passion, the caring. I had my prostate operation and was very worried about my future. I tried to bring up the subject with the nurses but no-one picked up my fear and dread. I felt so alone.
Sexuality represents a complex interaction between genetic, physical, psychological, social, cultural, spiritual and racial components. Although the literature contains many definitions, defining such a complex issue is difficult and perhaps restrictive. The terms 'body image' and 'sexuality' are frequently used interchangeably, although they are not the same. Body image is used instead of sexuality because of our difficulty and uneasiness with matters sexual. According to Lion (1982), nurses who are comfortable with their own sexuality and the sexuality of others, who have a sexual health knowledge base and who cultivate sensitive and perceptive communication skills can effectively integrate sex into the nursing process.

AIMS OF THE CHAPTER

Readers are encouraged to:

- Extend their knowledge about a broad range of issues associated with body image
- Gain some insight into their clinical practice through the use of the exercises in techniques of communication and assessment of clients' needs
- Empower their clients to raise sensitive personal issues of sexuality as they relate to the field of palliative care.

Sexuality is not merely the act of sexual intercourse. It is difficult to define because it has many meanings that are shaped and influenced by life experiences. We develop our understanding of sex and sexuality throughout life, picking up cues and influences from others and from the media. These influences lead us to develop our own conclusions about life, love, desirability, appearance and relationships. Sexuality encompasses body image, physical sexual responses, the way we perceive our appearance and attractiveness to self and others. Communication and relationships, self-image and self-esteem, and the sense of affirmation and acknowledgement that we experience from others in our everyday lives are all components of sexuality (Wells 2002).

There is evidence to show that health-care professionals fail to provide information and support to patients and partners when patients undergo treatment for gynaecological cancers (Juraskova et al 2003). As many as 70% of men with prostate cancer experience sexual dysfunction (Fossa et al 1997). Issues that should have been addressed remain unresolved when the patient is receiving palliative care but it is never too late to perform an assessment and plan care to ease distress and suffering. It is vital to understand that the location of the primary cancer or spread is only one indicator of sexual dysfunction. The quality of the pre-existing sexual relationship between patient and partner is equally if not more important. Men and women who are not in a committed relationship have to face the potential trauma of rejection by a new partner who learns of their illness. Some may avoid relationships because of the fear of rejection.

It is vital to understand that sex may be important or become more important to patients and their partners when they face advanced illness. Intimacy expressed through words, looks and gestures allows the expression of love. In a bitter-sweet way it serves to remind couples of what they have together but soon will lose. Illnesses, disabilities, fears and treatments inhibit sexual contact and desire. Health professionals must take this seriously.

Relationships and family dynamics are highly complex and difficult to understand. Although we should always try to help we must distinguish between the fixable and the unfixable. A family situation that appears intolerable to us may be acceptable to the family.

SEXUALITY AND PALLIATIVE CARE

For professionals, sexuality and palliative care do not immediately spring to mind as good bedfellows. When we consider why this is the case, it is usually because of our own discomfort in dealing with the subject. It is a difficult topic to deal with and our thoughts centre on the following:

- It is embarrassing
- I would not want someone asking me questions like that
- They are too old
- They are too ill
- I don't have the time
- I don't have the skills
- Other things are much more important at this time of life.

There may be more than an element of truth in the above responses but our patients may have concerns or worries about sex or sexuality that could easily be dealt with if we had the necessary skills and understanding to deal with them.

It is easy to assume that patients have a healthy understanding of their sexuality that developed at an early age and that they grew up with a healthy acceptance of who they are and what their bodies do. In spite of all the early education there still seems to be a problem surrounding sexuality, which continues into the professional lives of health-care professionals. Way back in 1980 Roper et al published their Activities of Living model of nursing, which has as one of its activities 'Expressing sexuality'. An examination of a selection of assessment documents and care plans often reveals that the 'Expressing sexuality' section has been removed or re-named as something less challenging, such as 'personal issues'. When it remains included in documents it may be left blank or filled in as 'not applicable' (Gamlin 1999). If we are to provide truly holistic care, the foundation of palliative care, we must offer patients and their loved ones opportunities to express their innermost fears about intimacy and love. Becker & Gamlin (2004) discuss these issues and offer practical solutions for enhancing patient care.

LEARNING ABOUT SELF

As we grow we learn about ourselves. The process of learning includes sucking, touching and smell. Mothers sometimes mistake a baby's attempts to gnaw his fists as a sign that he is hungry, when in reality he is making a discovery about himself. Shape, texture, wet and dry can be discovered orally and provide immense satisfaction for the infant. In the same way, infants use their fingers to explore the things around themselves, including their own bodies. Genital play is quite normal, but parents may become anxious about this if they do not understand its purpose. This in turn may lead to smacking the child for being naughty, which, besides upsetting the child, also informs them that they should not touch their genitals. The child learns that there are some areas of the body that are more acceptable than others.

If disapproval in relation to sexuality is repressive and restrictive throughout the growing years, children may develop a negative view of themselves, together with poor self-esteem. On the other hand, if they are given approval and allowed to continue healthy discovery of themselves, they are more likely to grow up with a more positive picture of their 'self' and with good self-esteem.

There is a very strong argument for censorship to protect young people from pornographic materials. Access to the Internet in general and to chat rooms in particular is a great cause of concern for parents. However, if children and adolescents are 'protected from' materials that have a sexual content because of parents' inability to face these issues, they receive powerful messages about sex and sexuality. Clearly, parents must always try to act in their children's best interests while providing them with a sound education.

The quality of sex education in schools is variable, with some teachers and governors believing that teaching about sex will encourage sexual behaviour. High teenage pregnancy rates and high rates of sexually transmitted diseases indicate that family and state sex education is failing our young and adolescents.

Our difficulty in facing things sexual persists into the education of health-care professionals. As a young student nurse, many years ago, I was sent to the library while my female fellow students attended a lecture on the anatomy of the female reproductive system. This implied that I did not need to know this information to be a nurse and that the female reproductive system was some-how embarrassing. In 2003 I was asked to present a sexuality workshop to a group of male palliative care volunteers. The female volunteers had already completed their workshop without their male counterparts.

When teaching about sexuality I always begin by asking about the group's previous educational experience in this area. Few students appear to have received any formal education about sexuality, including taking a sexual history or providing information to patients and carers. This is the same for nursing or multidisciplinary groups. Those who have attended workshops report that the content centred on human immunodeficiency virus (HIV) and homosexual practices. While this is, no doubt, important it represents a very narrow focus for sexuality education.

ADULTS AND ILLNESS

Regardless of how self-confident people are, serious illness may affect and distort this positive self-image. A look in the mirror may reveal someone with a different shape, bald, with skin and colour changes, clothes that are too big and whose looks are generally unappealing. The effects of illness, its treatment and medication take their toll on patients. Linked to other stressful factors, such as loss of earnings, strained relationships and a diagnosis of an incurable illness, they may become depressed, lethargic and socially isolated.

EXPRESSING SEXUALITY IN SERIOUS ILLNESS

Good communication skills are essential to support patients throughout their illness. Areas of their life that have not been problematic until now may become a source of concern, anxiety, fear and distress. Expressing sexuality may be one of these concerns. If it is not addressed by professional carers, patients and their partners may assume that this is an aspect of their life together that is now at an end.

This assumes that professional carers know what the potential problems may be, and that they have the prerequisite knowledge to discuss these confidently with patients! It may be useful to look at where the difficulties lie for nurses. If it is a belief that it is 'none of our business', who else will provide the patient with the relevant information? There appears to be an assumption that the patient will know intrinsically how to resolve these issues and that nurses should not interfere. However, patients may also assume that, because no one has discussed sensitive issues with them, it is because this is an area of their lives that is now at an end. They, too, are likely to be embarrassed and may not provide the relevant cues or ask questions about their situation.

If carers do not discuss issues because of embarrassment, this may say a great deal about how they perceive these areas and may reflect their upbringing and socialisation processes. Nurses carry out some extremely intimate tasks for patients, in spite of their embarrassment, because these tasks are not sexual in intent. However, there does seem to be a lack of knowledge among female carers around issues of male arousal. Contrary to popular belief, male patients do not deliberately have an erection while having an intimate task carried out. It occurs as a result of normal physiological processes that are beyond the control of the person involved. To then be castigated or ridiculed for an event that was not premeditated is unhelpful, highly embarrassing, demeaning, offensive and may prevent the patient from asking questions relating to intimacy.

Although the practice of men nursing women is becoming more acceptable, male nursing staff still find themselves prevented from nursing women. They are told that this is for their own good because a female patient might accuse the male nurse of rape or some other sexual misdemeanour. Of course, this is possible, but important issues arise from the situation. First, female nurses are not discouraged from nursing male patients. This is largely for practical reasons, as men only account for 8% of the UK nursing workforce. It is assumed that female patients do not like being cared for by male nurses because they will be embarrassed. It is also assumed that male patients will not be embarrassed but actually enjoy having intimate, invasive and uncomfortable procedures performed by female nurses. Again, practicalities must be considered, but it is time this cyclical and ridiculous argument was laid to rest. Patients – male and female – will meet nurses – male and female. While preserving patient choice, it is time that we stopped restricting certain nursing tasks to male or female nurses. Nurses should be prepared for the challenges of caring for patients, complete with their worries, fears and sexual hang-ups.

Ignorance on the part of professional carers is easier to address if they are otherwise willing to discuss intimate issues with patients. An understanding of male and female sexual responses, and the effects of illness on these, will assist the nurse to provide care and support in this area. It is also necessary to understand the effects of medication on libido, as this can influence the advice that is given.

EFFECTS OF ILLNESS AND TREATMENT ON LIBIDO

DEPLETED ENERGY RESERVES

Almost all patients with advanced cancer and non-malignant disease experience debilitating fatigue at some time during their illness. Fatigue is a complex problem with interacting physical and psychosocial components. Everyday tasks such as breathing, eating, grooming and excreting become onerous and difficult when fatigue is present. Physical and mental fatigue may in themselves make any sexual activity, particularly penetrative intercourse, difficult to even contemplate. However, research has shown that patients do enjoy being hugged and cuddled, even when seriously ill and dying (Leiber et al 1976). Health-care establishments and staff attitudes are rarely supportive of closeness and intimacy between couples.

It is likely that partners may feel miserable and rejected and the opportunity for misunderstanding is ever present at a time when open and sensitive communication between partners is essential to maintain love and intimacy. Professional carers often assume that patients in an older age group do not require this advice, as they are no longer sexually active. There are studies to show that many couples continue to have satisfying sexual relationships well into old age (Kaiser 1992).

There may be several reasons for reduced levels of energy in seriously ill patients. Excessive weight loss, as in cancer and cardiac-failure-related cachexia, causes extreme fatigue. Infection, especially when accompanied by an increase in body temperature, reduces the notion for physical intimacy and sexual contact. Even the common cold can prove to be a hindrance to the most ardent of lovers! Patients and their partners may be fearful and anxious about the outcome of their illness, or about whether they can tolerate the treatments for the illness, and these fears and anxieties may also reduce libido. If the couple stop communicating with each other as a result, then their ability to show affection may be reduced.

EFFECTS OF TREATMENT

The extract from *Cancer Ward* by Solzhenitsyn (1968) in Box 7.1 gives a graphic and moving account of the reactions of a young lady who discovers that she has breast cancer and must have a mastectomy.

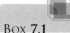

Box 7.1

Effects of treatment for illness

Asya and Dyoma had been friends through school. Dyoma was in hospital while his leg was operated on and Asya because of a breast lump.

'What is it, come on, tell me?' asked Dyoma. 'They are going to cut it off,' she cried. Dyoma tried to comfort Asya saying, 'Maybe they won't have to.' 'They will on Friday,' replied Asya . . . 'What have I got to live for?' she sobbed . . . 'Who in the world will want me now!' Dyoma tried to console her. 'People get married for each other's character,' he said. 'What sort of fool loves a girl for her character?' she replied angrily. 'Who wants a girl with one breast?'

Dyoma mumbled, 'Of course, you know, if no one will marry you . . . well of course, I will always be happy to marry you.'

'Listen to me Dyoma,' said Asya, looking straight at him with wide eyes. 'Listen to me – you will be the last one! You are the last one that can see it and kiss it. Dyoma, you at least must kiss it, if nobody else!'

Asya pulled her dressing gown apart and Dyoma kissed her doomed right breast. Nothing more beautiful than this gentle curve could ever be painted or sculpted. Its beauty flooded him. 'You'll remember? . . . You'll remember, won't you? You'll remember what it was like?' Asya's tears kept falling on Dyoma's close-cropped hair. When she did not take it away, he returned to its rosy glow, softly kissing the breast. He did what her future child would never do.

Today it was a marvel. Tomorrow it would be in the bin.

Solzhenitsyn 1968, p. 422–425

After surgery, particularly mutilating surgery, the apparent change in body image may result in the person not wishing to be seen by their partner and not wishing to participate in sexual activity. Sometimes women are encouraged, soon after mastectomy, to let their partners see the scar. There is an assumption that the partner has actually seen the woman's breast before, which may be quite wrong. There are many couples, young and not so young, who undress in the bathroom or in the dark and who make love in the dark, and who have never seen each other naked. Any insistence, however gentle, that the partner be shown the scar may have the effect of preventing other questions being voiced that would assist in promoting positive self-esteem and the coming to terms with altered body image.

Men who have had surgical treatment for bladder cancer or who are ostomates have had the nerve pathways disrupted, leading to an inability to have an erection. It may be possible for a prosthesis to be used, although at present in the UK there does not appear to be a wide acceptance of prostheses. More recently, drugs such as Viagra have given hope to men with erectile dysfunction. Men and their partners, in addition to a prescription, require careful support and ongoing support if they are to regain fulfilling sex lives. The tablet is only a small part of the therapy.

There are many ways of giving and receiving sexual gratification if penetrative intercourse is neither possible nor desirable, but patients may have never thought about them. There are booklets and books available from Relate (partner counselling) that can provide clear, factual information if there are no staff available or able to give such advice. CancerBacup provides an excellent range of literature to support all aspects of cancer and its consequences. We now seem to live in a 'leaflet culture'. We are given leaflets to explain our mortgage, insurance, guarantee, voting rights and holidays. Many of them are hard to read and understand and do little to further our knowledge. It is not sufficient merely to provide a patient with reading material. Familiarise yourself with the publication and be prepared to explain issues that may arise after the patient has had ample opportunity to read it.

Radiotherapy and chemotherapy also have effects on libido and feelings of wellbeing and may change body image. Some chemotherapeutic agents cause total hair loss, and hair loss is also associated with radiotherapy to the scalp area. After chemotherapy the hair generally grows back in but with radiotherapy patchy hair loss may remain. These situations cause distress to men and women and, coupled with other effects of illness and treatment, may reduce patients' desire or ability to be involved with their partners. Radical pelvic radiotherapy may lead to permanent vaginal fibrosis if no instruction is given on how to keep the vagina patent. If a vaginal dilator is given to the patient, it is often wrapped in a disposal bag. The message being given here is that the use of such a piece of equipment is 'dirty'.

CASE STUDY 7.1
Irene

Irene was a 42-year-old district nurse. She had a routine smear test and was shocked to discover that she had extensive cancer of the cervix and uterus. She had been having heavy, irregular bleeding but had put it down to the menopause, as her mother and sister had both experienced an early menopause. She was greatly supported by nursing and medical staff throughout her treatment and felt that they had always been open and honest with her. She had surgery, chemotherapy and radical pelvic radiotherapy, and her partner was a great help during the emotionally turbulent times. Jeff was 56 years old and they had been together for 4 years. There were no children.

On discharge from hospital, Irene was given a vaginal dilator with the instruction 'use it regularly'. Irene had never worked in a gynaecology unit and she was not sure what to do with the dilator. She kept it in the medicine cupboard in the bathroom. She and Jeff had been given no advice about resuming intercourse and decided to wait until Irene had a check-up at the hospital 6 weeks later. No pelvic examination was carried out at this time, although Irene was asked if everything was all right. There was still no advice about resuming intercourse so she and Jeff continued to abstain. She had to cancel her next appointment as she had a wedding to attend and it wasn't until several months after her treatment that she was seen again. By this time she had developed pain and discomfort in her vaginal area. On examination there was extensive fibrosis.

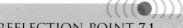

REFLECTION POINT 7.1

Thinking about Irene and her care

How would you, as Irene's nurse, have provided her with the information that would have prevented further problems from developing?

Simple instructions for using a dilator are as follows:

- Choose a time when there are unlikely to be interruptions
- Using a lubricant such as KY-Jelly, lubricate the dilator and place in the vagina while lying down in a comfortable position – this should be done very gently, but the dilator should be inserted as far as possible
- Leave the dilator in place for about 10–15 minutes, after which it should be removed and carefully cleaned and washed with unperfumed soap and water
- Do this daily until advised to discontinue.

If the couple both wish it, and if great gentleness is used, the partner's gloved fingers can be used instead of the dilator, to assist the process. I suggest gloved fingers to prevent damage (and possible infection) to the very sensitive vaginal mucosa. The other possibility is that, if fingers or dilators can be inserted into the vagina, then so can the penis. Again, great gentleness should be used and some couples may find it more comfortable to lie on their sides, just quietly, together. The use of appropriate lubricants can be discussed, which would avoid really sticky creams and ointments being inserted into the vagina. Vaseline, baby creams and oils and vaginal sprays should be avoided. Vaseline was never intended to be used for internal lubrication, and other creams, oils and sprays can set up irritation in the vagina, causing pain, itching and distress.

MEDICATION

Patients with advanced illness frequently take many medications that have an effect on sexuality. For example some medications have an effect on the nervous system, which is responsible for heightening sexual arousal. Consequently, those who take such drugs may experience a loss of libido. Explanations can be given to both partners, so that there is understanding on both sides. The man's inability to have an erection may be directly associated with the drugs he is taking rather than with the illness itself. Rather than providing an exhaustive list of medications that may affect sexuality, it is suggested that you review all the patients' medications. Be particularly aware of the effects of opioids, sedatives, anxiolytics, antihypertensives and diuretics. The *British National Formulary, Palliative Care Formulary* and your local drug information pharmacist will provide you with all the information you need. It may be possible to reduce or stop some medications or to provide an alternative.

IS SEXUALITY A COMPONENT OF PATIENT CARE?

It is easy to assume that a patient with an advanced or advancing illness may have far more important things than sexuality to think about, but it is possible to be wrong about this. The patient may have a number of concerns about sex/sexuality, for example anxiety about appearance and whether relationships with others will be affected by illness.

Case study 7.2
Robert

Robert was 26 years old and worked on a building site as a joiner's mate. He played football, went swimming and at weekends spent his evenings in the pub with his friends. He had a steady girlfriend with whom he had a sexual relationship. Apart from childhood illnesses, Robert had no experience of serious illness. Both his parents were alive and well. Robert began to feel lethargic and weary and was too tired to take an active part in sport. Eventually his mother persuaded him to see the doctor, thinking he might have anaemia. Robert had been too embarrassed to tell either of his parents that his testicles were swollen and sore. His GP suspected testicular cancer, which was confirmed by tests. Treatment, including orchidectomy, was undertaken but, prior to diagnosis, Robert's illness was quite far advanced, with metastatic spread to lungs and liver. Robert and his parents and girlfriend had been advised of his prognosis and knew that he was dying.

Robert was very preoccupied and staff assumed that he was trying to come to terms with having a life-threatening illness. He had been told that he could go home at the weekend. Robert was reluctant to go and asked if he could stay longer. Katy, his girlfriend, was really disappointed and asked the nurse to speak to him. The nurse chose a time when the ward was reasonably quiet and asked Robert if he had any unanswered questions about his illness. He became very embarrassed and said he knew all he needed to know about his disease but, after some hesitation, he said, 'It's Katy – she might want sex and I don't know if I can! And she might not want me near her at all and I couldn't bear that!'

This particular nurse was not very comfortable discussing sexual matters but was able to suggest that she would talk to Katy if Robert wished. She also offered the services of the stoma nurse, who was 'more into that sort of thing'! The outcome was that Robert went home to his parents' house and Katy went too.

When Robert came back into hospital, Sue, an auxiliary nurse, asked him how his weekend had gone. Robert cried and Sue closed the curtains. Sue held his hand but said nothing. Slowly Robert told Sue how close and loving he and Katy had been. 'After we made love we would hold each other and wake up still holding each other. Now I am skinny, smelly, dirty and weak – what else can go wrong'? Sue listened as Robert talked. She offered to come back when Katy visited. The three of them went to a quiet private room and Robert told Katy how he felt. They cried as Katy told Robert how much she loved him. After their next few days at home together Robert returned a different man. He said to Sue, 'Nothing happened in the trouser department but our love has grown again!'

For patients facing advanced illness numerous thoughts and fear may go through the mind:

- I look so awful
- She will not want to see me like this
- I used to look so good in these clothes
- Am I still attractive?
- I just want to be held – I don't want sex
- If we have sex I might pass it on
- My past sexual behaviour may have caused this
- I just can't face making love. It reminds me that we soon won't be able to do it any more
- I cannot bear the thought of her starting a new relationship when I die
- Am I allowed to have sex?
- Should I feel like this?
- Where can we go?

Questions and thoughts that may go through the mind of the partner may include:

- Will I hurt her?
- I don't find her as attractive as I used to
- I was going to leave her but it will look awful if I leave now
- If we have sex I might catch something
- My past sexual behaviour may have caused this
- I could never start another relationship when she dies
- I need sex and she is just using this illness as an excuse
- I have needs as well
- How can I convince her that I still love her?

Many jokes are based on sex and sexuality and most health-care staff are reasonably comfortable listening to or making jokes about sex. Sometimes, patients attempt to discuss their sexual concerns with staff. This may be done in a direct way, or may be presented in the form of cues that staff are supposed to be able to pick up. Box 7.2 gives examples of the latter.

In reality it seems that patients' worries are rarely discussed in a meaningful way in wards, departments or the community, despite the fact that a patient's sexuality is likely to be affected by advancing illness. Nursing models usually address sexuality in some way and the Activities of Living model (Roper et al 1980) is perhaps still the best known to nurses in the UK. A student nurse made the following comments in 1987.

We use Roper's model. We go through all of them in class and in theory it's all very good. One of these, of course, is expressing sexuality and that's important. But when it comes to doing it in class, what do you talk about? Helping women to look better after they've had a hysterectomy so their husbands will want to have sex with them? You spend ages on breathing then you get down to the end of the list, dying and expressing sexuality, and how we should talk to patients and get them to discuss their feelings, and that's it! No one ever does it! We write in our care plans, 'Encourage patients to express their feelings and anxieties' but it's never really approached.

Savage 1987

Box 7.2

Patients' attempts to discuss sexual concerns

- Ian, a 40-year-old man with advanced cancer, was sitting talking to his doctor, who asked him how he was feeling. Ian replied, 'Well I now find that I bend in the middle, doctor. What are you going to do about that?'

- John was a patient in an orthopaedic ward following a road traffic accident. He was making a good recovery and expected to remain in hospital for another 3 weeks. One night while speaking to Julie, his primary nurse, he told her he felt sexually frustrated. Julie felt a little embarrassed but did not take this as a sexual advance. She related John's comments to Chris, the senior house officer, who marched into the ward and said in a loud voice, 'Which horny git wants the bromide, then?'

- Brian was 46 years old and suffered from cancer of the penis. While in the bath one day he said to Sam, his nurse, 'I've been made redundant, you know, Sam.'

- Sally, a 68-year-old woman with lung cancer, looked in the mirror and said, 'There's definitely something wrong with this mirror. It gets worse every time I look in it.'

- Bill, a 28-year-old man with multiple sclerosis who was about to go home on weekend leave said, 'Well, we'll see if everything is working OK tonight.'

Although the quotation from savage appeared in a 1987 publication it is reasonably safe to assume that things have not changed very much. It is interesting to note that some NHS trusts that adopted the Activities of Living model have completely removed the section on 'Expressing sexuality' or have sanitised it by renaming it something less explicit (and less threatening?), such as 'Bodily appearance'. An examination of a range of nursing care plans reveals entries such as 'Mary likes to dress according to her sexual orientation' or 'Likes to wear own clothes and aftershave after his shower'. Then again, there is the ubiquitous 'No problems expressed'. Such entries suggest that these nurses have little awareness of the meaning of the concept and perhaps feel compelled to make an entry in the nursing assessment for the sake of completeness.

The following entries suggest some understanding, but the reader is left wondering what and how the patient was told, and what the patient's understanding was following such comments:

- 'Worried about stenosis following radiotherapy. Told to get a vibrator!'
- 'Counselled re sperm banking'
- 'Told about complications of treatment, including possible impotence'
- 'Given "Safe Sex" leaflet'.

It appears acceptable to some health-care professionals to talk to or give information to selected groups of patients. It seems acceptable and advisable to talk to patients after myocardial infarction before the return home, where they may resume sexual activity. Anxiety may be unnecessarily high in both patients and partners who fear reinfarction or death as a result of sexual intercourse. Thompson (1990) cites Ueno (1963), who claims that coitus accounts for fewer than 0.6% of cases of sudden death, most occurring in extramarital relationships. Overcoming the methodological challenges in such a study is difficult, but anecdotal evidence would suggest that the risk is low. It is worth reflecting on how many patients you have come across with postintercourse emergencies.

Men and women who have had cancer treatment that will affect their primary or secondary sexual organs may receive information. Women who have had a mastectomy or hysterectomy and men with testicular, prostatic or penile cancer may receive information, and possibly support, but it appears that, although cancer and cancer treatment can profoundly affect sexuality, support is not often offered. Fallowfield (1990) goes further to suggest that: 'ignoring such issues as sex in studies of patients who have undergone gynaecological or genitourinary or bowel surgery might result in a very incomplete assessment of the impact of treatment'. I agree with Fallowfield and would suggest that ignoring issues of sexuality in patients who have undergone any form of treatment for cancer might result in a very incomplete assessment of the impact of treatment.

Recently, when visiting a colleague in hospital who had undergone surgery for a hysterectomy a few days previously (she did not have cancer), I jokingly asked her if she had been given the 'predischarge chat'. She then proceeded to show me the leaflets and booklets she had received, and I asked what advice she had been given about resuming sexual activity. She told me that she had been advised not to have sex for at least 4 weeks and that, during that period, she should not become aroused. I suggested that it was time for me to leave in case my presence aroused her, as neither of us knew what would happen if we broke that hospital rule!

What prevents nurses from initiating discussions – and whose responsibility is it? Initiating a discussion about sex or sexuality is difficult to do for many reasons. Bor & Watts (1993) suggest that embarrassment, lack of training and a belief that sexuality is not relevant to a particular disorder prevent staff from approaching the subject with patients. In addition, Waterhouse & Metcalf (1991), citing Gross Fisher (1985), suggest that anxiety and conservative attitudes are significant factors. Not much changed in the next 10 years, according to Sutherland's unpublished survey (1995). There is clearly an important role for education if things are to improve. Perhaps the most important issue in this debate is that nurses and other health-care professionals expect the patients to initiate any discussion of this nature while the patients expect that the staff will do the initiating. Baggs & Karch (1987), Jenkins (1988), Krueger et al (1979), and Waterhouse & Metcalf (1991) support this. The debate is also clarified by these authors, who clearly conclude that there are patients who do want staff to talk about sexual matters and who do want staff to initiate discussions.

Another useful opt-out for the nurse is that the patient is too old or too ill but, as Leiber et al (1976) point out, there are some patients who have neither the ability nor the urge for sexual intercourse, yet intimacy and close human contact are desired. Their study concluded that patients with advanced cancer experienced, simultaneously with their spouses, an increased desire for physical closeness and a decreased desire for sexual intercourse. In a study concerning sexuality and the older cancer patient, Kaiser (1992) found that 63% of patients wanted more information on the impact of cancer on sexuality and that 54% wanted to discuss the issue with their physician. Patients rarely found that this need was met, despite the fact that loss of libido, impotence, decreased arousability and orgasmic difficulties may occur in patients with cancer.

It cannot be assumed that all patients share these feelings, but the literature is both helpful and challenging. It is helpful in that it shows that we should consider initiating discussions and challenging in that it does not tell us how to do it. Approaching a patient with a prearranged script is unlikely to be particularly helpful, but considering how a discussion could be initiated might reduce anxiety for the nurse and increase the benefits for the patients. This means that nurses should at least have some solutions for some of the problems that can arise.

PROBLEM-SOLVING APPROACH

Below are problems about which most nurses could give very simple information that would assist in ameliorating them, if they themselves were aware of some solutions. It is not possible to make the bad things that have

happened in patients' lives, because of the illness, become 'good' but information and advice may help with the process of adaptation and help to minimise some of their current distress. In providing information to health-care
professionals the author is not implying that all couples should be sexually
active in the middle of the crises that illness thrusts on them. However, I do
think it is reasonable that, if both partners wish it, they should be given
clear, appropriate, information that is not confused with myths and old
wives' tales.

WAYS OF HELPING

The patient with a large abdominal wound could be advised to adapt the preferred position for intercourse so that there is neither weight nor pressure on
the wound. If this is not possible, then a total change of position may be
required if the couple wish to have intercourse. Advice about stroking and
caressing other areas of the body should be included.

There are many myths about radiotherapy and the partner becoming
radioactive is just one of them. To prevent this kind of situation becoming a
problem, when patients are informed that they will be having radiotherapy
they should be told at the same time that this will not affect their partner in
any way.

In lovemaking, legs are used for balance and for erotic stimulation. As well
as the assault on body image and self-esteem, the loss of one or both legs can
profoundly affect the physical relationship. To achieve and improve balance,
cushions and pillows may be used. Pretty covers and soft textures may
enhance the experience and caressing other areas of the body can greatly
increase erotic stimulation, provided that it is what both partners enjoy.

Again, there are many myths surrounding hysterectomy, especially the one
that says a woman can no longer have intercourse after hysterectomy. For
some women, this may be seen as a blessed release. If they have never really
enjoyed sex with their partner, they may be quite glad that this is an aspect
of their lives that has 'legitimately' ended. The nurse who tells the husband
that 'Of course it's OK to have sex with your wife' will not be popular! In the
first instance, discussion should take place with the wife, on her own, at the
time surgery is planned, and her decision must be respected.

Women can be helped to enjoy sex if they and their partners have more
information on aspects of foreplay. If the illness is not immediately life-
threatening, this is the kind of situation that could be referred to a marriage
counsellor or therapist, provided it is what the patient wishes.

Pain is a powerful deterrent to physical intimacy. If it is constant, it should
be reassessed to discover the cause and to find if there are ways of reducing
it. The use of cushions and pillows to provide support for aching joints and
limbs may help and, while it may rob the act of lovemaking of some of its
spontaneity, it may be possible to 'plan' for it. This would allow for analgesia
to be effective and to reduce the experience of pain afterwards. If the act of
sex is associated with pain, it will rarely be anticipated with pleasure. Do

encourage couples to tell each other what they like and what they don't like. This applies to all the situations discussed. Partners are not all intuitive and may need direction from their spouse, especially in changing circumstances.

The gentleman who is unable to have an erection may well prefer to discuss this with a woman than with a man. This is because there is less of a threat to his manhood than there might be in discussing his situation with another man. Adapting to this problem takes some time, particularly if the possibility of impotence was not discussed in advance. This is a situation requiring a very sensitive approach and is not one that I would recommend for trying out the skill of discussing sex for the first time. A wide knowledge of other ways of giving and receiving sexual gratification is needed, otherwise, if only one suggestion is made and the patient or partner do not care to try it out, they may be left thinking that there is nothing else for them. If, however, there are health-care professionals reading this who are sufficiently confident to further develop their skills, they might wish to discuss issues around mutual masturbation and caressing and fondling. There are couples who have found that, since there is now no pressure to 'perform' they can take their time, and both can have an extremely enjoyable time doing so.

REFLECTION POINT 7.2

Helping patients with sexual problems

Take some time to be as creative as possible in finding some ways in which the patient and partner could be helped in the following scenarios

- The patient has a large abdominal wound

- A husband fears that he may become radioactive if he has intercourse with his wife, who has just completed a course of radiotherapy

- A patient has an above-the-knee amputation

- A lady who has had a hysterectomy believes she can no longer have sexual intercourse

- The patient has pain

- A gentleman who has been treated for prostatic cancer is unable to have an erection. He did not appreciate that this might be a result of his treatment.

Discuss these situations with a colleague and consider what advice could fairly easily be given and which situations are more difficult to deal with. What is it that makes a difficult situation 'difficult'? Would you consider referring any of the above to a specialist? If so, why and to which specialist?

Prostheses and implants may have a place for some patients, while others may find that glyceryl trinitrate patches sited at the penile–scrotal junction give enough of an erection for vaginal penetration to take place. Papaverine or alprostadil injected into the corpus cavernosum may also be appropriate for some patients. Specialist advice will be required for some of these.

However, the important thing in all these situations is the relationships involved. Assisting couples to talk to each other may be far more effective than advice on the nitty-gritty of sex. Keeping a sense of humour and using humour appropriately while giving advice can reduce the embarrassment to both patients and staff. Avoiding the trap of being coarse and crude, and remaining professional, can make the situation quite acceptable to couples.

SEXUALITY AND CONFIDENTIALITY

All health-care staff are taught the importance of confidentiality throughout their work and are told that it is a fundamental human right. Although rights are never absolute, the issue of confidentiality and sexuality merits special

Box 7.3

Learning exercise

Think of a patient you have known and cared for over a period of time. You are in a quiet, private environment where you will not be disturbed. The patient has made good progress in hospital and is to be discharged tomorrow. You have discussed all the usual matters like diet, exercise, outpatient appointments and resuming work, and you know that it would be in the patient's best interests if you gave them an opportunity to discuss any concerns about sex/sexuality. What will you say to your patient to initiate the discussion? You might say something like:

- 'Is there anything else worrying you?' This is very general indeed

- 'How are things between you and your partner?' This is a bit more specific

- 'Are you having problems of a sexual nature?' This may be too direct for many patients

- 'Some patients with a condition like yours have some questions/worries/concerns about sex/sexuality. I was wondering if you had any questions that you might like to discuss with me or with someone else?' This question is gently direct and might be met with 'Mind your own business, you smutty, offensive person!' or 'Well ... there is something, but it is a little embarrassing!'

It is very important that you do not attempt to memorise these approaches as if they were scripts; instead, you should consider how you would approach sexuality. After all, if you do not pick up the patient's cues or broach the subject yourself, there may be no opportunity to consider this aspect of life.

consideration. It is usual for a nurse to share most information received from a patient with colleagues. This practice is considered to be valuable, in that it helps all staff to be aware of their patient's problems and needs. While caring for a patient a nurse may learn about that patient's worries, concerns, anxieties and fears about sexuality. Before sharing such information with colleagues, it is essential that the nurse considers these two questions:

- Do I need to write this down?
- Do I need to tell my colleagues this information?

The 'knee-jerk' response to both these questions may be, 'Yes – I must record all information and I must tell my colleagues so that they can provide holistic care for the patient'. After careful consideration, however, it may be decided that the patient has told the nurse of their feelings and that there is nothing to be gained from telling the rest of the ward team. Such answers are rarely straightforward and the following scenarios could be used as a team-based learning exercise.

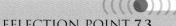

REFLECTION POINT 7.3

Scenarios for a team-based learning exercise

Jim is a 48-year-old sales executive who has been admitted to your ward with chest pain and hypertension. While talking to him in private one day, he tells you, his primary nurse, that he is worried he will not be able to satisfy his wife anymore. During a long discussion with him, you explain that his chest pain is not a heart attack and that, with a change in lifestyle, he should soon start to feel much better.

- Should the nurse write this down in the patient's notes?

- Should the nurse discuss this with colleagues?

Mary is a 64-year-old lady who had a mastectomy for breast cancer 6 years ago. She remained very well until about 6 months ago, when she developed multiple bony secondaries. While caring for her at home one Friday, she tells you how desperate she feels because her husband does not want to make love to her any more. You acknowledge her concerns and, because of a very heavy schedule, you apologise and tell her that you do not have the time to stay and discuss this with her now. You promise to return on Monday morning.

- Should the nurse write this down in the patient's notes?

- Should the nurse discuss this with colleagues?

FEEDBACK

Patients can expect that, in general, confidences will be kept, but confidentiality as an absolute right is debatable. What is important in the above examples is that the nurse receiving such personal and sensitive information must consider the consequences of keeping or of not keeping such confidences. As a patient, one might expect that information about sexual matters should not be discussed openly unless it will be of benefit to that patient to do so. If the nurse feels the need to discuss such issues with another member of the care team, there must be justification in doing so. In short, it may not be necessary to record or share information about sexual matters or concerns. If it is thought to be necessary, it should be done in the interest of the patient.

AFTER THE ICE HAS BEEN BROKEN

As previously acknowledged, initiating a conversation about sex and sexuality is likely to be difficult and embarrassing. Once the discussion has begun it is likely that the patient will want to express feelings and will perhaps want to ask for some information and advice. Responding to the first need requires good listening skills, which are discussed elsewhere in this book. It is very likely that you will be able to respond to the patient's informational needs without further assistance.

THE PLISSIT MODEL: A CONCEPTUAL SCHEME FOR THE BEHAVIOURAL TREATMENT OF SEXUAL PROBLEMS

The PLISSIT model (Annon 1976) can be helpful when caring for a patient who requires information about sexual matters, although it was originally developed for patients following myocardial infarction. This model has four aspects.

Permission

This involves the nurse giving permission to the patient to talk about sexual matters, either by raising the subject or by being available and accessible. It is very important not to assume that a patient will want a partner to be present, and it is vital that the patient's permission is gained before other persons are involved. Two contrasting examples illustrate how a nurse may give permission.

Andy is a 43-year-old man with acquired immune deficiency syndrome (AIDS) who is receiving palliative care. Jim is Andy's primary nurse. On a quiet evening after visiting time, Andy says to Jim, 'Carrying on a relationship when you've got this isn't easy, you know.' Jim says, 'I'll have a word with the doctor and perhaps we can get the social work appointment brought forward.'

On a similar duty, Kathy is in charge:

Kathy invites Andy to a quiet area of the ward and asks him if there is anything on his mind. 'Well things have been getting me down recently, you know, but it's a bit personal,' Andy replies, rather tentatively. 'It's a bit dif-ficult for you to talk about some of your concerns, but if there is anything at all that's worrying you, I would like to see if I could help,' replies Kathy.

Jim, for whatever reason, did not give Andy permission to voice his con-cerns. In contrast, Kathy indicated that it was permissible for Andy to tell her anything he chose. Clearly, if Andy were to respond, his relationship with his carer must be based on complete trust.

Limited information

Factual, general information about the patient's treatment and condition and how this may affect sexuality should only be offered after permission has been granted. This should include information being given in a positive rather than in a negative way. For example, 'It is perfectly safe for you to sleep in the same bed . . .', 'There is no problem in having family and friends nearby . . .', 'You will not harm your partner by kissing and cuddling, and it may help you to adjust to the shock you have both recently suffered . . .'.

General information about lubricants should be included. KY-Jelly may be part of the professional's vocabulary and of the senior-house-officer-leaving-party armoury, but it is not part of everyone's vocabulary!

Specific suggestions

This will depend on the questions and concern voiced by patients and their part-ners and on the particular illness. These responses are best if they are not pre-pared. You may need a knowledge of relevant anatomy, physiology, pathology and psychosocial responses to help with specific suggestions. There is no problem if you do not have every answer at your fingertips, so long as you find out quickly.

Intensive therapy

Occasionally, because of complex or pre-existing problems, patients may require specialist help. A patient may have suffered from a delayed sexual response or impotence before the illness was diagnosed and may benefit from the help of a sex counsellor or sex therapist. A clinical psychologist may be the best person to offer advice, while it is important to impress upon the spe-cialist that the patient's prognosis is limited. However, it is important to be aware that long-standing sexual problems may not be resolved rapidly.

HIV AND AIDS

Over the years, more and more people are dying from AIDS. This population and their partners, families and friends represent a part of the community that requires some consideration because of the problems they face during their illness and into bereavement.

Many lay people and health-care professionals automatically assume that the patient with AIDS is gay. Clearly, this is by no means always the case, but the person with AIDS is powerless to remove this label, which has been firmly attached by society and which has been attached where the patient is unlikely to see it. If they escape the 'gay' label they are just as likely to pick up the 'promiscuous' label, when in fact neither may be true.

Our society recognises and values the concept of kinship and its apparent hierarchical relationship to the intensity of grief. The member of staff who has been bereaved is likely to be awarded compassionate leave according to their relationship to the deceased, even though the personnel policy states that such leave is at the discretion of the manager. No account is taken of the actual relationship, so survivors from non-traditional (heterosexual) relationships can have great difficulty in obtaining understanding and support from their friends and family and from professionals. Therefore, they are at risk of developing a complicated or unresolved grief reaction. Also, when a homosexual person dies, the surviving partner may be excluded from the funeral and from inheriting from the deceased's estate.

Buckman (1988) offered these helpful words, intended for lay people who are helping a dying friend. They are equally helpful to those professionals who feel challenged when caring for a patient who has a different sexual orientation from their own.

It should be your objective . . . to help your friend to let go of life in his own way. It may not be your way and it may not be the way you read about it in a book but it is his way and is consistent with the way he lived his life. You can and should help your friend achieve that.

Buckman 1988

Box 7.4

Exercise: Let's look at attitudes

It is widely acknowledged that education must consider skills, knowledge and attitudes, and that attitudinal change can be extremely difficult. A prerequisite of attitudinal change is awareness and exploration. Before embarking on this exercise it is important to be aware that challenging attitudes can expose lack of knowledge and deep-rooted prejudice. It therefore requires considerate facilitation and respect for others. This exercise may be used in wards, departments and community settings. It does not assume or require any particular knowledge. It can be used in a unidisciplinary setting but has greater impact if a variety of disciplines can be encouraged to join in.

The exercise

It is best to begin by setting your own ground rules around issues such as confidentiality, use of strong language and respect for others. It is important that the group is not interrupted during the exercise.

Continued

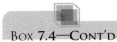

BOX 7.4—CONT'D

Each group member is given some 3″ × 5″ index cards and asked to write a few words that sum up any thought, feeling or attitude to sexuality that is present in society, in the home or in the work environment. Anonymity can be enhanced if everyone uses a pencil and prints their statements. There are no constraints about what may be written on the card, except that 'vulgar' language may only be used for a clear purpose. Some participants will appear puzzled, so you may wish to give some examples such as:

• Where I work, sexuality . . .

• The thought of two men . . .

• Sex is a private affair and should be left well alone . . .

• If they want our help they will ask . . .

• People should be allowed to . . . .

The individual does not have to believe or 'own' the statements, nor should the cards be signed. All the cards are then collected and shuffled thoroughly. Group members are invited, in turn, to select and read one card from the pile. They are invited to respond to the statements on the cards as they wish. If they would prefer not to respond to particular statements, regardless of the reason, they may return these cards to the bottom of the pile, without any explanation or justification, and select another one instead. When one person has responded, the remaining group members are invited to respond to the statement on that card as they wish. Supportive challenging is to be encouraged if the ground rules permit. As the exercise progresses, many attitudes will be discussed. Some group members may be surprised at their own and the others' reactions to the statements. The exercise should be brought to a close by generating an action plan, which emerges from the preceding discussion. Each group member is given a Post-it note and asked to write one action for the group to pursue. Again, a few examples may help:

• Invite the health-care adviser from the genitourinary medicine clinic to speak to staff about the latest AIDS statistics

• Collect up-to-date literature

• Attend a study day

• Contact health education department for current information on . . .

• Redesign our care plan

• Talk to one patient about sexuality.

If the action plan is ever to become a reality it is important to include a time frame and to agree on responsibilities.

Box 7.4—Cont'd

Example

- Invite the health-care adviser from the genitourinary medicine clinic to speak to staff about the latest AIDS statistics.

Action:

Peter James – Contact health-care adviser. Suggested date: week commencing 4/10/05

Sarah Winter – Organise duty rota and book seminar room

This may seem blindingly obvious, but remember, goals left to chance have no chance!

When you have finished the exercise you can collect the cards and use them with subsequent groups. You may like to invite the next group of medical students, complete with consultant and entourage, to participate in this exercise over their post-ward-round coffee and biscuits. It could well be worth it, even if you have to buy the coffee and biscuits!

SUMMARY

Health care in the UK has a long way to go before double beds become the norm in health-care institutions and sexual matters are openly discussed. Most of a couple's sexual relationship is, and will remain, deeply private. Health-care professionals must be prepared to create opportunities for patients and their partners to express their concerns and to deal with them with skill, sensitivity, tact and diplomacy. We owe it to the dying to enable them to make the best of the life that is left and, to the partners who will soon be bereaved, we owe the opportunity for cherished memories.

The literature, clinical experience and anecdotal evidence clearly indicate that little has changed over the past 30 years. Patient and their partners remain ignorant about issues related to sexuality. They do not receive sufficient high-quality information, nor are their fears, concerns or worries explored. I fear that, unless positive changes are made, the position will change little in the next 30 years.

What is needed is frank and open discussion between health-care professionals about how sexuality care can be improved. Nurses spend more time than other health and social care professionals with their patients. They have to become more comfortable addressing sensitive issues. Training and education that relies solely on didactic methods will not change practice. We must teach people to behave as we wish them to behave. Teaching methods that involve actor-patients have much to offer (Wakefield et al 2003). Participants are able to explore sexuality in a safe environment, knowing that they can scrutinise their own practice while obtaining honest feedback from the actors. This approach offers real opportunities to change practice, enhance care and improve quality of life.

REFERENCES

Annon J 1976 The PLISSIT model: a proposed conceptual scheme for the behavioural treatment of sexual problems. Journal of Sex Education Therapists 2:1–15

Baggs J G, Karch A M 1987 Sexual counselling of women with coronary heart disease. Heart and Lung 16:154–159

Becker R, Gamlin R 2004 Fundamentals of palliative care nursing. Quay Books, London

Bor R, Watts M 1993 Talking to patients about sexual matters. British Journal of Nursing 2:657–661

Buckman R 1988 I don't know what to say – how to help and support someone who is dying. Macmillan, London

Fallowfield L 1990 The quality of life: the missing measurement in health care. Souvenir Press, London

Fossa, S D, Woehre H, Kurth K H 1997 Influence of urological morbidity on quality of life in patients with prostate cancer. European Urology 31(Suppl 3):3–8

Gamlin R 1999 Sexuality: a challenge for nursing practice. Nursing Times 95(7):48–51

Gross Fisher S 1985 The sexual knowledge and attitudes of oncology nurses: implications for nursing education. Seminars in Oncology Nursing 1:63–68

Jenkins B J 1988 Patients' reports of sexual changes after treatment for gynaecological cancer. Oncology Nursing Forum 15:349–354

Juraskova I, Butow P, Robertson R et al 2003 Post-treatment sexual readjustment following cervical and endometrial cancer: a qualitative insight. Psycho-oncology 12:267–279

Kaiser F E 1992 Sexual function and the older cancer patient. Oncology 6(Suppl):112–118

Krueger J C, Hassell J, Goggins D B et al 1979 Relationship between counselling and sexual readjustment after hysterectomy. Nursing Research 28:145–150

Leiber L, Plumb M M, Gerstenzang M L, Holland J 1976 The communication of affection between cancer patients and their spouses. Psychosomatic Medicine 38:379–389

Lion E M 1982 Human sexuality and nursing. John Wiley, Chichester

Roper N, Logan W, Tierney A 1980 The elements of nursing. Churchill Livingstone, Edinburgh

Savage J 1987 Nurses, gender and sexuality. Heinemann, London

Solzhenitsyn A 1968 Cancer ward. Penguin Books, Harmondsworth

Thompson D 1990 Intercourse after myocardial infarction. Nursing Standard 4(43):32–33

Ueno M 1963 The so-called coition death. Japanese Journal of Legal Medicine 127:333–340

Wakefield A, Cooke S, Boggis C 2003 Learning together: use of simulated patients with nursing and medical students for breaking bad news. International Journal of Palliative Nursing 9:32–38

Waterhouse J, Metcalf M 1991 Attitudes towards nurses discussing sexual concerns with patients. Journal of Advanced Nursing 16:1048–1054

Wells P 2002 No sex please, I'm dying. A common myth explored. European Journal of Palliative Care 9:119–122

CHAPTER EIGHT

Complementary therapies in palliative care

Brenda Bottrill, Ishbel Kirkwood

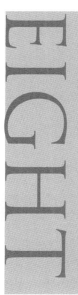

CONTENTS

INTRODUCTION

Complementary and alternative medicine (CAM) includes a large range of therapies, physical, psychological and pharmacological. The House of Lords Science and Technology Select Committee (2000) noted that: 'Some [therapies] offer complete systems of assessment and treatment; others complement conventional treatment with various supportive techniques. Some have well-developed regulatory systems, others are fragmented professions with little interdisciplinary agreement about regulation. A few have begun to build an evidence base, most have not.'

The most widely used complementary therapies among patients with cancer are the touch therapies (aromatherapy, reflexology and massage) and psychological interventions (relaxation, meditation and visualisation). The Select Committee proposed three groups of CAM therapies. Group 1 includes the most organised professions; Group 2 contains those therapies that most clearly complement conventional medicine. The committee felt unable to support therapies listed in Group 3 until there was research evidence of their efficacy.

The technological and pharmacological advances in recent years have given nurses a more clinical approach to their patients. Some complementary therapies have captured the interest of nurses who wish to re-establish a 'hands on', caring approach. Macmillan Cancer Relief (2002) cited aromatherapy, reflexology, massage, relaxation and meditation as the most popular patient therapies. 'To palliate' is to make the patient's condition seem less harsh by easing the symptoms without curing. The therapies included in this chapter adhere to that. They include relaxation, massage, aromatherapy and reflexology, as these are the therapies best known to the authors. We will, however, mention other therapies and topics, allowing a wider appreciation of the possibilities for patient care.

AIMS OF THE CHAPTER

The aims of the chapter are to:

- Enable readers to create a peaceful, relaxing environment for patients
- Recognise and treat stress
- Understand relaxation for use with patients and for self-care
- Use simple, relaxing techniques for patients for self-care at home
- Understand the most commonly used therapies – relaxation, massage, aromatherapy, reflexology
- Be aware of research into the use and efficacy of complementary therapies
- Have a basic understanding of psychoneuroimmunology
- Be aware of guidelines on use of complementary therapies and for nurses wishing to train in a complementary therapy.

The basic principles and aims of complementary therapies are shown in Box 8.1.

THE EMERGING ROLE OF COMPLEMENTARY THERAPIES IN ONCOLOGY AND IN PALLIATIVE CARE

Orthodox medical opinion is changing as evidence grows, showing effectiveness of some treatments in some conditions (British Medical Association 1993). A review of 26 studies in 13 Western counties revealed the average use

Box 8.1

Basic principles and aims of complementary therapies

- Relieve tension, pain and other symptoms

- Relax, revitalise and nurture

- Improve circulation and balance energy flow

- Support psychoneuroimmunological responses

- Release negativity and affirm the positive

of complementary therapies in palliative care to be 31.4% (Ernst & Cassileth 1998).

For complementary therapies to be fully accepted and integrated into palliative care, there is continued need for research. However, careful attention to appropriate trial designs is essential to the success of such studies because palliative care patients have limited physical and emotional reserves (Ross & Cornbleet 2003). Vickers (2000) noted the increasing quantity and quality of research in complementary medicine, a growing evidence base supporting the use of some complementary medicine treatments, consensus statements issued by conventional medical organisations recommending some complementary medicine treatments and increased practice of complementary medicine in conventional medical settings. Recently, osteopaths and chiropractors became the first complementary medicine practitioners in the UK to be regulated. Recommendations have been made for the statutory regulation of acupuncture and herbal medicine.

High quality, systematic reviews of some complementary treatments have been published recently, with the result that conventional medical bodies have supported the value of these treatments. The US National Comprehensive Cancer Network have included acupuncture, hypnosis and relaxation techniques in their guidelines on management of pain associated with cancer (Grossman et al 1999). Increasingly, conventional and complementary medicines are provided at the same site. Massage is offered in most hospices in the UK. Vickers (2000) noted that part of the effectiveness of complementary medicine has been ascribed to the therapeutic relationship between the practitioner and the patient and there have been increasing calls for more research into the clinical effects of caring, communication, patient empowerment and the meaning of illness.

RESEARCH INTO THE USE AND EFFICACY OF COMPLEMENTARY THERAPIES

The UK House of Lords Science and Technology Select Committee (2000) noted that very little high quality CAM research exists and recommended that CAM should attempt to build up an evidence base with the same rigour as is required in conventional medicine. However, the committee accepted that therapies that claim to relieve rather than cure certain conditions should be subject to less stringent standards of evidence.

The evidence base for the most widely used therapies for patients with cancer will now be briefly considered.

REFLECTION POINT 8.1
Research into complementary therapies

Should complementary therapies be subject to the same research rigour as other therapies? What might be gained and what might be lost by such an approach?

AROMATHERAPY

In an extensive review of literature relating to the use of aromatherapy by nurses, Maddocks-Jennings and Wilkinson (2004) found little empirical evidence to support the use of aromatherapy in nursing practice beyond enhanced relaxation. The authors recognised the potential for more collaborative research to explore clinical applications in more detail.

MASSAGE AND MASSAGE WITH AROMATHERAPY

Massage has been shown to reduce scores on scales measuring anxiety (Fraser & Kerr 1993) and to improve sleep (Richards 1998). Stevenson (1994) showed that in a group of patients, foot massage using Neroli essential oil and vegetable oil lowered clients' blood pressure and their heart rates. A quasi-experimental study compared the effects of massage, with or without the addition of a blend of essential oils, on patients undergoing cancer treatment (Corner et al 1995). This study's findings suggest that massage has a significant effect on anxiety and an even greater effect where essential oils were used. Massage was reported to be universally beneficial by patients in assisting their relaxation and reducing their physical and emotional symptoms. Wilkinson (1995) conducted research into the benefits to patients with advanced cancer of massage, with or without aromatherapy. The Rotterdam Symptom Check List (RSCL) and State–Trait Anxiety Inventory were used. Post-test scores for all patients improved. These were statistically significant in the aromatherapy group on the RSCL physical symptom subscale, quality of life subscale and state anxiety scale. Responses indicated that patients considered the massage or aromatherapy to be beneficial in reducing anxiety, tension, pain and depression. Wilkinson et al (1999) concluded that massage with or without essential oils appeared to reduce levels of anxiety but the benefits were clearly enhanced by the addition of Roman camomile essential oil as this seemed to improve physical and psychological symptoms as well as the patients' overall quality of life.

Preliminary results of a recent randomised study investigating the benefits of the use of hand massage or a relaxation tape showed significant reduction in preoperative anxiety of women with breast cancer. Both therapies appeared to offer similar relaxation benefits but 97% of patients preferred the hands-on therapy/massage (Kirkwood et al 1998).

REFLEXOLOGY

A recent reflexology audit by Milligan et al (2002) described a positive impact on quality of life and patient satisfaction but noted that reflexology was not readily available in Scottish hospices. The varying quality of reflexology research, to date, sets a challenge for practitioners and researchers to respond by developing a programme of rigorous studies to clarify some of the major issues, i.e. mechanisms of action and efficacy. If reflexology is to be integrated into mainstream health care, firm validated research must be established (Mackereth & Tiran 2002). There are several published, successful case histories of patients having reflexology, but no research studies to date. This current lack of validated research into the therapeutic values of reflexology and the mechanisms involved in its efficacy need to be addressed if its full potential is to be realised.

MEDITATION

In a randomised, controlled, clinical trial, Speca et al (2000) assessed the effect of a 'mindfulness, meditation-based, stress reduction programme' on mood disturbance and symptoms of stress in cancer outpatients. Treatment involved seven weekly sessions which had three components:

- Theoretical material related to relaxation, meditation and the body–mind connection
- Practice of meditation during the group meeting and at home
- Group processes focused on problem-solving and supportive interaction between group members
- A booklet was given as well as an audiotape of relaxation and guided meditation.

The treatment programme resulted in a 65% reduction in total mood disturbance, whereas the reduction in the control group was 12%. There was a reduction of 30.7% in total stress symptoms in the treatment group compared with 11.1% in the control group.

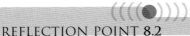

REFLECTION POINT 8.2

Education about complementary therapies

How do you educate yourself and your colleagues about complementary therapies?

GUIDELINES ON USE OF COMPLEMENTARY THERAPIES

Vickers (2000) noted a number of signs indicating that complementary medicine is becoming increasingly integrated and that similar clinical, scientific and regulatory standards are applied to it as are applied in other forms of health care. Such integration implies that clinicians agree on their roles and that patients feel that they are receiving care as part of a coordinated service.

National guidelines have been developed by a joint project between the National Council for Hospice and Specialist Palliative Care Services and the Prince of Wales Foundation for Integrated Health (Tavares 2003). These national guidelines have been drawn up for the use of managers, health professionals and others responsible for the development of complementary therapy services with the aim of encouraging good practice and enabling the development of high-quality services. Based on the best available evidence, the guidelines bring together the different issues and questions that organisations face when considering the development of complementary therapy services in supportive and palliative care. The focus is mainly on cancer, although information is given about clinical issues for people with motor neurone disease, Parkinson's disease and multiple sclerosis.

The Department of Health has set up a team to investigate the licensing and regulation of complementary therapists. It is likely that the therapies used by nurses, for example, aromatherapy and acupuncture will be scrutinised. The National Institute for Clinical Excellence, which assesses the clinical and cost effectiveness of drugs and treatments, has also published guidelines on complementary therapies in palliative care (Duffin 2002). One key recommendation is that NHS and voluntary sector service providers should make high-quality information available to patients about complementary therapies and services.

CREATING AN ENVIRONMENT IN WHICH TO WORK

It is helpful to create a peaceful environment when conducting complementary therapy, taking account of all the senses. The ideal is a quiet room, decorated in light colours, with comfortable, supportive chairs and foot rests so that patients can sit or lie back with their feet raised. It can be enhanced by books, a music centre and an outlook on to a garden, so that plants, trees and birdsong can be appreciated. If patients are confined to bed, make them as comfortable as possible, well supported and warm. Relaxing music can be used if the patient wishes. If the window looks on to a garden or trees, a little fresh air accompanied by nature sounds is helpful in achieving relaxation. The patient's choice is paramount. These are only suggestions.

The senses can be stimulated or calmed by the environment:

- **Sight**. All colours have an effect on how we feel and have helpful attributes and vibrations. Some of these effects are listed in Table 8.1. Sunlight through the window is welcoming, flowers are always available and are uplifting, a tank with fish has a calming effect.
- **Smell**. Aromas can evoke memories and feelings and are therefore very personal. Aromas of food, toiletries or cleaning fluids can affect a patient's emotions, as everyone perceives smells differently. This subject is discussed in more detail below.
- **Hearing**. Music can be helpful in creating any mood, e.g. quiet and peaceful, uplifting and bright, sombre and deep. There are various relaxing musical tapes available; also the therapist's own relaxation tapes, which I have found useful for group members to use on their own. The familiar

TABLE **8.1**

Attributes of colours

Brown	Grounding and nurturing
Red	Physical energy, blood stimulant
Orange	Courage
Yellow	Emotional balance/wisdom
Gold	Uplifting, as in sunlight
Pink	Love
Green	New life
Blue	General healer
Turquoise	Protective
Indigo	Mental clarity
Purple	Meditation
White	Purity

voice of the therapist helps when it is more difficult to relax without the support of the group. Some patients prefer nature sounds, e.g. water falling, waves rushing inshore, whale sounds, birdcalls, wind rustling leaves. Songs can sometimes be too emotionally evocative to create a quiet mind. Generally there is a vast choice of easy listening and light music from which to choose. Peace and quiet is sometimes preferred.

- **Touch**. Touch to the patient is discussed in more detail below. Touch by the patient is very important and is demonstrated by the number of soft toys and favourite items that patients have beside them. The soft touch of an animal's coat has a relaxing effect and some patients gain comfort from stones, crystals and talismans.

- **Taste**. In creating a particular space for peace, taste is perhaps not a relevant point but it is very much part of the hospital stay. Nutrition plays a key role in palliative care and appetite is so often poor when patients feel low. It is important to stimulate taste buds with small portions of enticing and nutritious food. Smell and colour play their role in this also.

((((●))))

REFLECTION POINT 8.3
Creating a relaxing environment

Taking account of the thoughts listed above, how could you best create a helpful environment in which to work?

STRESS

In palliative care, nurses often help patients to cope with a slow deterioration, probably interspersed with acute episodes and hospital admission. This ongoing situation brings with it extra problems and stress relating to family, home, employment, finance and mobility. Symptoms of stress are shown in Table 8.2.

Stress may be intermittent or persistent. It can be described as anything that makes abnormal demands on the human body. It is not inherently bad, and a certain amount may enable us to reach goals, develop abilities and discover our strengths (Selye 1974). The problems occur when stress and tension become 'distress' and, under this now destructive force, breakdown occurs.

In the distant past the energy triggered by adrenaline (epinephrine) secretion was used to fuel the 'fight or flight' response, thus allowing the body to quickly return to normal resting function, i.e. sympathetic–parasympathetic balance. The stresses mentioned above still trigger the production of adrenaline but this 'fight or flight' response is inappropriate and the energy has no physical outlet, leaving feelings of frustration, with all the attendant symptoms (Table 8.3).

TABLE 8.2
Symptoms of stress

Physical	Mental	Emotional
Nausea/diarrhoea	Panic attacks/loss of control	Fear: of the unknown, of dying
Tachycardia, hypertension	Racing thoughts	Shock
Eating disorders	Anxiety/depression	Exhaustion
Hot or cold sweats	Loss of concentration	Emotional withdrawal
Headaches	Paranoia	Anger
Muscular pain and tension	Memory loss	Loss of self-esteem/confidence
Tachypnoea/dyspnoea	Disorientation	Guilt, grief
Dry mouth and throat, loss of voice, grinding of teeth	Poor coping strategies	
Insomnia		

It is in this state that patients can benefit from practising relaxation techniques or receiving relaxing therapies, giving the body a chance to recover.

RELAXATION

Relaxation techniques go back to ancient times. In recent medical history the work goes back to Edmund Jacobsen in the 1920s and 1930s. He connected increased emotional stress to muscular contractions and tension. His work concluded that conscious relaxation of muscles would quieten the emotions. This is also a principle of yoga. Jacobsen started the technique called 'progressive muscle relaxation' of consciously tensing and releasing muscle groups in a sequence through the body (Jacobsen 1938). Other studies have been carried out, but Benson & Klipper are best known for continuing this work. In 1976 they published *The Relaxation Response*, basing their method on yoga and inducing a state similar to that achieved in meditation. Figure 8.1 illustrates the general direction of relaxation.

RELAXATION ACTIVITIES

Try the relaxation activities described below.

TABLE **8.3**

Patients' experiences of stress release

Physical	Mental	Emotional
Increased energy	Able to cope with illness/ treatment/domestic affair	Feeling renewed
Relief from nausea	Relief from anxiety/racing thoughts	Feeling soothed, calm & reassured
Relief from muscular tension	General wellbeing Relief from panic attacks	Pampered feeling Happier, brighter
Pain relief	Self-confidence restored	Hopeful
Improved breathing technique	Pleasant, dreamlike thoughts Relaxed/refreshed	
Improved sleep pattern		
Improved circulation and warmth		

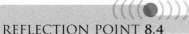

REFLECTION POINT 8.4

Thought patterns

Experiment with the power of thought over the physical and emotional body sensations.

- Recall an event or a personal encounter that was difficult for you

- Remember your feelings at that time and observe your bodily reactions

- Don't dwell on those thoughts for too long. Let them go and recall another situation where you were really happy. It may have been in a place you enjoy and/or with friends

- Again, observe the bodily reactions and the change in feelings. Be aware of how your thought patterns can affect your bodily functions and feelings

In practices of relaxation, meditation and visualisation, we are using this knowledge to achieve a state of harmony, health and wellbeing.

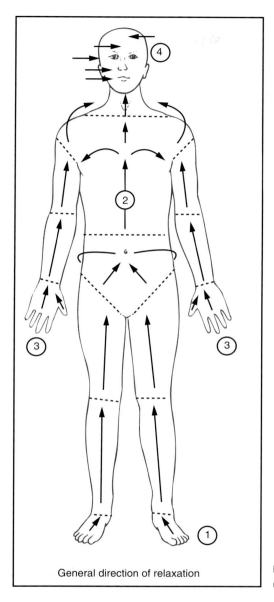

General direction of relaxation

Figure 8.1 The general direction of relaxation.

Using the breath

- While sitting in your chair, take an easy breath in and sigh your breath out. Feel the letting go as your body sinks and relaxes into the chair

- Go on breathing normally. Your body has spontaneously relaxed and the following inhalation will be naturally deeper because of the deep exhalation

- Try not to slump too much, because good posture for breathing creates space for each breath

- Observe your natural breathing. Has it changed? How? Observe the muscles that have relaxed and others still held in tension.

Energy block release

Benson & Klipper's (1976) method of progressive muscle relaxation is popular in medical circles. The authors' preference is practise the short sequence known as 'energy block release' prior to relaxation because it not only begins to unlock tight muscles and joints by gentle movement and stretch but also allows energy (life force) to flow within the body.

The sequence of energy block release is as follows:

1. Take shoes off and let your feet feel free. Stand up.
2. Flex and extend ankles and do slow rotations.
3. Alternate rising on to the ball of each foot (as if treading grapes).
4. With parallel feet, stand hip-width apart with knees bent as far as comfortable. Place hands on thighs. Circle knees slowly clockwise, then anticlockwise.
5. With parallel feet, again hip-width apart, bend knees alternately as if walking but keep heels on the ground. This eases hip joints.
6. Legs slightly wider apart than hip width, feet turned out at 'ten to two'. Knee bends alternately from side to side ease ankles, calves, knees and thighs.
7. Rub hands till really warm, place on sacroiliac joints then do pelvic circles one way then the other with feet hip-width apart.
8. With arms hanging loosely, feet hip-width apart, rotate spine keeping head and neck in line.
9. Keeping feet hip-width apart, bend sideways, using the out-breath to bend, letting go into the stretch. Inhale to come up, repeat on the other side.
10. Breathe in, shrugging shoulders to ears, then sigh out and drop shoulders to release.
11. Dropping the head so that the chin rests towards the chest, very easily roll the head round to listen to the right shoulder then return through the centre point to listen to the left shoulder, then return to centre. Breathe in and lift the head back into a comfortable upright position.
12. Gently shake arms and hands.
13. Think of the trunk of the body as the trunk of a tree, with the feet as roots and the branches as the nervous and circulatory systems flowing out to the fingertips. Cross your hands at your wrists and gently raise your arms as if taking off a sweater. As your arms comfortably stretch above your head, feel the height of your trunk and spine and visualise the flow of sap within the tree as if flowing within your spinal column. See yourself as a newly sprouting and flowering spring tree. Use your

sigh out to let your arms float down again a little in front of you, being careful not to stress the shoulders. Stand and breathe gently, observing how you feel. Observe any changes in yourself. Repeat once or twice, resting, breathing, observing in between each stretch, then sit down comfortably.

These exercises usually bring spontaneous laughter from patients, helping the relaxation process, and can be varied with patients according to their medical condition, mobility and comfort.

REFLECTION POINT 8.5
Effects of the energy block release sequence

Has the sequence deepened and expanded your diaphragmatic breathing naturally? Do you notice warmth or tingling in your hands and face? How would you describe how you are feeling following the sequence? It can take a few sessions before changes are observed. Practice should always be pleasurable and never a strain.

VISUALISATION

Visualisation is used by therapists to help patients form clear pictures within their minds when in a relaxed state. Gentle music can be helpful in evoking the images. Although guided visualisation has a place, we find that patients' own spontaneous visions are so varied and personal that they are more powerful in achieving the end result of relaxation, aiding their coping abilities.

Examples of images that people have found helpful are mostly taken from nature, e.g. water, sea, sand, trees, birds and mountains. Some experience free movements, such as dancing, swimming and flying. Happy childhood memories are also recalled. Images of health have been used as an aid to recovery. In cases of tumours some people find it helpful to use a focused image, such as lymphocytes attacking and defeating the tumour, others do not. Alternatively, one can imagine a light switching on, dispelling the darkness, using positive thought and giving no energy or space to negativity. This feeling of wellbeing after relaxation is produced by the release of endorphins in response to positive thought and pleasant images. For those who find visualisation difficult, self-suggestion by words (affirmation) is an alternative, e.g. 'I am lying in a silk cocoon and nothing will disturb me.' Affirmation can help and support patients in gradual steps towards their goals. These must be attainable in reality or disappointment and negative feelings arise.

DEEP RELAXATION

Nurses should try this technique for themselves before helping patients to achieve this deeper level of relaxation. It can be carried out sitting in a chair or lying on the floor or in bed. Make sure you are warm and comfortable and your body is supported. A pillow under your head is helpful to bring the neck in line with the body, and a pillow under the knees helps release both the hips and lumbar spine when supine. Allow a few moments to breathe gently and naturally.

1. Take the hands to the solar plexus and diaphragm area and focus on that area for a few moments, enabling the upper abdomen and lower chest to rise and fall in diaphragmatic breathing.

2. When you have done this for a few moments take your hands back to any position that is comfortable and let your breathing be gentle and natural. Use this natural breathing as you move through the body, trying to make it feel more comfortable following the out-breath. Let go a little bit more as you go through each muscle group, starting at the feet and moving up to the head.

3. Take your awareness down to your toes, feet and ankles. Move them only as much as you need to make them comfortable and on the out-breath release tightness and experience softness and warmth as if the feet were melting into the floor or bed.

4. Repeat this sequence throughout the whole body, moving gradually upwards to the head and face. Experience the feeling of wellbeing as the face glows.

5. Enjoy this relaxed feeling for a few moments and then begin to reawaken the body. Starting with hands and feet (you may feel them very light or heavy), gently bring them back to life. Have a lovely, soft stretch like a cat on a sunny windowsill. Stroke your eyes and face with your hands. If you are lying down, bend your knees and curl up on your side before you sit up. If you are sitting have another stretch. Open your eyes and give your limbs a gentle rub, taking plenty of time to reawaken.

Coping with emotions during relaxation

During patient relaxation sessions there can be a resistance to relaxing because some people are afraid of letting go, thus releasing feelings and becoming tearful. This occasionally happens and the nurse or therapist must be prepared for and sensitive to the release of emotions, for example crying, hysterical laughing or nervous coughing. This can happen in a group or in a one-to-one situation. It is for this reason we prefer group relaxation sessions to be led by two facilitators: one to lead and take care of the group and the other to meet individual needs and supply emotional support. Sometimes people can become uncomfortable or wake up suddenly and need to be reassured of their surroundings. We are often called to see patients following the delivery of bad news and our part is to provide a private and soothing environment while the patient comes to terms with the shocking reality of their diagnosis/prognosis. Relaxation is not appropriate when intense, volatile emotions need an outlet. However, such emotions need to be expressed, not repressed, and patients attending counselling alongside relaxation make good progress.

We recognise that from a medical point of view these cases follow a radical programme of treatment. From the complementary therapy angle we do not expect to effect a cure, therefore our input can also be termed palliative as we are helping to allay symptoms and aid the patient to control the ongoing stresses of life.

Case study 8.1
Wendy

Wendy, a 54-year-old woman who was treated for carcinoma of the breast, was referred by the nurse counsellor some time after discharge and attended the relaxation class. The following is her own description of relaxation.

After having been in hospital my biggest problem was insomnia, something I had never experienced before and something that began to take over my life. I dreaded going to bed at night and panicked because I wasn't sleeping. I wandered around doing household chores. There seemed to be nothing else for it other than the dreaded sleeping pills. However, this was a road I did not want to go down. Then there was a glimmer of hope. It was suggested that I go to a relaxation class. Sceptical at first, I attended my first class and the benefits were immediate. Here was something I could do for myself after all. I could never have believed that I could be so relaxed, I didn't even know where my hands were. Everyone in the group had different experiences, all positive. As the music played, afterwards I became very light and flew like a bird over the waves and soared on the air currents. I visited happy haunts and danced there. My sleeping pattern has improved tremendously, and I don't need pills anymore. I don't dread going to bed or panic if I'm awake. Part of my daily routine is to take my tape to a quiet corner and relax with it for half an hour. To be able to do this is a gift that I have been given which I'm sure will sustain me in all kinds of situations throughout my life. Every cloud has a silver lining.

Case study 8.2
Maureen

Maureen, a 47-year-old lady, was shocked by her diagnosis of ovarian cancer. She attended the relaxation class while receiving chemotherapy.

I was told I had ovarian cancer, and a course of chemotherapy would follow. After the initial feeling of devastation, I decided that I wanted to help myself and not leave it all to the medical profession. I joined the relaxation class 3 weeks after my operation. The relaxation was of great help, giving me a feeling of great happiness. At night sleep came more easily as the relaxation tape helped to switch off my anxieties. I also used it instead of painkillers, both for headaches and postoperative pain.

Continued

CASE STUDY 8.2—CONT'D

I used the relaxation technique twice daily for the first 8 weeks. After that my great need for relaxation appeared to diminish, i.e. pain had disappeared, sleep came more easily and I had started to live again. I still continue to set aside time to relax deeply at least twice a week, often using the tape. I believe a healing process takes place during this period of great peace.

TOUCH

Few nurses consider what may be conveyed by touch. It can help alleviate tensions and anxieties associated with illness, either as a means of communication or relaxation. In the UK, touch is rarely used outside personal or familial relationships. In the past, nurses touched those in their care more than they do today. The increase in technology has meant that nurses are more often in contact with equipment than with patients. The touching that does take place is often associated with a procedure or task rather than to show feeling or help comfort a patient. In palliative care, touch is particularly relevant as patients may have faced the ravages of modern-day treatment, creating an altered body image. It is important, however, that nurses recognise individual differences in tactile communication and consider the patients' need for space and privacy if they so wish. Barnet (1972) identified groups of patients who benefit most from touch. These include people with altered body image and lowered self-esteem, those who are dependent, anxious or dying. Touch is in itself a form of communication, which enhances verbal communication, conveying empathy. Watson (1989) states: 'It is an expression of the nurse's participation in the other's experience of suffering.'

In our experience, some patients with tumours express feelings of being unclean. This highlights the importance of touch to support the undermined self-esteem. It is particularly so in clinically isolated patients, who benefit from the reassurance of hands-on care. There are, however, those who have created barriers against the spontaneity of bedside touch. They may accept more easily the idea of premeditated touch, in a structured way, in the form of a massage. The action then is less likely to be misconstrued, ambiguity and anxiety are reduced and the touching is fully accepted.

MASSAGE

References to massage are numerous in Greek and Roman literature. It grew in popularity in the 19th century through the influence of Per Henrik Ling, whose system of Swedish massage has lasted right up to the present day. In

1894, the Society of Trained Masseurs was formed. They were the founder members of the Chartered Society of Physiotherapy (Hudson 1988). However, massage was used less by the physiotherapists with the advent of more fashionable electrical apparatus and modern drugs. Its use was thought to be pampering rather than therapeutic. Today the value of massage is gradually being recognised as a complement to conventional medical treatments.

Massage, like touch, is a means of comforting someone who is ill, helping to relieve any unpleasant symptoms. Instinctively we 'rub better' an injured area of the body as a mother would do to her child who had fallen. The simple act of rubbing or massaging increases the blood flow, relaxes tense muscles and conveys to the person, non-verbally, that you care. Gentle massage strokes are soothing, help the patient to relax and improve the quality of rest and sleep. In a relaxed state the release of physical tensions can lead to the release of emotions that may relate to the illness or anxieties associated with it, which have been stored for a long time. In our experience, this letting go of the emotions occurs when the muscles that tighten to hold in the emotions are massaged; for example the muscles in the shoulder girdle, lower back and face, when the 'stiff upper lip' relaxes. The whole body can be relaxed by massaging a small area, for example the hands, face, head or feet.

Nurses who have worked in haematology will appreciate that treatment, including bone marrow transplant, can last for several months with regular hospital admissions. It can be very hard on the patients, who become neutropenic and are low in body and spirit. They must be nursed in near isolation for many weeks at a time. They need a great deal of encouragement to keep going and I am moved by their courage and determination. It is a distressing time for the relatives, who try to keep cheerful for the patient's sake.

The role of the relaxation therapist is to help patients through this treatment regimen. Because they are neutropenic they cannot attend a group session so the therapist works individually with them, using primarily a gentle way of touching feet (following ward protocol). This technique has an extremely relaxing and calming effect on the whole body and can ease pain in the back, limbs and head. Significantly a change in patients' breathing pattern can be noted part way through the session, when a spontaneous sigh occurs and the deep, rhythmical, relaxing diaphragmatic breathing takes over. Sometimes patients choose to have soothing music and sometimes peace and quiet. The patient's own moisturising lotion is used to massage the feet so that nothing foreign is introduced into the controlled environment. One drop of lavender essential oil is sometimes placed on tissue to give a subtle aroma. Its properties are antiseptic, relaxing and balancing. These patients are very vulnerable to infection and the chemotherapy leaves the skin, especially on the hands and feet, very dry.

Patients may fall asleep during massage, particularly of the extremities. The hands, feet and face contain many acupressure points, which, during massage, will receive a gentle stimulus.

As with all relaxation therapies, a quiet room is preferable but it is possible to create a pleasant environment at the bedside. Nurses with no massage qualifications can simply hold and stroke the forehead, hands or feet. Using oil or lotion, allow the hands to gently mould to the area being touched. A gentle circling motion, using the pads of the fingers, can be introduced using only light pressure. Relaxation can be assisted by ensuring that the patient is warm. A heated towel wrapped around the feet is beneficial. Encourage the patient to slow the breathing by placing a hand on the solar plexus.

Byass (1988) suggests that massage can have a positive effect on relationships between ill people and their relatives or friends. Communication barriers can develop for many reasons, ranging from fear to a desire to protect each other from the truth of the situation. To teach a family and friends the basic massage strokes can promote rebonding and empathy between giver and receiver. Overeagerness to be able at last to do something could mean touching too deeply or firmly. Therefore, nurses or therapists should check their touch on themselves. When tight muscles are touched for the first time, the temptation to touch deep and hard should give way to a gentle hold, allowing the warmth from the hands to reach the muscles and help to relax them. If a patient is discharged with a carer or relative to give gentle massage, it is wise for them to keep in touch with the nurse or therapist trained in massage. Time spent teaching carers is time well spent. Passing on the skills of massage empowers them to enter the healing process, whether the healing is into life or death.

CONTRAINDICATIONS TO MASSAGE

Although massage is possible in the majority of consenting patients, there are some conditions where massage would be inappropriate. These include areas receiving or recently treated with radiotherapy or whole-body irradiation prior to bone marrow transplant, areas that have infectious skin conditions (because of the risk of spread), areas that have still to heal or have recent scar tissue, which is very fragile, and areas with diagnosed or suspected tumours. Patients who have deep venous thrombosis, petechiae or purpuric spots are also unsuitable for this treatment. Massage would be possible with medical guidance if the following conditions existed: jaundice, low blood count, thrombocytopenia, skin rashes or cardiovascular conditions, for example varicose veins.

POTENTIAL PROBLEMS DURING MASSAGE

In ward situations, nurses should be aware of problems that may arise during massage so that these can be avoided.

- Intimate or private conversation should be avoided. Suggest a quiet period without conversation to facilitate the massage benefits. However, before some people can deeply relax it is a necessary part of the therapy that they have freedom to express their anxieties.

- Always state which items of clothing are to be removed.
- Try not to massage in an isolated or locked room; check that someone knows your whereabouts.
- Personality clashes can sometimes happen between nurse and patient; such a combination would certainly not create a relaxed state.
- Although trained to deal with difficult situations, nurses are not counsellors; therefore seek help if you are unsure of how to deal with a patient's revelations during massage. However, a necessary attribute of the nurse or therapist is to be a good listener.

Although there are countless articles on the benefits of massage, nurses require good, sound, research-based studies on which to build their knowledge. The lack of coordination in nursing research has meant that opportunities for building on previous studies have been lost. However, as research projects are entering the lives of most nurses, it gives everyone with an interest in complementary therapy care an opportunity to prove its worth. Work that is based on single case histories is now accepted as valid evidence.

Case study 8.3
Helen

Helen is a 45-year-old woman, recently diagnosed with acute myeloid leukaemia. She writes:

When I was admitted to hospital and diagnosed with acute myeloid leukaemia, the doctors and nurses I spoke to all emphasised how helpful a positive mental attitude would be in assisting my recovery. As I am generally quite optimistic, I was prepared to fight the illness and work on maintaining a positive attitude, but it can be very hard work. There are times when inner resources become depleted. When I was offered the opportunity to have a relaxation foot massage on the ward, it seemed worth trying. As a regular, twice-a-week event, it became a very useful way of recharging my batteries and, especially on a bad day, brought a sense of perspective to all that was happening to me. It has also been pleasant to have someone non-medical, but still knowledgeable, to talk to. The use of aromatherapy oils (one drop) enhanced the massage process. The scent made the whole room a therapeutic place for some time after the massage session. I feel that relaxation has definitely helped me get through my treatment in a much better mental state.

Helen was admitted for two courses of harsh chemotherapy and continued to practise her own relaxation and health-promoting lifestyle to aid her recovery between visits. She is now in remission, and hopeful.

●●●●●●

CASE STUDY **8.4**
Grace

Grace is a 37-year-old woman. She writes:

When I was first given my diagnosis of breast cancer, I was an emotional wreck, having panic attacks, with very little self-confidence and experiencing a feeling of doom and devastation. In the ward, while recovering from my operation, I experienced having my feet gently massaged. It is like someone pulling the plug out and letting your worries disappear down the drain. I was left feeling so relaxed that I almost couldn't have cared less what was happening around me. My body felt heavy but light at the same time and I felt myself entering a peaceful space, tranquil and yet energising at the same time. Whatever thoughts had been spinning around my head had stopped, the butterflies in my stomach had disappeared and I felt an incredible inner strength. I changed over a very short time from a nervous wreck to a calm, relaxed, composed patient. Words do not do this amazing treatment justice. It has to be experienced to realise the full potential. (It has been noted that the difficulties experienced by the staff cannulating the veins of patients was made easier when patients received a relaxation foot massage.) I also attended the relaxation group and was helped by the techniques and the calming voice of the therapist. I have changed into the positive and self-assured person that I now am. While in hospital I also practised tai chi, which strengthened my calmness and helped me to cope better.

Grace also described her fear of 'the dreaded chemotherapy' and needles, which she also had to undergo, and how using her relaxation tape she became so relaxed during this procedure as to appear asleep. Staff were amazed at the transformation. She also participated in a weekly support group, addressing issues of an emotional and psychological nature, during the course of her treatment. She still attends the weekly relaxation class for patients who have returned to work and, recently, very unluckily had to undergo a biopsy and received a second diagnosis of melanoma. She admitted that her ongoing relaxation practice and receiving the foot massage was helping her through this second trauma.

A year ago I could not have coped so well. I would have gone to pieces but I am managing to stay calm and positive.

AROMATHERAPY

Aromatherapy is a popular therapy for nurses to use. It is truly holistic, using essential oils from plants in a controlled manner as a form of treatment. We will give a general overview of this therapy before applying it to palliative care.

The essential oils are concentrated liquids extracted from the leaves, stems, flowers, fruit, bark and roots by several methods (Worwood 1992). The most common methods are distillation and simple pressure.

If an essential oil would be adversely affected by distillation, it is subjected to extraction by solvents or, more recently, condensed carbon dioxide, which produces a more true-to-nature fragrance. All essential oils are very volatile. They are therefore stored in little glass bottles with a dropper fixed in the neck. This facilitates measurement, acts as a safety device and helps to prevent evaporation.

Rene Gattefosse, a French chemist who coined the term *aromatherapie* in 1928, became fascinated by the therapeutic properties of essential oils after discovering, by accident, that lavender essential oil was able to rapidly heal a severe burn on his hand. He also found that many of the essential oils were more effective in their totality than were their isolated active ingredients or their synthetic substitutes. This rings true in today's health care, where the side effects of modern drugs are an ever-increasing problem.

Marguerite Maury brought aromatherapy to the UK, applying the research of Dr Jean Valnet to her beauty treatments. She created an aromatic complex adapted to the client's temperament, health and lifestyle. This personal prescription is still used today, matching the therapeutic properties of the oils to the patient's condition. It is therefore important that the nurse therapist using aromatherapy should be familiar with the patient's past and present medical history.

Aromatherapy can be used in several ways:

- **Vaporisation**. This is an effective way of dispersing the aromatic molecules into the atmosphere. A small burner used in a room with the appropriate oils can create a relaxed or invigorating atmosphere or ease breathing in chest infections. Vaporising a blend of oils creates a relaxed atmosphere, which usually provokes an immediate response from the patient entering the room. As well as being enjoyable, it creates a talking point for the nervous or anxious person, who may be unfamiliar with the therapy.

- **Baths**. This is one of the most pleasurable ways of using essential oils, adding between three and six drops of the oil of your choice when the bath is full. Again it can be relaxing or stimulating, depending on the oils used. Mixing the essential oil with a tablespoonful of milk before dropping in the water aids dispersal.

- **Shower**. Oils can be applied in the shower after the wash. Between one and three drops of oil dropped on to a wet flannel and rubbed on the skin are a substitute for those who don't have the luxury of a bath.

- **Steam inhalations**. These are used mainly for chest, sinus and throat infections. Two drops of essential oil are dropped into a bowl of almost boiling water. The head is bent over the bowl with a towel covering it to hold the steam in. This vapour is breathed for up to 5 minutes.

- **Neat application**. This is not usually recommended but there are a few exceptions. Lavender oil can be applied directly to burns, insect bites and cuts. Tea tree oil can be applied neat to spots, athlete's foot and verrucas. Lemon oil is effective in the treatment of warts.
- **Internal use**. This method of application, whether oral, intravenous, rectal or vaginal, requires special training and experience of an aromatologist. In France, however, medical practitioners and physiotherapists practise this internal route.
- **Massage**. This is the method of application favoured by aromatherapists in the UK. Massage training is included in aromatherapy training. A blend of essential oils suited to the patient's condition is mixed with a base or carrier oil, preferably cold pressed to retain nutrients that are destroyed during the refining of some vegetable oils. In their raw, natural, unrefined state, oils such as olive, almond and sesame seed contain vitamins, minerals and essential fatty acids that in themselves nourish the skin. Aromatherapists would use one to three drops of essential oil in 5 ml of base or carrier oil as a recommended concentration. In palliative care, one drop of essential oil in 5 ml of base oil is recommended. If the patient has sensitive skin, a little patch test of the blend can be carried out on the inside of the arm and observed for reddening or itching. If there is a reaction within 10–15 minutes, the patch test should be removed with plain vegetable oil. Massage with essential oils allows the skin to absorb the aromatic molecules, which are transported in the circulation to the system or organs for which the oils have an affinity.

ESSENTIAL OILS CHEMISTRY

Lawless (1992) noted that essential oils chemistry, in general, consists of chemical compounds that have oxygen, hydrogen and carbon as their building blocks. They are subdivided into hydrocarbons, which are almost exclusively made up of terpenes, and oxygenated compounds, which are mainly esters, aldehydes, ketones, alcohols, phenols, oxides, acids, lactones, sulphurs and nitrogen compounds.

The common terpene hydrocarbons include:

- **Limonene**, which is antiviral and found in 90% of citrus oils
- **Pinene**, which is antiseptic and found in pine and turpentine oils
- **Chamazulene** and **farnesol**, which have outstanding anti-inflammatory and bactericidal properties.
  Oxygenated compounds include:
- **Esters**, which are probably the most widespread group found in essential oils and have fungicidal and sedative qualities
- **Aldehydes** have a sedative effect with powerful antiseptic properties and are generally found in lemon-scented oils

- **Ketones,** which are some of the most toxic constituents of essential oils, give the oils their potency and must therefore only be used by someone familiar with the chemistry. Ketones are often found in plants that are used for upper respiratory complaints to ease congestion
- **Alcohols,** which have good antiseptic and antiviral properties with an uplifting quality
- **Phenols,** which are generally bactericidal and strongly stimulating, but can be skin irritants
- Among the oxides, by far the most important is **cineol,** which stands in a class of its own, with a powerful expectorant effect, and is the principal constituent of eucalyptus oil.

An understanding of essential oils chemistry is a necessary part of professional aromatherapy. Essential oils are the life force of the plants from which they come. The many therapeutic properties attributed to a single oil attract scepticism but this diversity of properties and actions reflects the chemistry of the oil. When two or more oils are blended together, the synergy created is more than the 'sum of parts', i.e. the chemistry from each plant joins, enhancing their effect, and makes the blend more active than when used singly.

ESSENTIAL OILS AND CHEMOTHERAPY

At present, the use of essential oils with patients having chemotherapy is not recommended. This contraindication has not been substantiated by any research but while no one seems to know what chemical interaction takes place between essential oils and chemotherapy drugs, it is wise to err on the side of caution. McNamara (1994, pp. 46–47) suggests: 'It seems most unlikely that essential oils could override the impact of cytotoxic drugs, and therefore inhibit the body's response to chemotherapy.'

As mentioned above, the current practice is to avoid massage on areas receiving radiotherapy. Two oils have been researched in French hospitals by Penóël & Franchomme (1990), with positive results. Niaouli and tea tree oils were applied as a thin film over the area to be irradiated; this helped to prevent burning and scarring. This is one of the areas where the application of essential oils without massage could be useful.

Many patients enjoy the aroma, and indeed their interest in the oil has led them to enquire about it and to purchase their own. The aroma from an oil burner or electric vaporiser may not be agreeable to other patients in a shared room. Therefore, a drop of oil suitable to the patient can be dropped on the nightclothes or pillow without invading the others' privacy. Because of their potent aromas, the essential oils can evoke memories, as already mentioned. These memories can be pleasant or otherwise, and therefore the use of such oils on patients is a personal experience. Some orthodox treatments can disturb the olfactory system, and smells that have been enjoyed in normal circumstances can now be perceived differently. With over 150 oils to choose from, it shouldn't be difficult to select one that will give pleasure. Most

TABLE 8.4

Actions of essential oils

Regulators	Sedatives	Stimulants	Euphorics
Geranium	Roman camomile	Peppermint	Grapefruit
Bergamot	Lavender	Rosemary	Ylang ylang
Frankincense	Sweet marjoram	Eucalyptus	Clary sage
Rosewood	Neroli	Juniper	Jasmine
Rose	Sandalwood	Tea tree	Patchouli
	Vetiver		

patients welcome the pleasing aromas as a diversion from the everyday routine aromas experienced in hospital.

Aroma alone can have a subtle but real effect on the mind and, via the mind, on the body. Inhaling the oils also has a direct effect on the body, as some part of the oil will be absorbed via the lungs and into the bloodstream. The oils in Table 8.4 are shown only for interest and not as guidelines for patient use.

Essential oils are now sold quite freely to the general public. There is no way of knowing the source of the oil, or its chemistry, and whether or not it has been adulterated to meet minimum standards. Cheap oils usually indicate poor quality. Therefore, it is wise to find a retailer where the oils come from a reputable supplier. Oils are like wine. There are good years with a healthy yield and bad years with a poorer yield. Reputable suppliers use their specialist knowledge to supply the best oils available.

CASE STUDY 8.5
Christine

Christine was a 57-year-old retired shop manageress. She was single but had a supportive man friend whom she saw each week. Her sisters were very close and extremely supportive.

Christine had breast cancer. Initially a lump was removed; this was followed by a mastectomy. Two years later a lump was removed from the other breast and chemotherapy followed for 2 years with biopsies to check on condition. Christine's room in the hospital was easy to find by the aroma from her essential oils, which she loved. This love of the oils led her to me (BB) for therapy. The oncologist agreed to Christine's therapy and her treatment began in January, and continued almost every 2 weeks until her death in July.

Usually, I massaged where Christine felt her need was greatest, often on her upper back, arms, hands, face and feet. The massage was always carried out using a gentle technique with holding, stroking movements. The selection of oils used were bergamot for its uplifting qualities, Roman camomile for its antispasmodic and stress-reducing properties, sandalwood for relaxation and as a urinary tract tonic and lavender as a general mood enhancer and to improve Christine's sleep pattern. Neroli was always used on the face as she enjoyed the perfume and it has good rejuvenating qualities. The dilution was 1%, with one drop to each 5 ml of carrier oil. Christine enjoyed her visits and looked forward to them. She listed what she thought the benefits of her sessions were:

- It gives me a definite sense of wellbeing
- It makes me feel more relaxed and less anxious about my own condition
- I felt I was doing something positive for myself and getting benefit from it
- It took about 4 weeks to really feel good but now I feel totally different
- It has helped to bring back my confidence
- The relaxed atmosphere while aromatherapy is being done is helpful.

Christine always left with a feeling of wellbeing, which I shared also.

Complementary therapists work under the instructions of medical and nursing staff and in concert with them. New knowledge on the safe and beneficial marrying of complementary therapies with conventional medical treatments is constantly coming to light.

REFLEXOLOGY

How beautiful upon the mountains are the feet of him that brings good tidings, that publishes peace.

Isaiah 52:7

Few people pay much attention to their feet, which take a severe beating in their path through life. They are delicate structures a fraction of the body size, which support and transport the entire body weight. Little notice is given to self-inflicted foot problems, which can cause problems elsewhere in the body (Dougans & Ellis 1992).

Many reflexologists believe that reflexology originated in China some 5000 years ago, although concrete proof is elusive. Perhaps this knowledge was left aside in favour of acupuncture, which emerged as the stronger growth. This knowledge of foot reflex therapy might have been lost to antiquity had it not been for the enquiring medical minds of the late 19th century and early 20th century. The Europeans expanded on the research of their predecessors but credit must go to the Americans for putting modern reflexology on the map.

Dr William Fitzgerald, an American ear, nose and throat specialist, found, through knowledge that he gained in Europe and in his own research, that pressure he applied to the fingers created a local anaesthetic effect in the arm and shoulder right up to the face, ear and nose. This enabled him to perform minor surgical procedures using his pressure technique. He divided the body longitudinally into 10 zones (Fig. 8.2). A line is drawn down the centre of the body with fine corresponding zones on each side of this line. The zones are of equal width and extend through the body from front to back, Fitzgerald's theory being that parts of the body within a zone will be linked with one another by the energy within that zone. Dr Fitzgerald gave lectures on his zone theory and gathered around him a circle of practitioners. Unwittingly, he gave Native American folk medicine respectability. Diagrams of the zones of the feet appeared in the first edition of his book.

Eunace Ingham, an American masseuse, charted the zones in relation to the effects on the rest of the body, until a map of the body evolved on the

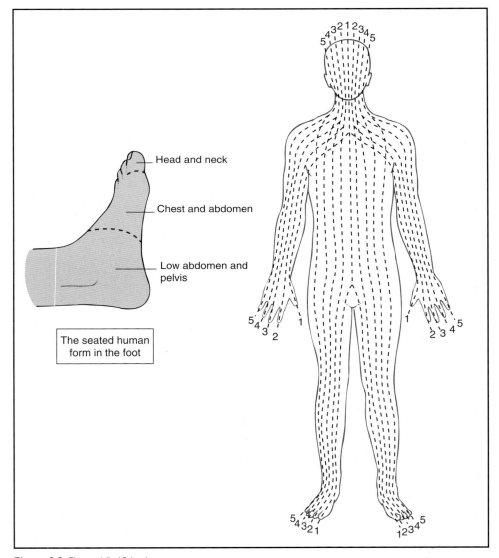

Head and neck

Chest and abdomen

Low abdomen and pelvis

The seated human form in the foot

Figure 8.2 Fitzgerald's 10 body zones.

feet. She developed a special subtle method of massage, which is now taught as the cornerstone of this work. To date, most reflexologists work on the theory of the zones described by Dr Fitzgerald but there exists a strong link between reflexology and acupuncture. As acupuncture and reflexology are concerned with balancing energy flow to stimulate the body's own healing potential, a greater number of therapists are now combining reflexology with meridian therapy to provide a more comprehensive and effective treatment.

PERFORMING REFLEXOLOGY

Reflexology can be performed with the patient lying or sitting. Most therapists face the soles of the feet and prefer the head to be raised slightly so that facial expressions can be observed. The therapist should be aware of the patient's medical history, medications and general health state. The feet are observed for deformities, calluses, bunions and enlarged toe joints. As already mentioned above, the feet represent a microcosm of the body and every bump or crevice aids the therapist in building a health picture. The initial touch of the therapist's hand is important: it is reassuring to the patient. A gentle massage before treatment relaxes and warms the feet, allowing the patient to become accustomed to and feel comfortable with the feet being touched. Treatment consists of finger pressures traversing across the zones on the feet. The thumb is the finger mainly used but the index finger can also treat smaller areas. The treatment usually starts on the toes and works downwards on the foot until all the systems and organ-related zones have been worked on. Some discomfort may be felt in a zone; this can vary in intensity from a pinprick sensation to a deeper, intense pain. It is detected by the finger in various ways; for example, a change in tissue tone, a small pea under the skin, or granules like sugar. It is usual for the therapist to move away from a painful zone to allow the patient to relax but return later in the treatment to give that zone a gentle stimulus to help rebalance the organ or system that is out of tune. Some people are extremely sensitive to reflexology, experiencing light-headed sensations or discomfort in the organ or system being treated. The therapist is alert to these symptoms and holds the feet gently until the sensation passes.

BENEFITS OF REFLEXOLOGY

Reflexology is ideally suited to patients who are shy, private people or whose lifestyle has no space for touching another individual. The feet being distal to the body makes treatment less invasive. For the therapist, it can feel a bit like performing body maintenance.

Reflexology treatments can improve the quality of life of terminally ill patients. Alleviation of pain makes the patient feel more relaxed and comfortable. There is functional improvement of the organs of excretion, including the skin and lungs, and improvement of bowel and bladder sphincter control. It is a therapy that is acceptable to patients who have a poor body image through radical surgery, obesity or emaciation or who, for one reason or another, would prefer to keep their clothes on.

Reflexology rebalances and maintains body energy via the feet, which, over the years, have lost out in the popularity stakes. However, with increasing interest in holistic healing practices comes the realisation that feet play a fundamental role.

LIMITATIONS OF REFLEXOLOGY

Reflexology does not discriminate. People of all ages can derive benefit from it. However, as with all therapies, it has its limits, beyond which its practice is ineffective. There are some conditions that contraindicate its use, for example deep venous thrombosis, acute infectious diseases, conditions where surgery is indicated, gangrene or extensive mycotic infections of the feet and an unstable pregnancy. In insulin-dependent diabetes, blood glucose checks should be performed following reflexology as treatment can stimulate the pancreas, thus reducing the insulin requirement. Children are receptive to the therapeutic stimuli, as are elderly people, whose bodily functions are toned with treatment.

THE PRACTICE OF YOGA IN ANGINA PATIENTS

Yoga was introduced into palliative care as part of a lifestyle change and stress-management programme for patients suffering from angina. The facilitating team include a clinical psychologist, cardiologist, physiotherapist, nurse, dietitian and yoga/relaxation teacher.

The practice of yoga – postures, breathing control, relaxation, chanting, meditation and visualisation – all play their part in returning the body to health, happiness, wholeness, balance and wellbeing. Individuals can learn to practise yoga for themselves or be taught in groups as a therapeutic experience. The improvement in blood oxygen saturation is significant in angina patients who practise yoga.

TESTIMONIES OF ANGINA PATIENTS ATTENDING WEEKLY YOGA CLASSES

Below are some comments from three men on the benefits to their wellbeing of attending yoga classes.

A. Since taking yoga class I feel more able to relax on a bus or at a meeting or when walking – I now 'walk tall' with shoulders relaxed. Even more beneficial, I have changed [at the age of 70] my breathing pattern and through this I can counteract my 'stress' feelings more easily. I feel quite rejuvenated after the class and enjoy the company too.

B. As a regular in our group I reach total relaxation very quickly. On return [from complete relaxation practice] I have a deep feeling of warmth, peace and wellbeing with all previous stress and worry completely gone. It is difficult to believe that only 30 minutes have elapsed. The reaction is also evident in the others because there is a general sense of contentment and reluctance to get up and go home.

C. I have attended the weekly class for yoga, relaxation and meditation for the last 4 years. I can truthfully say that this class has done wonders for the angina from which I suffered and also for my general health. As a result I am a far more relaxed person and able to cope better with the stresses of everyday life. The feeling of wellbeing experienced after a class is quite remarkable and I am now able to do things that I thought were completely gone. For example, 4 years ago I could hardly lift a golf club and now I play regularly, two rounds per week, which is only an example of the benefits from the yoga, relaxation and meditation class.

The original angina management course that these patients attended for 10 weeks is a lifestyle change course of which yoga and relaxation is only a part. Aerobic exercise with a physiotherapist, and stress management and pacing strategy learnt with a psychologist, played a major part in the physical and mental tasks and recreations that patients are able to achieve. This course is based on work by Dr Dean Ornish (1990).

Clinical areas where complementary therapies could be beneficial are shown in Box 8.2.

PSYCHONEUROIMMUNOLOGY

The biopsychosocial model of health psychology maintains that biological, psychological and social processes are integrally involved in physical health and illness (Suls & Rothman 2004). Maier et al (1994) described four interacting information-processing systems in humans: the mind (the functioning of the brain), the endocrine system, the nervous system and the immune system. These four systems continually communicate with each other and the health model incorporating all of these systems has been termed psychoneuroimmunology (Keller et al 1994). These systems interact to maintain health, fight disease and delay death. Three of the systems, nervous, endocrine and immune, have receptors on critical cells that can receive information via messenger molecules from each of the other systems (Dantzer 2001, Raison & Miller 2001, Trautmann & Vivier 2001).

Eric Kandel (1998), Nobel Laureate in physiology and medicine in 2000, explained the process used in the body to convert electrical activity in the brain, which represents thoughts, into longer lasting changes in the body. 'The regulation of gene expression by social factors makes all bodily functions, including functions of the brain, susceptible to social influences' (Kandel

Box 8.2

Areas where complementary therapies could be used

- Stroke units
- Intensive therapy units
- High-dependency units
- Macmillan units
- Geriatric departments
- Before and after surgery
- HIV units
- Antenatal care
- Respiratory units
- Rheumatology
- Oncology
- Hospice units
- Rehabilitation units

1998, p. 460). For example, stress, social support and emotions have been shown to play important roles in the progression and management of cardiac disease and cancer (Anderson 2002, Smith & Ruiz 2002).

Oakley (2004) noted that 'an increase in hope and decrease in despair and hopelessness – all functions of the mind – may be critically important factors in our improved health and longer life'. Research supports this statement. A prospective study of coronary heart disease and optimism found that a more optimistic outlook lowers the risk of coronary heart disease in older men, while there was a link between pessimism, hopelessness and the risk of heart disease (Kubzansky et al 2001). A 30-year study showed that a pessimistic style is significantly associated with morbidity (Maruta et al 2000).

Oakley (2004) described four coping skills that are learned and not innate:

- Knowledge of the world and environment
- Inner resources and beliefs
- Social support/interpersonal relationships
- Spirituality.

Psychoneuroimmunology is an area in which new knowledge is continually being developed. Where thoughts are stress related, complementary therapies are relevant on account of their relaxing and uplifting effect. Siegel (1986) states: 'The immune system is controlled by the brain either indirectly through hormones in the bloodstream or directly through nerves and neuro-chemicals. Our state of mind has an immediate and direct effect on our state of body. We can change the body by dealing with how we feel.' He used two major tools to change the body state, namely emotions and imagery. We would like to suggest that by working with the body using complementary therapies, yoga and relaxation, one can effect a change in negative patterns of emotion and thought.

Deep diaphragmatic breathing can also have an effect on the immune system by stimulating the flow of lymph. The cisterna chyli (deep receptacle for lymph from the lower body) is sited deep in the body at the diaphragm and can be touched by deep breathing, which stimulates the flow, with an inner, massaging effect. Other ways of stimulating lymph flow are exercising the limbs, skin brushing, drinking plenty of water and special lymph drainage massage techniques, for example the Vodder system of manual lymph drainage (Wittlinger & Wittlinger 1940). Using a selection of these tools, a feeling of wellbeing is achieved, which would scientifically be expressed as the natural release of endorphins, triggered by positive thought and action.

Simonton et al (1978) first used positive visualisation therapy with good effect on cancer patients. Louis Proto (1990) stated: 'There is a connection between low energy states and disease.' This underpins the belief that stress depletes energy and therefore the body's normal ability to resist infection or breakdown. Le Shan (1989) discussed psychological changes necessary to mobilise the immune system. He moved from asking what was wrong with the patient to what was right with the patient. What was their most natural way of being, relating and creating? What kind of life and lifestyle would make them glad to get up in the morning and glad to go to bed at night? What would give them the maximum enthusiasm and zest for life? Some patients following this programme successfully increased their life expectancy. In a study that was carried out over 15 years, Greer et al (1990) found strong evidence that women who responded to cancer with a 'fighting spirit or denial' were significantly more likely to be free of recurrence for a longer period than were women showing other responses.

We have moved from a consideration of how stress can depress the immune system to a discussion of mental, physical and emotional strategies that boost and mobilise the immune system. As we have seen, complementary therapies play their part in this. Both Le Shan (1989) and Gawler (1984) utilise and pursue the practice of meditation in healing. This brings us full circle back to our therapies of gentle yoga, relaxation, breathing and meditation.

SELF-HELP FOR THE NURSE

All carers need to care for themselves if they are to deliver a good standard of care to their patients. We each come to work with our life's experiences, ups and downs, and it is especially hard to be focused if our own life is disturbed.

Experience has shown that those who tire easily do not take care of themselves. Be aware of the need for methods discussed above, always remembering to use the breath. Exercise also helps to dissipate the stresses encountered. It need not be strenuous. Walking briskly, taking in plenty of fresh air, swimming and badminton, are all pleasurable ways of exercising. Perhaps you choose to relax in less active ways, such as reading, listening to music, going to the theatre, even taking a hot bath or receiving a relaxing massage. Some hospital trusts are now providing entrance to leisure complexes for employees. With target deadlines and high standards to be met, stresses can build up all too easily.

Therefore, employers should encourage their employees to make use of these facilities. Whichever you choose for yourself, taking care of your own needs helps to keep your life in perspective, ensuring that there is a balance between giving and receiving.

PATIENT SELF-HELP

In palliative care, patients feel at the mercy of medical intervention, whatever their disease. Empowering them in their own care helps to restore their self-esteem. Patients could be encouraged to do some gentle exercises, such as those described above, keeping within the boundaries of their capabilities.

Walking each day when the weather permits tones muscles, eases joints and improves the circulation. Relaxation can be undertaken either in a group setting, as some hospitals have, or at home, following the nurse's or therapist's guidelines. Again, some hospital units have complementary therapists available on a day-care basis. If a patient wishes to have a particular therapy and the health-care team agrees that it is an appropriate adjunct to care, the patient will have an appointment on a regular basis and progress is monitored and reported. Information is given to patients about support agencies, all of which employ caring staff who will respond to the level of need. Often, patients' appetites are impaired and sensible eating within their own limitations is advised. Social activities can again be picked up, as mingling with others whose company is enjoyed can both relax and stimulate. Laughter shared in company can reduce anxiety levels (Mallett 1995, Robinson 1977).

Dr Patch Adams promotes laughter as a therapy in the USA. He demonstrates this by taking a group of volunteers to less fortunate areas of the world dressed in comic suits, building bridges through laughter.

There are many other therapies available and those wishing to do so can refer to the section on further reading at the end of this chapter.

GUIDELINES FOR NURSES IN USING COMPLEMENTARY THERAPIES

Any nurses interested in training for complementary therapy should enquire whether the course is recognised by the governing body of the particular therapy and whether proof of completion is provided. The standardisation of training in aromatherapy, reflexology, hypnotherapy and homeopathy is currently under review, so it would be wise to gain the best qualifications possible. The Royal College of Nursing (RCN) indemnity insurance lists activities for which a nurse is covered, provided satisfactory training has been undertaken. It includes aromatherapy, reflexology, massage, acupuncture and homeopathy. The practice of a complementary therapy by any nurse should follow the Nursing and Midwifery Council code of conduct (2004a) and guidelines for the administration of medicines (Nursing and Midwifery Council 2004b, p. 9). There may also be local guidelines set down by whichever authority you work for. In 2003, the launched guidelines on integrating complementary therapies into clinical care.

As nurses are the professional carers most suited to providing complementary therapies, consideration must be given to the time-consuming aspect. Therefore, gaining the full support of peers, line managers and medical personnel is essential. It would be sensible to have agreed times with colleagues set aside for the therapy where the nurse can be fully attentive to the patient without anxiety about the ward workload. On the other hand, employing a professional therapist would free the nurses' time for other essential ward duties, which might benefit the patient. This may be better than trying to incorporate a complementary therapy into an already busy schedule. We represent both aspects of this care – one of us being a nurse and complementary therapist, the other a practising complementary and relaxation therapist.

REFLECTION POINT 8.6

Who should administer complementary therapy?

Should complementary therapies be administered by nurses or by other therapists to free up nurses for other duties? Discuss with a colleague the advantages and disadvantages of each position.

Last, but not least, consider whether the proposed therapy is in the patient's best interests and is an appropriate adjunct to care. If so, gain informed consent from the patient and relatives. In the present climate of litigation, nurses must be aware of the consequences of their actions. Therefore, research-based material to reinforce the therapy and provide evidence of its benefits would help nurses to justify their actions, should this be necessary. To date, the demand for therapists has overtaken the amount of research currently available that proves their validity. The small-scale pilot studies undertaken have failed to build on earlier work, leading to duplication in many cases. The way forward is for nurses to ensure that their therapy is research-based, or to be involved in a research study using their own therapy. Proof of a therapy's efficacy will aid the trend towards its increased use.

The Royal College of Nursing have a complementary therapies nursing forum. It provides newsletters so that the committee can make contact with the membership, report on activities and share information. There are workshops and conferences nationwide, which are well attended by an ever-increasing membership. At the time of writing, membership is 8789. The forum has published guidelines for nurses who wish to train in a complementary therapy and a Statement of Beliefs for those practising the therapies.

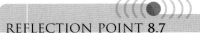

REFLECTION POINT 8.7

Clinical supervision in complementary therapy

Why might you need clinical supervision when practising complementary therapies? How do you access it?

This chapter is intended to stimulate interest in complementary therapies, giving an insight into their roots and into the potential for their use in palliative care. We hope to inspire nurses with a holistic awareness to bring touch and the associated therapies into nursing practice, hopefully helping patients to a better quality of life throughout their illness.

Macmillan Cancer Relief (2002) publishes a comprehensive directory covering complementary therapy services in the UK. The reader may be pleasantly surprised, as we were, to discover how widely theses services are offered in palliative and cancer care.

REFERENCES

Anderson B L 2002 Biobehavioural outcomes following psychological interventions for cancer patients, Journal of Consulting and Clinical Psychology 70:590–610

Barnet K 1972 A theoretical construct of the concepts of touch as they relate to nursing. Nursing Research 21:102–110

Benson H, Klipper M Z 1976 The relaxation response. Avon Books, New York

British Medical Association 1993 Complementary medicine: new approaches to good practice. Oxford University Press, Oxford

Byass R 1988 Soothing body and soul. Nursing Times 84(24):39–41

Corner J, Cawley N, Hildebrand S 1995 An evaluation of the use of massage and essential oils on the wellbeing of cancer patients. International Journal of Palliative Nursing 1:67

Dantzer R 2001 Can we understand the brain and coping without considering the immune system? In: Broom D M (ed.) Coping with challenge: welfare in animals including humans, vol. 7. Dahlem University Press, Berlin, p 102–110

Dougans I, Ellis S 1992 The art of reflexology. Element Books, Shaftesbury

Duffin C 2002 Complementary therapies set to face closer scrutiny. Nursing Standard 16(17):7

Ernst E, Cassileth B R 1998 The prevalence of complementary/alternative medicine in cancer: a systematic review. Cancer 83:777–782

Fitzgerald W, Bowers E F 1917 Zone therapy. Health Research, Mokelumne Hill, CA

Fraser J, Kerr J R 1993 Psychophysiological effects of back massage on elderly institutionalized patients. Journal of Advanced Nursing 18:238–245

Gawler I 1984 You can conquer cancer. Hill & Coutent, Melbourne

Greer S, Morris T, Pettingale K W, Haybittle J L 1990 Psychological response to breast cancer and 15 year outcome. Lancet 335:49–50

Grossman S A, Benedetti C, Payne R, Syrjala K 1999 NCCN practice guidelines for cancer pain. Oncology 13:33–44

House of Lords, Science and Technology Select Committee 2000 Sixth report into complementary and alternative therapies. House of Lords, London

Hudson C M 1988 The complete book of massage. Dorling Kindersley, London

Jacobsen C 1938 Progressive relaxation, 2nd edn. Chicago University Press, Chicago, IL

Kandel E 1998 A new intellectual framework for psychiatry. American Journal of Psychiatry 155:457–469

Keller E E, Shiflett S C, Schleifer S J, Bartlett J A 1994 Human stress and immunity. Academic Press, San Diego, CA

Kirkwood I et al 1998 Unpublished research carried out at Western General Hospital, Edinburgh

Kubzansky L D, Sparrow D, Vokonas P, Kawachi I 2001 Is the glass half empty or half full? A prospective study of optimism and coronary heart disease in the Normative Aging Study. Psychosomatic Medicine 63:910–916

Lawless J 1992 Encyclopedia of essential oils. Element Books, Shaftesbury

Le Shan L 1989 Cancer as a turning point. Gateway Books, Bath

Mackereth P, Tiran D 2002 Clinical reflexology: a guide for health professionals. Churchill Livingstone, Edinburgh

Macmillan Cancer Relief 2002 Directory of complementary therapy services in UK cancer care: public and voluntary sectors. Macmillan Cancer Relief in association with Cambridge Publishers, Cambridge

McNamara P 1994 Massage for people with cancer. Cancer Support Centre, London

Maddocks-Jennings W, Wilkinson JM 2004 Aromatherapy practice in nursing. Journal of Advanced Nursing 48:93–103

Maier S F, Watkins L R, Fleshner M 1994 The interface between behaviour, brain and immunity. American Psychologist 49:1004–1017

Mallett J 1995 Humour and laughter therapy. Complementary Therapies in Nursing and Midwifery 1:73–76

Maruta T, Colligan R C, Malinchoc M, Offord K P 2000 Optimists vs pessimists: survival rate among medical patients over a 30 year period. Mayo Clinic Proceedings 75:140–143

Milligan M, Fanning M, Hunter S et al 2002 Reflexology audit: patient satisfaction, impact on quality of life and availability. International Journal of Palliative Nursing 8:489–496

Nursing and Midwifery Council 2004a The NMC code of professional conduct. Nursing and Midwifery Council, London

Nursing and Midwifery Council 2004b Guidelines for the administration of medicines. Nursing and Midwifery Council, London

Oakley R 2004 How the mind hurts and heals the body. American Psychologist 59:29–40

Ornish D 1990 Programme for reversing heart disease. Ballantine, New York

Penoël D, Franchomme P 1990 L'aromatherapie exactement. Roger Jollois, Limoges

Proto L 1990 Self healing. Piatkus, London

Raison C L, Miller A H 2001 The neuroimmunology of stress and depression. Seminars in Clinical Neuropsychiatry 6:277–294

Richards K C 1998 Effect of back massage and relaxation intervention on sleep in critically ill patients. American Journal of Critical Care 7:288–299

Robinson V 1977 Humour in nursing. In: Carlson C E, Blackwell B (eds) Behavioural concepts and nursing intervention, 2nd edn. J P Lippincott, Philadelphia, PA, p 191–210

Ross C, Cornbleet M 2003 Attitudes of patients and staff to research in a specialist palliative care unit. Palliative Medicine 17:491–497

Royal College of Nursing 2003 Complementary therapies in nursing, midwifery and health visiting. Guideline 002 204. RCN, London

Selye H 1974 Stress without distress. Hodder & Stoughton, London

Siegel B 1986 Love, medicine and miracles. Arrow Books, London

Simonton C, Simonton S, Creighton J 1978 Getting well again. Tarcher, Los Angeles, CA

Smith T, Ruiz J M 2002 Psychosocial influences on the development and course of coronary heart disease: current status and implications for research and practice. Journal of Consulting and Clinical Psychology 70:548–568

Speca M, Carlson L, Goodey E, Angen M 2000 A randomised, wait-list controlled clinical trial: the effect of a mindfulness, meditation-based, stress reduction programme on mood and symptoms of stress in cancer outpatients. Psychosomatic Medicine 62:613–622

Stevenson C 1994 The psychophysiological effects of aromatherapy following cardiac surgery. Complementary Therapies in Medicine 2:27–35

Suls J, Rothman A 2004 Evolution of the biopsychosocial model: prospects and challenges for health psychology. Health Psychology 23:119–125

Tavares M 2003 Guidelines for the use of complementary therapies in supportive and palliative care. National Council for Hospice and Specialist Palliative Care Services and the Prince of Wales' Foundation for Integrated Health, London

Trautmann A, Vivier E 2001 Immunology. Agrin: a bridge between nervous and immune systems. Science 292:1667–1668

Vickers 2000 Recent advances, complementary medicine. British Medical Journal 321:683–686

Watson J 1989 Human caring and suffering. A subjective model for the health sciences. Colorado Associated University Press, Boulder, CO

Wilkinson S 1995 Aromatherapy and massage in palliative care. International Journal of Palliative Nursing 1:21

Wilkinson S, Aldridge J, Salmon I et al 1999 An evaluation of aromatherapy massage in palliative care. Palliative Medicine 13:409–417

Wittlinger H, Wittlinger G 1940 Textbook of Dr Vodder's manual lymph drainage, vol. 1: Basic course. Haug, Heidelberg (translated, revised and edited by R H Harris, 1990)

Worwood V 1992 The fragrant pharmacy. Bantam Books, London

FURTHER READING

Barraclough J (ed.) 2001 Integrated cancer care: holistic, complementary and creative approaches. Oxford University Press, Oxford

Botting D 1997 Review of the literature on the effectiveness of reflexology. Complementary Therapies in Nursing and Midwifery 3:123–130

Clarke S 2002 Essential chemistry for safe aromatherapy. Churchill Livingstone, Edinburgh

Davis P 1988 Aromatherapy A–Z. C W Daniel, Saffron Walden

Gawler G 1995 Women of silence. Hill & Coutent, Melbourne

Hewitt J 1977 The complete yoga book. Rider, London

Keable D 1985 Relaxation training techniques: a review. Part 1, What is relaxation? Occupational Therapy April: 99–101

Keable D 1985 Relaxation training techniques: a review. Part 2, How effective is relaxation training? Occupational Therapy July: 201–204

Mackereth R, Tiran D 2002 Clinical reflexology: a guide for health professionals. Churchill Livingstone, Edinburgh

Munro R, Nagarathna R, Nagendra H R 1990 Yoga for common ailments. Gaia, London

Price S 1991 Aromatherapy for common ailments. Gaia, London

Price S, Price L 1995 Aromatherapy for health care professionals. Churchill Livingstone, Edinburgh

Rankin-Box D 1995 The nurse's handbook of complementary therapies. Churchill Livingstone, Edinburgh

Siegel B 1990 Peace, love and healing. Rider, London

Wilson A, Bek L 1981 What colour are you? Aquarium Press, Wellingborough

Wright S G 1995 The competence to touch: helping and healing in nursing practice. Complementary Therapies in Medicine 3:49–52

WEBSITES/DIRECTORIES

The House of Lords Report on Complementary and Alternative Medicines: www.parliament.the-stationery-office.co.uk/pa/ld199900/Idselect/ldsctech/123/12301.htm

Aromatherapy Organisations Council: www.aocuk.net

Macmillan Cancer Relief (2002) Directory of complementary therapy services in UK cancer care. Macmillan Cancer Relief in association with Cambridge Publishers, Cambridge

ADDRESSES

Association of Reflexologists
27 Old Gloucester Street
London WC1 3XX

Bristol Cancer Help Centre
Grove House
Cornwallis Grove
Clifton
Bristol BS8 4PG
www.bristolcancerhelp.org

British School of Reflex Zone Therapy
Marks Orchard
Whitbourne
Worcester WR6 5RB

Complementary Therapies Special Interest Group
Royal College of Nursing
20 Cavendish Square
London W1M 0AB

International Federation of Aromatherapists
IFPA House
82 Ashby Road
Hinckley
Leicester LE10 1SN

Life Foundation School of Therapeutics
Body, Heart and Mind Technology
15 Holyhead Road
Upper Bangor
Dyfedd
North Wales

Macmillan Cancer relief
89 Albert Embankment
London SE1 7UQ
020 7840 7840
www.macmillan.org.uk

Maggie's Centre
The Stables
Western General Hospital
Crewe Road
Edinburgh EH4 2XU
(psychological support and relaxation only)

National Association of Complementary Therapists in Holistic and Palliative Care
32 Milner Road
Selly Park
Birmingham B29 7RQ

RCN Complementary Therapies in Nursing Forum
20 Cavendish Square
London WIM OAB
www.rcn.org.uk

Royal Marsden Hospital
Fulham Road
London SW3 6JJ

The Prince of Wales Foundation for Integrated Health
12 Chillingworth Road
London N7 8QJ

Wordsworth Cancer Support Centre
PO Box 20–22
York Road
London SW11 3QE

CHAPTER NINE

Supporting the family and carers

Rosemary McIntyre, Jean Lugton

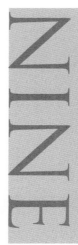

INTRODUCTION

Many definitions exist but none captures adequately the diverse and dynamic social entity that is 'family'. While the importance of the family within palliative care is increasingly recognised, the family as a *concept* is a very slippery fish to catch (Parkes 2002). Families vary in size and composition and despite the fact that individuals within a family can share many characteristics, often the differences between them can seem more obvious than the similarities.

At its simplest, and for the purposes of this brief chapter, the family will be whoever the individual identifies as such, whether or not a biological or legally recognised relationship exists. Whatever definition one might choose to apply, there is little doubt about the profound influence that the family has on its members and upon society as a whole. Almost 30 years ago the potency of this influence was captured in the following quote:

The influence of the family stands in a peculiarly central, crucial position. It faces inward to the individual, outward toward society, preparing each member to take his place in the wider social group by helping him to internalise its values and traditions as part of himself. From the first cry at birth, to the last sigh at death, the family surrounds us and finds a place for all ages, roles, and relationships. It has enormous creative potential, including that of life itself and when it becomes disordered, it is not surprising that it possesses an equal potential for terrible destruction.

Skynner 1976, cited in McCormack 1997, p. 191

AIMS OF THE CHAPTER

The content and activities in this chapter will enable the reader to:

- Explore the implications of advanced illness for the patient's relatives and carers
- Analyse the potential contribution of conceptual and theoretical frameworks to underpin practice in family-focused palliative care
- Discuss the role of the family in supporting patients with advanced illness
- Analyse two case studies that represent differing clinical and psychosocial challenges and care settings, systematically assess the families' needs and propose interventions appropriate to the situation and the context of care.

THE FAMILY UNDER CHANGE

Until the latter part of the 20th century, family life in the UK followed accepted conventions, with the 'traditional' nuclear family comprising children living with both natural parents, who were married to one another, often with extended family members living close by and involved in their daily lives. This traditional view is now being challenged on the basis that it no longer describes the 'typical' experience of family life in the UK. Indeed, some might argue that in the past the stereotypical family structure has allowed negative aspects of family life, such as spousal and child abuse, to be concealed behind the closed doors of the family home.

Societal changes that have influenced family structure and function include increased geographical mobility and changes in traditional gender roles and patterns of employment. Increasing globalisation and migration have led to the multicultural society that we now have in the UK, bringing diversity and dynamism to family and community life. Other societal changes include a reduction in the influence of formalised religion within families, reduced social stigma associated with cohabitation, separation and divorce, and a more gradual softening of attitudes towards same-sex partnerships (Whyte 1997).

Contemporary family life in the UK reveals increasing numbers of families liv-ing in diffuse relationships with more children living in one-parent households or in reconstituted 'step'-families. Recent advances in reproductive medicine also mean that single parenting can be an active choice and the growing acceptance of gay and lesbian parenting now evident in America is likely to follow elsewhere.

The evidence that supports these trends does not, however, go unchallenged and it has been suggested that the reported decline of family life in Britain has been much exaggerated by the media (Baggaley 1997). Baggaley suggests that a shift in the population profile has in fact skewed the statistical evidence, resulting in falsely inflated ratios of single parent families. Population statis-tics in the UK reveal increasing numbers of households with *no* dependant children, and there are now more households comprising elderly people, young single adults living alone or in groups, or couples who have delayed child-bearing for career or other economic reasons. If these 'all-adult' house-holds were removed from the calculation, leaving only those with children in them, then the relative ratio of children living in single parent families would be significantly lower than has been published (Baggaley 1997).

Despite the reported 'terminal decline' of marriage, it still remains a popu-lar life choice. Also, while the UK the divorce rate is now running at over 40%, the remarriage rate also continues to increase. The reconstituted families that result from these trends are, however, vulnerable to breakdown because of the emotional and economic impact of the complex relationships and living arrangements that result (Baggaley 1997). Nevertheless, despite the ongoing debate, the traditional nuclear, kinship-based, heterosexual family with its prescribed roles and enshrined legal, economic and religious systems has now been challenged and the 21st century family is recognised to be a flexible social entity that can express itself in a wide variety of forms and ways (Kissane & Bloch 2002, Yates 1999).

RELEVANCE TO PALLIATIVE CARE

Strong bonds of affection and long enduring emotional ties may occur both within the traditional framework of 'the family' or within other relationships where there is a deep and reciprocal emotional commitment. Having an understanding of the patient's family context, in terms of family structure and close relationships, has particular relevance in palliative care practice. Palliative care nurses today need to respond to the needs of people from a range of family forms, some that are traditional and others that might not con-form to the conventional view of family.

Nurses hold a unique position in terms of their prolonged contact with patients, whether within the hospital or community setting. Efforts to estab-lish a more holistic view of patient care have not yet succeeded in all care set-tings and including the family within the focus of care remains challenging for some practitioners (Whyte 1997). Illness creates a highly charged emotional climate and the family will need support on a number of levels (Twigg & Atkin 1994). Vicarious suffering is common in those facing the impending loss of a loved family member and relatives need help in mobilising their own coping resources and in accessing the services and resources needed to help them face the challenges that their situation presents (Yates 1999).

FAMILY DYNAMICS

In dealing with a life-limiting progressive illness, shifts and negotiations in family roles will occur and difficulties can be encountered as family members try to respond to fluctuating and often subtle changes in the ill person's condition. This fluidity and adaptation of family roles involves hard work and negotiation on the part of the family members, often resulting in significant stress (Kristjanson & Ashcroft 1994).

The dynamic and interdependent nature of the family has led it to be linked to systems theory, whereby a system is 'a complex of elements in mutual interaction'. When this definition is applied to families, it allows us to focus our attention on interactions among family members rather than merely observing individual family members separate from their wider family context. The term 'family system' therefore describes the dynamic and reciprocal nature of the family unit. The strong interdependence that operates between family members, and the individual and collective influence for good or ill that family members have upon each other, is represented below using the powerful image of a mobile.

> Visualise a mobile with four or five pieces suspended from the ceiling, each gently moving in the air. The whole system is in balance. Steady yet moving. Some pieces are moving rapidly; others are almost stationary. Some are heavier and appear to carry more weight in the ultimate direction of the mobile's movement; others seem to go along for the ride. A breeze catching only one segment of the mobile immediately influences the movement of every piece, some more than others, and the pace picks up with some pieces unbalancing themselves and moving about chaotically for a time. Gradually the whole exerts its influence on the errant parts but not before a decided change in direction of the whole may have taken place.
>
> Allmond et al (1979), cited in Wright & Leahey 2000, p. 37

Drawing further on this analogy, Wright & Leahey (2000) consider the individual parts of the mobile and the ways that their relationships to each other affect its overall functioning. The relative size, position and closeness or isolation of different parts of the mobile within the overall system and with each other is also considered. The mobile analogy encourages us to see the family as a complete unit, albeit made up of individual people. As in the case of the mobile, complex interactions and 'subtle reciprocities' will operate within the family and these can be profoundly disrupted by serious illness in a close family member (Wright & Leahey 2000).

SYSTEMS AND SUBSYSTEMS

While each individual family member is a complex system in their own right, each individual, in turn, forms a subsystem that exists within the family system. Also, specific affiliations operate within families, resulting in a number of subsystems such as the 'couple unit' or 'father–child' or 'mother–child' alliances. These subsystems profoundly influence the interactions that operate within the family. In the wider context, external to the family unit, the family system is surrounded by external links (suprasystems) such as friends, church, school or neighbourhood (Wright & Leahey 2000). Understanding the complex interconnectedness of individuals and of whole-family systems can facilitate a more holistic and inclusive approach to palliative care.

ILLNESS EXPERIENCE OF FAMILIES

Serious illness in a family member is a change that affects the whole family in terms of its relationships and interactions (Pittman 1988). When a serious illness affects a family member, the whole family 'system' has to be reorganised in order to take over or provide help with the roles and responsibilities previously undertaken by the sick person. The changes in roles and relationships that results from serious illness can cause significant stress to both the patient and the carers. For example, the ill person may be distressed to find themselves dependent upon the children they have cared for as a parent and children may lack confidence in taking over responsibilities that were until recently the parent's.

In a study of the social networks of women with breast cancer (Lugton 1997) it was found that cancer not only impacted upon the identity of the patient but also affected the identities of their families and close social contacts. Whyte (1997) also suggests that, while a crisis such as a terminal illness touches all members of a family, each individual family member will be affected differently. For example, it has been suggested that women and men may react differently to stress (Magni et al 1988, Thoits 1987, Wilhelm et al 1997). In a Taiwanese study, higher levels of stress were found in mothers during a child's illness, which may have resulted from the mothers being the primary caregivers of the ill child (Yeh 2002).

Carers may be elderly and in poor health, and elderly couples are often mutually dependent in a range of ways, so that illness in one of the couple could cause the intricate structure of the relationship to collapse. However, in a study of older carers, Garry & Arthur (2001) reported that the elderly carers in their study wanted to continue to care for their sick relative for as long as possible they expressed pride in the way they looked after their ill spouse or sibling. This confirms the finding of others that caring is not inevitably an unremitting burden but for some it can be a rewarding experience that maintains family bonds (Grant et al 1998)

Thomas et al (2002) explored the emotional work that is undertaken by family carers of people with cancer. Their study focused on four points in the cancer journey: at diagnosis, after the first treatment, at recurrence and when the focus has moved to palliative care. The researchers described the caring as being made up of a combination of practical tasks and emotional work. The emotional work revolved around being positive, maintaining hope, sustaining normality and sharing their loved one's struggle against the disease (Thomas et al 2002).

In advanced non-malignant illness, the diagnosis of 'dying' or 'terminal illness' may not be conferred in the precise way it normally is with cancer, and the resultant uncertainty will affect the patient and family. In a study of families caring for a child with cystic fibrosis, it was found that long-term care in chronic illness of this type requires the nurse to share the extended illness trajectory with the family, also helping family members to travel it together. This requires considerable emotional investment by the nurse (Whyte 1997).

Family carers' right to receive support from health-care professionals is increasingly being acknowledged. The underrecognition by nurses of the needs of informal carers has been highlighted (Nolan et al 1995). National strategy now also confirms that informal carers need to be assessed in their own right rather than as being part of a needs assessment of the patient (Department of Health 1999). In a study of support needs of cancer patients' relatives, Eriksson et al (2001) found that family carers needed both emotional and informational support to help them cope with their caring role. This research confirmed that emotional support from health professionals included conveying acceptance and responsiveness, listening to concerns, demonstrating understanding and showing concern for the family's welfare. Informational support needs for families included information about the causes and management of symptoms, how to care for the patient, the likely prognosis, how to respond to sudden changes in the patient's condition and services available to assist them. The researchers suggest that emotional support cannot be given as systematically as can information, and nurses should therefore remain alert to the family's need for emotional support, making themselves available for ad hoc discussions with relatives (Eriksson et al 2001).

Support for families who are caring in the community was investigated by Ramirez et al (1998), who noted that, in the UK, while 90% of terminally ill people spend some time in hospital and 55% of deaths occur there, most of the final year of a patient's life is spent at home. This study also showed that 75% of seriously ill people receive care at home from informal carers. In 70% of cases the principal carer is the spouse, in 20% the main carers are the children and in 10% of families friends are the principal carers. About a third of terminally ill people receive care from one close relative only. Fewer people with non-malignant terminal illness have access to informal carers, reflecting the older age at death of these patients. This study also showed that district nurses are involved in the terminal care of half of the cancer patients and a quarter of dying patients who have non-malignant conditions (Ramirez et al 1998).

Whatever the care setting, families dealing with a dying relative need practical, psychosocial, financial and spiritual support and they also need access to information and support. For example, family and friends appreciate practical instructions from district nurses or Macmillan nurses on how to care for the sick person. Ramirez et al (1998) also noted that family carers describe feeling useless when they are not taught basic nursing care. However, relatives' greatest support comes from seeing the patient being well cared for with symptoms adequately controlled (McIntyre 2002). Relatives also need to be regularly updated on the patient's condition and care.

In the potentially alienating atmosphere of hospital, relatives seem to need reassurance that the special status of their dying loved one will be recognised. When relatives see staff showing warmth and friendship towards the patient they feel greatly comforted. In such an emotional climate, if relatives have to leave the patient's bedside for a spell, they are reassured that there will be someone who really cares about their relative until they return.

McIntyre 2002, p. 208

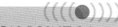

REFLECTION POINT 9.1
Effect on the family of the patient's illness

Reflect on recent experiences of care where the stability of the family as a unit was positively or negatively affected by the patient's illness. What effect did this have on family members, the patient and the professional carers? What implications were there in these situations for care provision?

THE EXPERIENCE OF STRESS

When a family faces the challenges of a terminal illness in one of its members, there are many potential stressors. There is the anticipated loss of the person, threats to the existing relationship, the pain of seeing a loved person deteriorating and suffering from the symptoms of their illness, the helplessness in terms of being able to make the sick person better and the stress of assuming additional duties and new roles within the family. Some of these stresses can be reduced more readily than others. For example, distressing symptoms can be alleviated by high-quality palliative care but the pain of impending loss is less amenable to amelioration.

Family caregivers often have to balance competing needs and priorities and they may need support from health professionals to help them to recognise and mobilise their own resources and gain access to externally available resources (Shyu 2000). There are often mutual expectations of support and responsibility within families, which can be difficult to achieve within the context of serious illness. The literature would appear to suggest that some families are able to adjust more effectively to illness than others. Robinson (1992) found that adjustment was better in families where there was flexibility in roles, where there was direct and consistent communication between family members and where there was tolerance of individualism within the family.

Some consensus exists that particular 'types' of families seem to be able to cope more effectively with stress and illness. Kissane & Bloch (2002), in their study of grief in families, identified characteristics of families that had been found to cope most effectively. Families found to be 'effective copers' were described as being 'cohesive', 'emotionally expressive' and with 'low levels of conflict'. Another family type was described as 'conflict resolving'. The behaviour pattern found in these families was to remain cohesive and emotionally expressive, even when experiencing moderate conflict. This study also described 'hostile families', where maladaptive responses to adversity reflected the family's inability to function as a team in the face of challenge. 'Hostile families' were found to demonstrate high levels of conflict, low levels of cohesiveness and low levels of emotional expression (Kissane & Bloch 2002).

The relevance of this to palliative care is that, by exploring patterns of interactions and reactions within the family, by recognising family strengths and providing information and facilitating communication, nurses can empower and support families to deal with the serious illness of their family member. Such support restores coping abilities and helps the individual to clarify problems and make decisions. By employing a family nursing approach it is possible to acknowledge and address these diverse factors (Wright & Leahey 2000).

OVERVIEW OF COPING THEORY

Coping represents a response to the subjective experience of stress. Coping can function in a number of ways. A coping response can seek to remove the *source* of the stress, or to reduce the *impact* of the stress, or it can seek to help the individual to *adjust* to the stress. Although now over 20 years old, the transactional theory of stress and coping offers an important contribution to our understanding of stress and coping (Lazarus & Folkman 1984). Transactional coping theory describes coping as a dynamic process that occurs between the person who experiences the stress, the situation they find themselves in and the environment. Sources of stress vary widely and the nature and degree of stress that is experienced by any given individual will depend

Box 9.1

Female caregiver

There are large numbers of female caregivers in the UK who simultaneously face the demands of caring for ageing parents and for their own children. Societal expectations are that female relatives will function as primary caregivers and women can experience multiple stresses and emotional conflicts as they try to respond to the array of demands placed upon them. Family caregivers bear a considerable physical and emotional burden, and often experience health problems attributable to the stress of caring, and their own support needs can go largely unrecognised. Within the hospital setting, female relatives frequently function as the main point of contact between the family and the staff. Moreover, many of these women will have been the patient's main caregiver at home and will be dealing with the emotional repercussion of the final admission. Having had to witness the physical, and sometimes also the mental deterioration in the condition of a loved one has been judged to be the most stressful aspect of the care-giving experience for close relatives. Distress of this magnitude has significant implications for care (McIntyre 2002).

upon that person's perception of the threat that they consider they are being presented with.

Central to transactional coping theory is the notion of 'cognitive appraisal'. This describes the individual's evaluation of potential threat or harm. The term 'primary appraisal' describes the initial evaluation that is made of a stressful situation, when the individual assesses the nature and level of threat that they consider they are being presented with, and the demands (physical and psychosocial) that the stress places upon them. If, following primary appraisal, the person concludes that a threat or challenge does indeed exist, then 'secondary appraisal' will follow. Secondary appraisal enables possible coping strategies or resources to be evaluated in terms of their potential value in 'coping with' the stressful situation. The appraisal–reappraisal loop continues as the person utilises, reviews and monitors their potential to remove threat at source or considers the steps that can be taken to manage the negative impact of the stressor.

Coping strategies can be either 'problem-focused', which usually involves direct action aimed at removing or reducing the source of the threat, or 'emotion-focused', which, while not removing the stress, can reduce the distress that is experienced (Lazarus & Folkman 1984). The terms 'active coping' and 'palliative coping' have been used to parallel problem-focused and emotion-focused coping respectively (Bailley & Clarke 1989).

It should be noted that, while emotion-focused (or palliative) coping strategies do not directly remove the stress at source, these strategies may well be the only options available to the individual. Emotion-focused coping strategies are particularly important in advanced and incurable illness, as such situations are not amenable to amelioration by problem-solving strategies. In such situations denial and rationalisation can be used to enable the individual to perceive situations in less threatening ways (McIntyre 2002). Social support, in the form of support from others, can also facilitate coping, aiding emotional adjustment and raising self-esteem. Finally, while strategies such as smoking or taking alcohol to relax may have unwanted health consequences, these behaviours may for some represent a 'palliative' approach to coping. Folkman's transactional theory has more recently been reviewed and modified in a study of stress and coping in care-giving partners of men with HIV/AIDS (Folkman 1997). However, the basic tenets of their original transactional theory continue to have relevance to this chapter.

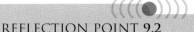

REFLECTION POINT 9.2
Problem-focused and emotion-focused coping strategies

Can you suggest some examples of problem-focused and emotion-focused strategies that have been employed effectively by patients and family members who are dealing with imminent death within the family? Can you remember any examples of less effective strategies that were used and suggest why these may have been selected?

HEALTH BELIEFS AND BEHAVIOUR

Deeply ingrained within each of us is a network of beliefs and attitudes around health, illness and death that can be termed 'health beliefs'. Our beliefs about health profoundly influence health behaviours and will determine how we respond to illness and death within the family. While not new, the theory of health beliefs has evolved and continues to offer insight into the ways that individuals and families respond to health and illness (Smith et al 1987).

Of particular interest to this chapter is the influence that the family can have on developing our beliefs about health, illness and death and the impact that these can subsequently have on our health behaviour in later life. Early experiences shape our values, beliefs and attitudes in a wide range of areas, and the family, and in particular our parents, provide a framework of reference against which we develop our own values and beliefs about health. The term 'health behaviours' covers a wide range of activities that can impact on health. Some have potential for a positive impact on health and wellbeing while others may have a negative effect. Positive health behaviours might include physical activity, good dietary habits, disease prevention such as immunisation and health screening and strategies to promote work–life balance. Negative health behaviours might include cigarette smoking and excess food or alcohol intake.

When making health-related decisions, individuals will normally consider the potential cost and benefits (physical, psychological, social or economic) of adopting or rejecting particular health-related behaviours. Health beliefs are what underpin judgements about the perceived seriousness of certain illnesses and about our own susceptibility to developing those illnesses. This is particularly so when the illness is cancer (Yates 1999).

Social class, culture and religion can also affect health beliefs and behaviour. For example, people from disadvantaged backgrounds are more likely to smoke and are less likely to eat a nutritious diet. As a result, such people are more susceptible to a range of illnesses, including cancer, and will die younger than those from more privileged backgrounds (Smith et al 1987). Remaining positive in the face of cumulative adversity is very challenging and not surprisingly the result can be an unfortunate cycle of negative health behaviour and consequent ill health.

It is also known that an individual's current health behaviour is relatively insensitive to the threat of longer-term negative consequences. This is seen in the high levels of smoking among young people, who do not perceive themselves to be at risk, at least for the foreseeable future, of developing smoking-related diseases such as lung cancer. Gender influences also operate in the area of health beliefs and behaviours. The influence of gender on health beliefs and behaviour is confirmed by the prevailing tendency of men to avoid presenting for health care or screening. (Chaplin & McIntyre 2001).

Religious influences also affect health beliefs in a range of ways. While we now live in an increasingly secular society, there are different faith groups that believe that good health is a gift from God and that our own behaviour has less significance in this regard. Some also see illness and suffering in terms of atonement for sin or even as a path to spiritual growth. Ingrained attitudes to illness and death can mean that for some the very word 'cancer' carries stigma, thus inhibiting communication and delaying diagnosis and access to treatment and care (Smith et al 1987).

Health professionals' own health beliefs can cause them to make unhelpful judgements about people who have illnesses such as lung cancer or liver cirrhosis and sufferers can be stigmatised and blamed for having brought the illness on themselves. The prevalence of these attitudes needs to be acknowledged and confronted so that culturally sensitive care is provided.

LOCUS OF CONTROL

The term 'locus of control' refers to the extent to which individuals normally see themselves as being powerless in the face of adversity or able to control events that affect them in life.

Locus of control is described as being either internal or external. People described as having an internal locus of control tend to view themselves as active agents who are self-directing and able to exercise some control over events that affect them. Conversely, those with an external locus of control believe that events are beyond their control and see their fate as largely determined by external forces. Locus of control orientation has been linked to information-seeking behaviour, in that those with an internal locus of control are more likely to actively seek out information (Steptoe et al 1991).

It has already been established in the literature that relatives of dying patients who have unmet needs for information experience significant stress. Control and mastery appear to exert a positive influence on coping outcomes and can result in reduced levels of psychological or physical ill health arising from stressful encounters (McIntyre 2002, Seale 1993). By acknowledging the vulnerability that terminal illness can generate, it should be possible, by offering information, education and support, to enhance the patient and family's sense of control and therefore decrease their feelings of powerlessness and alienation (McIntyre 2002, Steptoe et al 1991).

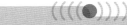

REFLECTION POINT 9.3
Health beliefs and locus of control

Having now read a little about the theories of 'health beliefs' and 'locus of control', can you relate this to your own attitudes and beliefs regarding health, illness and death? Where did your own health beliefs originate? What factors or situations might make you feel helpless or empowered and why? Can you now relate this understanding to the ways that others might behave and react in the face of illness or death? Can you see the close links with coping theory?

FAMILY NURSING PROCESS

The section that follows will offer only a brief summary of the main principles of family nursing practice as an in-depth exploration of the growing body of knowledge in this important area is beyond the scope of a short chapter such as this. Readers wishing to explore the theoretical basis of family nursing practice further are recommended to consult texts that focus specifically on these areas. Detailed and comprehensive coverage of this important area is provided by Whyte (1997) and Wright & Leahey (2000). The family nursing process represents a cyclical problem-solving approach to family-focused care. It mirrors the stages in the nursing process to include assessment, planning, intervention and evaluation (Fig. 9.1).

STAGE 1: ASSESSMENT

The assessment process in family nursing includes structural assessment, developmental assessment and functional assessment. Each can only very briefly be reviewed here and, as stated above, readers are urged to read fur-

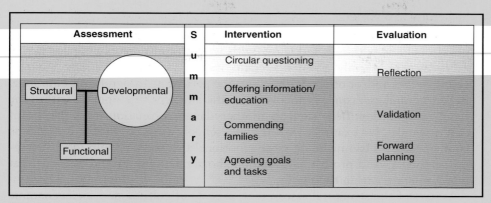

Figure 9.1 The family nursing process

ther in this area (Whyte 1997, Wright & Leahey 2000). An overview of the Calgary family assessment approach is given in Figure 9.2.

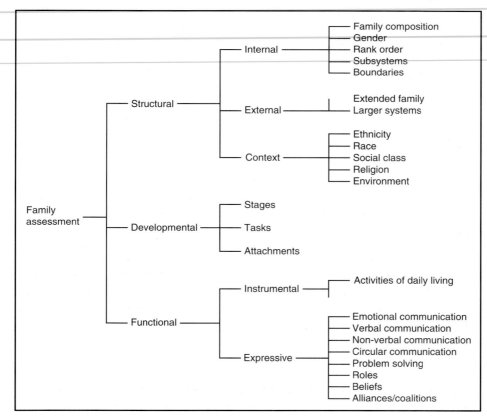

Figure 9.2 The Calgary model of family assessment

Structural assessment

This aspect of family assessment looks at the family unit in terms of the people it contains within it and those with whom family members interface in everyday life. Family members could include parents, children, siblings, grandparents and/or others with whom the patient has a significant emotional tie. Structural assessment can allow specific alliances that operate within the family to be identified, such as mother–daughter relationships; significant external links, for example with friends, school, work or church, can also be confirmed. This can highlight close emotional ties and can help identify support networks and provide information about relationships and tensions that might operate within the family.

As part of the structural assessment, aspects of cultural and socioeconomic background can be explored so that specific needs can be identified and met. Such knowledge is vital to ensuring culturally sensitive care and can also be helpful in ensuring that the patient and family's rights to access to benefits, support and resources are identified. Information about the layout and location of the patient's home may also form part of structural assessment, as such information can assist in determining care needs. Gathering this information should, however, be a sensitively handled and appropriately paced process tailored to suit the individual situation and the particular people concerned (Wright & Leahey 2000).

Developmental assessment

A developmental family assessment rests on the premise that the family as an entity will go through 'life cycles' or developmental stages just as individuals do. Family life cycles involve a series of transitions, starting with young adulthood, moving on to the joining of families with a new couple setting up home and/or marriage. The next cycle involves families with young children, then follows families with adolescents and then the stage of 'launching the children and moving on'. 'Families in later life' represents the last stage in the family life cycle (Wright & Leahey 2000). Assessing the family's current developmental stage can highlight current issues and stresses that might be affecting that particular family at that point in time. Such issues might include childcare needs, concerns about a pregnant daughter or the care needs of an aged parent.

Developmental assessment can identify life events for the patient and family such as birth, illness, divorce or death in the family, and any implications these might have for care and support can be assessed. Significant life events such as serious illness and/or death of a family member clearly herald a major transition for the whole family A sensitively conducted developmental assessment can also identify the family's current awareness of and adaptation to impending death in the family, including the degree of openness in communication that operates within the family around awareness of death. Ongoing assessment in this area will enable subtle shifts in awareness and in the relationships within the family to be identified and responded to so that appropriate support can be provided.

Functional assessment

Functional assessment provides a helpful framework for the palliative care nurse when identifying needs and planning care. Some insight into the beliefs and values that operate within the family around health, illness and death can be helpful. This can offer some insight into the ways that the family members are perceiving and responding to their current situation and can lead to a more empathic understanding of what is going on for that particular patient and family.

Assessing the family's usual communications style is also important in this regard. Patterns of communication vary widely within families. At one end of the spectrum families might favour free expression of intense emotions and may be openly demonstrative in their behaviour towards each other and to those external to the family. At the other side of the spectrum are those families whose family norms determine a more reticent manner, with minimal display of emotions and reserved, contained behaviour. Where the family members fall on this continuum will have implications for the care and support needs of that patient and family, and for the health professionals who care for them. Assessing the family's customary ways of coping with adversity can help identify the coping strategies they might currently be drawing on and may reveal the support they might need to help them mobilise additional coping resources (McIntyre 2002).

Family boundaries Linked to the above, it can also be useful to establish the nature of the boundaries that exist around families, and the extent to which these boundaries are or are not permeable to external intervention. Some families will resist any attempt to breach their boundaries, seeing this not as support but as an unwelcome intrusion, while others are very receptive to 'external' support. Having some insight into the ways that these boundaries operate can help nurses to understand and accept, without judgement, the family's views and decisions. It can also allow social support needs to be assessed and can inform judgements about which interventions and resources might be appropriate and acceptable to a particular family. The relevance of these boundaries to palliative care practice can perhaps be demonstrated with reference to the Marie Curie Nursing Service, which provides direct nursing care, normally overnight when a family member is caring for a dying relative in the home. While large numbers of patients and families highly value this service, seeing it as a crucial coping resource, others find it difficult to accept having an 'outsider' overnight in their home.

Whatever the care setting, functional assessment will allow an evaluation to be made of the level of functioning in activities of daily living. Functional impairment in the patient such as loss of continence, inability to move independently, deterioration in mental function or an increase in pain will profoundly influence the needs not just of the patient but also of the caring family. Functional assessment can inform decisions about the amount and type of care and resources that are required. When care is being provided in the patient's home the potential for caregiver strain is particularly high. Family carers may themselves be frail and elderly and assessment of their functional capacity is also crucial to establish their capacity to continue with care and their own needs for care, support and resources.

It has been established that 60% of patients with advanced cancer have expressed a preference to die at home. It is also known that a well-functioning family can support the patient in achieving this wish (Whyte 1997). However, while dying at home represents the ideal for some, it should never be forced on patients and families, as it places significant demands on the care-giving family. Family caregivers may or may not have the physical or emotional resources needed for round-the-clock end-of-life care. Any evidence of escalating care needs in the dying patient will require close monitoring and proactive intervention if the patient's wish to die at home is to be supported and crisis admission to hospital or hospice is to be avoided. In the profoundly challenging situation of palliative care, the needs of the family, and in particular the main caregiver, should be included in ongoing functional assessment and care planning.

Principles of family assessment

If family assessment is to became an established aspect of palliative care, nurses may need to challenge their own beliefs that (1) they don't have the time, the skills or the resources to do this or (2) if they have extended dialogue with the family they might open up a can of worms that they are subsequently unable to deal with. If nurses could embrace the single belief that 'illness is a family affair' they would acknowledge that from diagnosis to death the family is influenced by, and will in turn influence, the illness and the suffering associated with the illness (Wright & Leahey 2000). We also suggest that, while in-depth family assessment might be desirable, and indeed essential in specific areas of family nursing practice, it is quite possible to conduct a useful family assessment in around 15 minutes. Remember that in any case nurses have privileged conversations with patients and families and can quite naturally amass a lot of important information in the course of carrying out care.

For comprehensive coverage of family assessment, the reader is recommended to read further around this important area. Suggested sources to consult include Kissane & Bloch (2002), Whyte (1997), and Wright & Leahey (2000).

KEY INGREDIENTS IN FAMILY ASSESSMENT

Five key ingredients of a brief (15 minute) family assessment have been identified as:

- Good manners
- Therapeutic conversation
- A genogram (and, if relevant, an ecomap)
- Therapeutic questions
- Commendations (Wright & Leahey 2000).

Good manners

Good manners are not always included in the communications that nurses have with patients and families. Good manners in this regard would require that reciprocal introductions are conducted at the start of each span of duty and the nurse always addresses the patient and family by name, while conveying equality. Good manners also include explaining any procedures and ensuring that communications are honest and are respectful. There is evidence that when a climate of courtesy operates this will build the family's trust in the staff and the nurses in turn will experience improved job satisfaction from providing family care (McIntyre & Chapman 2001, Wright & Leahey 2000). While continuity of contact with professional carers is easier to achieve within community nursing practice, efforts should be directed in all care settings to achieve the optimum level of continuity of care.

Therapeutic conversation

Therapeutic conversations are described as purposeful and time-limited interactions that rely very heavily on the nurse's use of active listening skills. These conversations can be integrated within task-driven care but they must always demonstrate respect. In the course of these interactions the nurse can be drawing upon the valuable lay knowledge and expertise of the patient and family about the illness and its management.

Genograms and ecomaps

These tools can support structural assessment by allowing a range of important information about the patient and family to be presented in a simple pictorial form. When constructed from a brief interview, a genogram will normally contain essential information only. A good starting point might be to record information about the patient and main family members – ages, health status, occupation (or school grade). Later in the interaction, more sensitive questions can be asked about areas such as religion, ethnicity or marriage.

An ecomap is a simple diagram that can help identify key links and support networks for the patient and family, such as church, friends, neighbours or workmates. Useful questions to access this information might be 'Who or what, outside the immediate family, acts as a resource or a support to you?' and/or 'Who or what outside the immediate family is a source of stress to you?' This could give some indication about how diffuse or rigid the family's boundaries are and how open they might be to external support and resources. Families are normally happy to engage with the staff in compiling this information, seeing this as a commitment on the part of the nurses to consider the family's needs along with the patient's. Once completed a genogram can act as a potent visual reminder to staff to 'think family' when providing palliative care (Wright & Leahey 2000). Figure 9.3 shows the conventional symbols used in a genogram and Figures 9.4 and 9.5 show a sample genogram and ecomap.

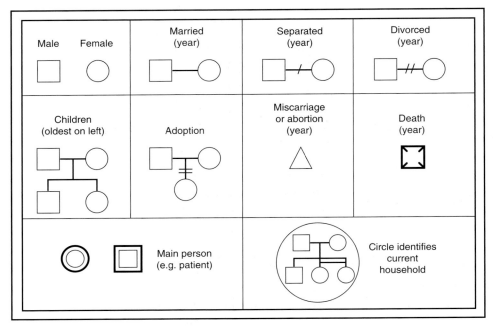

Figure 9.3 Main symbols used in a genogram

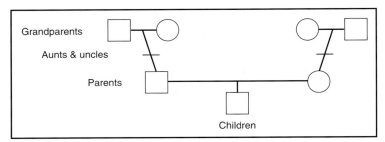

Figure 9.4 A sample genogram

Therapeutic questions

Within a brief family meeting it might be useful for the nurses to have identified some relevant questions that they would ask family members so as to
involve them in the care. Questions will vary with each care setting and family but examples might include:

- Which of your family and friends would you wish/not wish us to share
  information with? (This can identify key alliances, resources and conflicts)
- Within the family, who do you believe is most distressed at this time?
  (This can help to identify those with greatest need for support and/or
  intervention)

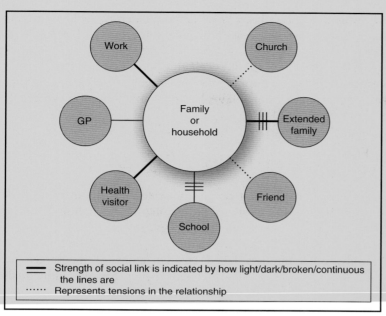

Strength of social link is indicated by how light/dark/broken/continuous the lines are
...... Represents tensions in the relationship

Figure 9.5 A sample ecomap

- What is the single biggest challenge right now for the family? (Allows beliefs about the illness to be explored)
- What could we be doing that would be most helpful to you and the family right now? (Clarifies expectations and increases collaboration)
- What is the most burning question for you at this moment in time? (Identifies issues of greatest concern) (Wright & Leahey 2000).

Commending strengths

In dealing with severe, life-limiting illness and with impending loss, families can very readily feel defeated and hopeless. Commending the family is crucial to giving carers a more positive view of themselves and of their caring efforts. Affirming the family in this way represents a powerful, effective and enduring therapeutic intervention and has the capacity to lift the spirit and enable the family to draw on their strengths and abilities. Commendations must never be patronising but should always be sincere and individualised, drawing on the evident strengths and positive qualities of that family or family member. Some commendations might be 'Your husband has been extremely well cared for by you and the family' or 'It's really very helpful to us that you can tell us just what he needs'. Families will also treasure any small kindly remarks or commendations that are offered about their ill loved one, as these confirm for them that the staff can see the *person* in the patient. Showing that the patient is valued in this way might, where appropriate, just need a simple statement such as 'We can see that your Dad is a very special person – we have grown fond of him too while he's been here'. Given sincerely, such comments can bring significant comfort and reassurance to the relatives (McIntyre & Chapman 2001).

Nurses can and do reduce families' physical, emotional and spiritual distress by engaging with them in therapeutic communications. This is true whether in an extended interaction, a brief interview or even a sentence (Wright & Leahey 2000).

ANALYSIS OF CASE STUDIES

Earlier in this chapter you read about family dynamics and the impact of illness on families and the theories of stress and coping, health beliefs, locus of control and family nursing. Drawing on this background knowledge, you are now asked to analyse two case studies, which describe the Paterson family and the Macleod family. Both families faced the challenge of incurable and advanced illness. Your analysis should highlight issues for the individuals involved and for the care that might be provided.

CASE STUDY **9.1**
The Paterson family

Meg and Richard Paterson, both 42 years old, had two daughters, Beth aged 14 and Megan aged 12, and a son, Jake aged 7. After Jake was born, Meg had trained as a fitness instructor. This let her work part-time in her main area of interest, sport and leisure. Meg's job provided discounted family membership to the Health Club and the whole family were fitness enthusiasts. Richard was a bus driver who had to work long and irregular hours in order to make a decent wage. Richard's father had died 5 years before from a heart attack. His mother lived just 2 miles away and visited often.

Meg's mother had died of breast cancer when she was 5 years old and she was raised jointly by her father and her paternal grandmother, a deeply religious woman who was then a widow. Meg's grandmother had died 10 years previously from a stroke and a year later her father had married again. Since then, Meg's relationship with her father and his wife (Claire) had been courteous but distant and they visited each other fairly infrequently.

Onset of illness
Meg routinely carried out monthly breast self-examination and it was in this way that she discovered a small, painless lump under her arm. Within 2 weeks she had been seen by her GP and referred for mammography and biopsy. Carcinoma of the breast with nodal involvement was confirmed and within 10 days she was admitted for surgery. Meg sought detailed information on the pros and cons of the various treatment options and then opted for a mastectomy with axillary clearance to be followed by daily chemotherapy given over 4 weeks, with long-term hormonal therapy.

Richard's mother looked after the family while Meg was in hospital for surgery and later as she struggled through her therapy. The children were not told much about their mum's illness and although they knew it was serious they accepted this. Meg was tearful at times over her hair loss and general exhaustion but she was determined to get well and gradually the family began to pick up the threads of their lives again.

Recurrence and interventions

Two years after her surgery, Meg became unwell with breathlessness and acute back pain and it was confirmed that she now had metastases in her lungs and spine.

Meg was referred to the oncologist (Dr Brice), who suggested a single dose of radiotherapy for the spinal pain and chemotherapy three times a week over 3 weeks for the chest problem. Meg and Richard felt that they had little to lose and perhaps something to gain from the treatment. At this point they met Joyce, the oncology nurse specialist.

Over the next 2 weeks, Meg had her treatment and, although it was clearly taking a heavy toll, she was determined to get through it. Although her breathing was a little easier, she still had a lot of back pain, and she was profoundly fatigued and very low in spirit. After Meg's assessment, Joyce requested an urgent case review, as she felt that decisions must be made urgently about Meg's future treatment and care.

Shifting the focus of care

Meg, Richard, Dr Brice and Joyce met and, after a tearful discussion, all agreed that active treatment should stop forthwith. From this point on the emphasis would be on promoting Meg's comfort and her quality of life.

Richard was totally devastated but Meg was determined to be strong. Although she was anxious about how the children were to be prepared for what lay ahead, she was very definite that she did not want to die at home, as she feared the effect this might have on the family. Admission to a hospice was also declined, as she felt that the hospice atmosphere might be too 'religious' for her liking!

Meg's last 2 weeks were spent in the general surgical ward where she had been treated. The children came to visit each day with Richard's mother. Richard had contacted Meg's father, who visited the hospital daily. Meg was very pleased that her Dad was taking a closer interest in her and in his grandchildren.

Richard remained at Meg's bedside night and day until she died.

Case study 9.2
The Macleod family

The Macleod family consisted of Susan, aged 30, and her husband David, 32, their son Andrew, aged 7, and daughter Mary, aged 18 months. Prior to Mary's birth, the family had led a fairly normal life. Andrew was settled at his school and doing well. David worked as a computer technician. However, Susan had had to give up her part time job as a care

Continued

assistant at a local home because of health problems. She had been hoping to return to work after Mary was born, as her mother Linda, who lived nearby, had offered to babysit for her. Susan did not relate well to her only sister or her parents-in-law, and her father was dead.

Susan's baby girl, Mary, had been born with major congenital heart abnormalities. She had heart surgery to relieve the worst of the symptoms but the doctors said that no further surgery could be attempted until she was older. Because of the seriousness of the heart defects, Mary's prognosis was very uncertain. The children's hospital where Mary was to receive specialist treatment was some distance from where the family lived and appointments with the specialist paediatrician were at fairly long intervals. The local hospital monitored the situation on a more frequent 'as needed' basis. When Susan and Mary were discharged home from hospital, the plan had been that they would receive support from the specialist hospital, the local hospital, GP, health visitor and community paediatric nurse.

It was important that the care should be holistic, rather than focused purely on Mary's medical needs. However, smooth coordination of services proved difficult because of the involvement of two hospitals and difficulties in getting respite care. Also, Mary was prone to recurrent chest infections, which caused Susan to be very anxious, and it was difficult to judge whether or not Mary should be admitted to hospital each time this occurred.

Family members' reaction to Mary's illness

Susan

When Susan and Mary were discharged from the specialist hospital, the health visitor noted that Susan was extremely anxious, especially at night, when she worried that Mary might die. She constantly went to her cot to check on her. The paediatric nurse showed Susan how to resuscitate Mary should this be necessary. Mary had frequent admissions to the local hospital. Less frequently, she had follow-up appointments at the specialist hospital. On the dietitian's advice, Mary was fed with special formula milk, which was rich in nutrients. The health visitor visited the family every week, supported and advised Susan and monitored Mary's weight gain, which remained surprisingly good. Susan took Mary to see one of the GPs whom she felt had a special interest in Mary. She herself attended another GP with whom she felt able to discuss her own problems. Susan was an intelligent woman, determined to fight for the best possible care for Mary. Sometimes she expressed anger and frustration with her problems. She attended some sessions of a postnatal depression group at the health centre.

Susan found it increasingly difficult to cope and respite care became a priority. The health visitor approached the local children's centre and a multiprofessional meeting was held there with the social worker, centre staff, health visitor and community paediatric nurse. Mary was given a place in the centre's baby room. This proved to be a helpful move. Susan had a little time to herself to rest and to do her household chores. As Mary grew older, she found the nursery environment stimulating and, from being rather fretful in the beginning, became much happier and a firm favourite with the staff. It was also decided that Susan should have a home help. When Mary was 15 months old, an overnight placement with a carer was found for her on a weekly basis, to give the family respite.

David

David was also very anxious about Mary's condition and tried to support Susan as much as possible. However, he was at work during the day and thus it was Susan who had to cope most of the time. Worrying about Mary did affect David's work and sometimes he had to take time off when Susan was unable to cope or when Mary was admitted to hospital.

Andrew

Before Mary's birth, Andrew had been the only child and had received a lot of attention from both his parents. He responded to the birth of his sister with a mixture of love and a little jealousy that he had to share his parents' attention. However, Mary's condition soon demanded more and more of her parents' attention and David began to feel a bit left out. His life had changed enormously. Of course, he still went to school, but mum and dad did not have so much time to help him with his homework and they talked constantly about Mary and her problems. It was difficult for him to explain to his friends why his sister was in hospital so often and why they could not visit his house if they had colds.

Linda

Although Linda had been looking forward to the birth of her grandchild and wanted to be involved in babysitting, when she realised the seriousness of Mary's condition she became reluctant to help in case something happened to Mary while she was in her care.

Although Susan realised that Mary's heart condition was serious, Mary's sudden death following a short admission to the local hospital was a great shock and was very hard for her family to accept. Susan was angry, as she felt that Mary should not have died.

The questions set out below may assist you in your analysis.

Structural assessment

Take a few minutes to compile a brief profile of each family that identifies the patient and shows key relationships, including children, parents and grandparents.

Now add some outline information to show their relationships to each other and their current status in terms of health, illness or death of a family member (with cause). (A genogram is very useful for this as it is quick to do and offers 'at a glance' summary information about the family unit. See Figure 9.4 for an example.)

Developmental assessment

Given the ages of the Paterson and Macleod family members, and the current life events for each family at this point in time, what challenges might these families be facing right now as a result of their current situation?

What impact might this have on relationships within the family and with their external family and social networks? (An ecomap can illustrate what you know about the family's main links, alliances and boundaries. See Figure 9.5 for an example.)

Functional assessment

What clues are contained within each of the case studies about the patient's and family members' health beliefs, values and coping styles?

How might these factors influence the way that these individuals might respond to the illness and what might this mean for the care we as health professionals provide?

IMPLICATIONS FOR PRACTICE

Having now made this very preliminary assessment of each family, consider the following questions:

- What immediate implications might there be for the provision of palliative care for these families?
- What priorities have you identified for the ongoing assessment and care needs of each family and for particular family members?
- What resources do you think could be made available to support these families?
- How might you evaluate the care that is provided for these families?
- What contribution might the family nursing approach have to offer for each of these families?
- Can you see any application for this approach within your own care situation?

LEVELS OF FAMILY NURSING PRACTICE

Wright & Leahey (2000) describe three levels of practice at which health professionals might engage with families. They describe these as (1) the family as context, (2) interpersonal family nursing and (3) family systems nursing (Wright & Leahey 2000). McCormack (1997) considered the relevance of each of these levels of engagement in family nursing practice within different UK health-care contexts.

'Family as context' is where the family is viewed as a valuable resource in terms of providing nurses with essential background to the patient but the family members are not, in themselves, regarded as being within the normal focus of care. McCormack (1997) likens this level of practice to the situation within the UK when nurses are dealing with relatives in the acute hospital setting.

'Interpersonal family nursing' describes the health-care practice where the health professional spends time not just with the patient but also with one or more family members. The focus of contact with the family is, however, mainly in recognition of their potential to support the patient and their care. The family in this case is viewed as a resource and as such is the secondary focus of attention for the health professional. McCormack (1997) parallels this level of intervention with the practice of health visiting or psychiatric nursing practice within the UK.

'Family systems nursing' is the third and most complex level of family nursing practice. In this approach it is the family, not the individual patient, that is the unit of care. Interventions are geared towards supporting the family to bring about any changes that might be required within the family system. Family systems nursing recognises the reciprocity that operates between the patient and family and acknowledges the impact that illness can have on all family members (Wright & Leahey 2000). This advanced practice requires specific educational preparation if practitioners are to develop the complex skills needed to practise competently. Those most likely to operate at this level include clinical nurse specialists and other highly experienced practitioners who work intensively with families during crisis (McCormack 1997).

PRACTISING FAMILY-FOCUSED PALLIATIVE CARE

Nurses who provide palliative care will normally be operating at more than one level of practice at any given time depending on their role, the situation and the care setting. For example, seeing the family as the source of important background about the patient (family as context) will continue to hold value in informing the care we provide. Also, when we bring the family into our focus of concern when offering holistic palliative care, this is congruent with interpersonal family nursing. Expert practitioners such as the palliative care clinical nurse specialist will employ more complex and advanced skills, often while working within the patient's home. These advanced practitioners may operate at the level of family systems nursing, continually assessing and responding to the changing needs of each family member (McCormack 1997).

Crucially, and at whatever level they practise, nurses should acknowledge the contribution of the family to the care of the patient and respect the family's potential to function as a crucial coping resource for the patient. Nurses must also recognise the vulnerability of family members themselves so that appropriate resources can be implemented to support the family in their difficult and distressing situation (Wright & Leahey 2000).

FAMILY-FOCUSED COMMUNICATIONS

Family communications must be individualised and should be based on a comprehensive and ongoing assessment rather than a 'one-off' information-gathering process. Evidence from the literature confirms that relatives within the hospital setting are reluctant to approach staff so nurses should take active steps to convey their availability and be willing to approach the relatives directly (McIntyre 2002). Supportive interventions in palliative care rely on the effective use of communication strategies such as active listening, sensitive questioning and reflecting, so that family members' concerns are elicited and insight into their needs is gained.

The technique of 'circular' questioning may sometimes be used where a communication block within the family is causing distress. Circular questioning draws on the principles of 'cybernetics' whereby phenomena are described in terms of a feedback loop involving a circular, bidirectional and dynamic pattern of action – consequences – action. An everyday example of such a loop within family communications might be 'wife criticises husband – husband withdraws – wife criticises husband' (and so on).

In seeking to break the negative loop, the individuals can be asked to try to interpret the situation from the other's perspective. For example, in palliative care, a husband might be asked 'Try looking at this from your wife's point of view – what do you think her major concerns are right now?' or a patient might be asked 'You say that you don't want the children to know about your illness – what do you think the children are making of what's going on right now?' Such strategies can be used with all parties present and can sometimes help to unblock difficult situations like collusion. However, they should be used very judiciously and sensitively and only where support can be provided during the reorientation within the family relationships that more open awareness can bring about. This brings us to briefly consider the various contexts within which awareness of death operates.

AWARENESS CONTEXTS

Communications within palliative care reveal a complex web of coping strategies being employed by those caught up in the impending death. A pivotal issue is whether, and by whom, the forthcoming death is acknowledged and accepted, as this will profoundly influence the nature of the communications that take place (McIntyre 2002).

Some 40 years ago, Glaser & Strauss (1965) coined the term 'awareness contexts' to represent a continuum at one end of which is 'closed awareness', where all concerned fail to acknowledge the fatal prognosis. At the opposite end is 'open awareness', where open dialogue about the impending death occurs between all parties. Between these polar positions lie the intermediate states of 'suspicion awareness', characterised by the family and caregivers being aware of the prognosis and the patient having unconfirmed suspicions, and 'mutual pretence', where all are fully aware of the prognosis but all elect to pretend otherwise (McIntyre 2002). It should be noted that these positions are not fixed and that people can move in and out of different awareness contexts. Within the shifting trajectory of advanced illness, helping families to reframe their understanding of the situation and each other's perspectives, and setting realistic goals can reduce uncertainty and can support coping.

Although the literature underscores the value of open, honest communication, the suggestion that 'open awareness' is universally preferred has been challenged. The habitual communication patterns of some families might make open disclosure inappropriate for that particular family, and in these situations there might be tacit agreement within the family to avoid open discussion of the prognosis (McIntyre 2002). Indeed, according to Shea & Kendrick (1995), forcing the truth on those who do not want it is as inexcusable as preventing honest discussions. These authors urge us not to underestimate people's inner resources and, while we should avoid deceit, they suggest that the truth 'need not be breached with a fist of steel but should be embraced by a velvet glove' (Shea & Kendrick 1995).

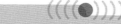

REFLECTION POINT 9.4

Awareness contexts

From your own practice, can you identify a family where closed awareness operated? Was this a positive or negative situation for the family? How did it affect the patient? How did you adapt your approach to care to manage this situation? How did you feel about this?

PRACTICAL ADVICE AND INFORMATION

Offering practical advice on care-giving and providing timely and accurate information can support coping in family members. Commending the care-givers' efforts can build confidence in their caring role. Nurses must be sensitive to signs of increasing physical and emotional vulnerability in family members, especially as the illness progresses and the family member becomes increasingly embedded either in providing care within the home or in extended, often overnight, presence at the patient's bedside in the hospital or hospice setting. Such relatives are already under significant stress, often compounded by environmental and communication difficulties that can be amenable to change. This area was studied by one of us, whose study focused on improving support for families of dying patients in hospital (McIntyre 2002). A brief synopsis of McIntyre's action research study, together with some key findings is offered in Box 9.2.

RESEARCH EXTRACT – SUPPORT FOR THE FAMILY IN THE ACUTE SETTING

Jan's story

Jan was a 40-year-old schoolteacher and mother of two children aged 7 and 9. Over the past week she had been staying in the ward most of the day and also overnight with her dying mother. When her mother was admitted to hospital the previous week with acute breathing difficulties, her death looked imminent. At the time of interview, although Jan's mother's condition

Box 9.2
Research study: Support for families of dying patients (McIntyre 2002)

Study outline

McIntyre's action research study had two main data-gathering phases separated by an extended intervention period. The first phase of the study involved individual interviews with 44 relatives of dying patients in eight acute hospital wards and with two staff nurses drawn from each of the eight study wards. The Phase I interview data from the nurses and the relatives fed into the intervention. The intervention phase of the study was launched by a 2-day workshop that was attended by all 16 of the participating nurses.

During Day 1 of the workshop, the Phase I relatives' and nurses' interview data were fed back to the nurses. Day 2 of the workshop took the form of a communication skills workshop. The nurses used the insights gained from the research data to determine what changes were needed in their own clinical area. An evidence-based workshop manual, which also included the interview data, was provided for each ward team. Working with their own ward teams, the nurses then developed standards for improving family support during terminal illness. During the implementation and subsequent audit of the standards, significant changes in practice were made and facilities for families were improved. An example of one of these standards and its audit tool are provided as Appendices 9.1 and 9.2.

Following the intervention and audit, a second round of interviews took place with the nurses and a new sample of relatives. Data from this second round of interviews and audit data from the study wards provided the framework for the final comparative evaluation of change.

Insights gained from the study

The most striking insights from this study related to the reciprocal nature of the stress that is experienced by relatives of dying patients and the nurses who provide care in acute hospital wards, and to the transactional nature of the relatives' and nurses' coping responses. Support strategies often yielded reciprocal benefits in that measures taken to support relatives were found also to support the nurses and to reduce their reported levels of stress. This was most powerfully revealed in relation to nurse–relative communication, where nurses' approach strategies to the family altered significantly over the course of the study, and to the provision of improved facilities for relatives' comfort and privacy.

The Phase I findings had highlighted barriers to effective nurse–relative communication. These barriers were evident in the discomfort mutually experienced by nurses and relatives when approaching each other in the ward. Relatives commonly felt inhibited about approaching nurses, whom they perceived to be 'too busy' to be interrupted. Many relatives also reported not knowing whom they should approach and when; consequently, significant unmet needs for information and support were reported.

The nurses' discomfort about communicating with relatives also stemmed from several sources. Their perceptions that relatives had 'high expectations' of them had an intimidating effect and the anticipation of failure that this generated caused them to avoid initiating contact with relatives. Nurses also felt constrained by lack of privacy when communicating with relatives; they also felt that they lacked knowledge about the relatives' awareness of their loved ones' prognosis and lacked confidence in their own communication skills. The Phase 1 data confirmed that the nurses experienced much stress when dealing with relatives in the hospital and that they themselves had significant unmet needs for support.

Research into practice

The effect of the intervention was to dismantle some of these barriers in quite fundamental ways. When the relatives' feelings and experiences were illuminated through the Phase 1 data and were presented back to the nurses, this had a truly galvanising effect. The impact of the data, and the experiential communication workshop that followed, caused the nurses to re-evaluate their own communication skills and reassess their potential to change aspects of the environment of care and the way that they practised. This allowed the nurses to reappraise the threat that family-focused care presented. As a result, new coping possibilities emerged and their personal comfort in their role increased. Nurses now routinely initiated the approach to relatives, they adopted the 'named nurse' approach, thus ensuring that continuity of contact was offered. In this more relaxed climate, nurse–relative dialogue flourished and warmer relationships were established. Phase 2 data from both relatives and nurses confirmed a reduction in the level of reported stress in both relatives and nurses.

The transactional nature of coping

The crucial importance of providing a private area where relatives could rest and receive information and support from staff was revealed in both the nurses' and the relatives' accounts. There was evidence to suggest that such a facility not only supports the relatives during an emotionally intense experience but also acts as a potent coping resource for nurses. When nurses were able to offer such amenities to the relatives this gave them significant satisfaction, and they were also able to communicate with families within an appropriate environment. The nurses reported a reduction in their stress and in the use of distancing behaviours; they also reported enhanced and warmer communications with relatives.

This study confirmed that a comfortable and private room designated for relatives' use represents a crucial coping resource for both relatives and staff and has significant potential to enhance the quality of care and communication during terminal illness. Furthermore, when the crucial areas of communication and facilities were improved and nurses felt better able to deliver high-quality care, the positive feedback that this generated provided the impetus needed to implement improvements in other areas of family care and support.

Dynamic relationship of denial and hope

Another compelling message from this study relates to the dynamic characteristics of denial and hope. Denial, often viewed as a rather negative concept, can operate as an important coping strategy that most individuals

Continued

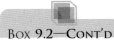

Box 9.2—Cont'd

employ in fluctuating measure and with considerable insight in the time leading up to the death of a loved one. From the interviews it was clear that, for some patients and families, to mutually and openly acknowledge the imminence of death can require a shift within the family relationship that is of such profound significance that for some it represents a step beyond what they can contemplate. For such families, while there might be tacit acknowledgement of the reality of death, mutual pretence continues to the end. In these circumstances, nurses should respect the family's choices, while being available to facilitate dialogue if that is what is wanted. In other families, where open disclosure of the prognosis is preferred, nurses must be very sensitive to the needs of the now grieving patient and family, with all the implications this has for their need for privacy, support and comfort.

remained very poor it had stabilised somewhat. The text below represents the dialogue that took place when Jan was asked about her experiences while in the ward and during her overnight stays.

Researcher: *How often are you visiting at the moment, Jan?*

Jan: *I'm here more or less all of the time. Ken [the patient's partner] and I are taking it turn about to stay overnight. I try to be here as much as possible. I've been off work all last week, but I intend going back tomorrow morning. I'll stay overnight and then go to work straight from here tomorrow. I'm a schoolteacher and I've got classes and they [the pupils] are only a few weeks away from exams. Even if it's only for a couple of hours I'll go in to school to take some classes. The head teacher and all the rest of the staff are very helpful and understanding. I can come and go as I please. But I do feel that I want to go in. And I know that I can get back here quickly if I need to. Next week I intend to come backwards and forwards [to the hospital] and go in to work in between.*

Researcher: *When you are here in the ward, how welcome and comfortable do you feel?*

Jan: *I feel very very welcome and very comfortable. The surroundings are pleasant and the nurses are all very cheerful and understanding. They can't do enough for you.*

Researcher: *What are they doing that you find so helpful?*

Jan: *Well, they [the nurses] are talking to me. They are asking me how my mum is and asking how I am. I would say over the past few days I feel that they are concentrating more on me – well, maybe not more on me, but just as much on me and my wellbeing as caring for my mother. They're excellent.*

Researcher: *How comfortable were you when you stayed overnight?*

Jan: *Very comfortable. As long as my mother is settled and sleeps through the whole night, I can sleep through the whole night as well. I am sleeping on a Z-bed in beside her. Right in beside her, next to her bed. My husband and I have obviously talked about my mother's condition and we are both pretty aware that the majority of people die through the night and I would just hate her to be alone. I feel better knowing that I can be here through the night.*

Comment and analysis

Jan offers a 'typical' example of many female relatives in that she is faced with the competing demands of children, work and a dying relative. The second paragraph in the exemplar reveals Jan's inner conflict as she tries to respond to the rival claims that are being made on her.

Jan drew on a number of coping resources to help her deal with these difficulties. As her husband worked from home, this relieved her of some of the worry associated with the home and children. She also enjoyed a supportive relationship with her husband that proved crucial to her coping efforts. Jan was a professional woman who enjoyed a fair degree of autonomy and could rely on supportive relationships at work. She had the security of knowing that she need not fear for her job. Nevertheless, her commitment created a degree of tension that she planned to resolve by combining attendance at work and hospital. Jan's network of social support confirms findings that middle class, well-educated people have better access to coping resources and can therefore employ more efficacious (problem-focused) coping strategies (Pearlin & Schooler 1978).

Jan's experiences reflected the emotional climate in the ward and the ward environment. She felt comfortable and accepted in the ward and describes how the nurses talked to her and showed concern for her wellbeing. A connection had been established between Jan and the nurses, causing her to say 'I feel secure', thus confirming the nurturing potential of such relationships. In that ward climate Jan was also free from concerns about feeling 'a nuisance' or 'in the way'.

Facilities provided for Jan's comfort during her long vigil helped her to cope with the situation. She describes feeling rested and comfortable, which contrasts with the overwhelming exhaustion reported by many relatives. The support Jan derived from being physically close to her mother is also evident as she repeats the phrase 'I'm right in beside her'. Reports that relatives derive support from being accommodated close to their dying loved one have emerged in this study and in the literature (Hull 1989).

While facilities for physical comfort such as a bed, a room to rest in and regular refreshments represent 'palliative' measures, the support that they provided strengthened this relative's coping efforts when coping resources were severely taxed. In Jan's case, being able to sleep in comfort alongside her mother relieved her stress and ensured that she was sufficiently rested to resume her professional commitments. For Jan these interventions facilitated the use of problem-focused coping strategies.

By facilitating close contact between the dying patient and family in these final days, the potential to reduce future regret was optimised. Jan sums up her feelings thus: 'I would just hate her to be alone. I feel better knowing that I can be here.'

EVALUATION OF FAMILY-FOCUSED CARE

Evaluation of family focused care must be an ongoing process that is individualised for that family, is collaborative in approach and involves the patient and family. Asking the family what has been most or least helpful can empower patients and families to have an input into their care. Reviewing progress with the family, such as a distressing symptom brought under control or improvements in communication, can reduce powerlessness and build the family's confidence in the care. Affirming the patient's and family members' worth in appropriate and respectful ways also forms part of the evaluation process. Forward planning is part of the evaluation cycle and allows active input by the family to future goals of care, thus increasing the patient's and family members' feelings of security and control.

IMPLICATIONS FOR FUTURE PRACTICE

The challenge for health-care professionals is to display sensitivity to the diverse culturally derived needs of families in our care. This is vital within the practice of palliative care.

Yates (1999) challenges us to tap into the rich source of 'lay knowledge' that exists within families. This author reminds us that health professionals only get to glimpse what close family members know, in great detail, about the patient's context and private world with all its tacit understandings and meanings. Nurses are also challenged to acknowledge that their 'scientific knowledge' is in no way superior to the 'lay knowledge' of the patient's family (Yates 1999). The implications for professional practice are that traditional approaches to providing family support now need to be reviewed as truly family-focused care requires:

- Critical self-reflection on the part of nurses to improve their understanding of the constraints that operate in provision of family-focused care

- Advanced communication skills to support the families in their search for meaning in the devastating circumstances that they face
- A broader social and political agenda to support the changes that are needed in service delivery (Yates 1999).

Mutual respect is fundamental to family-focused care. This requires sensitive communication and influencing skills, and the ability to manage conflict and promote agreement when dealing with families. Health professionals need to be prepared to remove the power differential that can operate in health care by establishing a climate of collaboration and equality when working with the family (McIntyre 2000, Whyte 1999).

APPENDIX 9.1: SUPPORT FOR THE DYING PATIENT'S FAMILY IN HOSPITAL – PROPOSED FRAMEWORK FOR WARD AUDIT

Relatives' communication with nursing staff

- Do nursing staff initiate and then regularly maintain contact with relatives for communication and emotional support?
- Is a private area available where relatives can receive information and support?
- Do relatives have access to a named nurse during each duty span?
- Do relatives receive a daily update from nurses on the condition and care of their loved one?

Relatives' communication with medical staff

- Are relatives able to meet with an appropriate member of the medical staff for information and advice and are such meetings either spontaneously provided or arranged within 24 hours of the relatives' request?

Facilities for privacy, comfort and rest

- Are dying patients and their relatives cared for in a single room if desired?
- Is there an area for relatives to have periods of rest away from the bedside?
- When staying overnight at the bedside are facilities such as a folding bed or recliner chair and blankets offered to enable relatives to rest?
- Are regular refreshments provided or made available?
- Do relatives have convenient access to toilet and washing facilities?

Social and spiritual support

- Where appropriate are relatives referred to the hospital social worker for financial or other advice?

- Around the time of the patient's death:
  - Are relatives comforted within a private setting by a member of staff who is known to the family?
  - Is information about spiritual advisors and death registration procedures provided if this is required?
  - Are the patient's belongings returned in a sensitive, appropriate manner?

Interprofessional communication

To facilitate coordinated multidisciplinary family support:

- Do measures/procedures exist to ensure that nurses are made aware of the family's knowledge about and acceptance of the prognosis?
- Is a nurse present when relatives receive information about their loved one's prognosis?
- Are referrals and meetings with other members of the care team (and their outcomes) recorded and accessible to nursing staff?
- Are members of the care team given opportunities to attend courses or study days on care of the dying and bereaved and on aspects of communication and counselling?

Source: Based on findings from McIntyre 2002.

APPENDIX 9.2: STANDARD FOR FAMILY SUPPORT IN HOSPITAL

Standard reference: REN 3 S
Topic: Terminal nursing care
Subtopic: Care of relatives
Care group: Relatives of terminally ill patients
Standard statement: Relatives/significant others of terminally ill patients will be offered the maximum physical, psychological and spiritual support during the terminal stages of the patient's illness

Structure	Process	Outcome
Facilities for comfort and privacy		
The Unit can offer: S.I A private room designed specifically for relatives' use	The nurse will undertake to: P.I Maintain the room and equipment in a clean, comfortable condition	O.I Relatives have access to a designated room within which their needs for privacy and support can be met
S.2 Provision of furniture to enable relatives to rest during the day and night in comfort and privacy	P.2 Inform relatives of their access to: • the relatives' room • facilities for rest during the day and night	O.2 All members of the multidisciplinary team are aware of the range of facilities in the unit and will utilise these as required
S.3 Facilities for making refreshments	• facilities for making tea and coffee	O.3 Relatives of dying persons can obtain rest, sleep and refreshments in a private area that is close to the patient
S.4 A reclining chair or Z-bed for relatives who wish to stay overnight at the bedside	P.4 Provide a reclining chair for relatives who wish to stay overnight at the bedside	O.4 Relatives who wish to stay overnight can rest in a recliner chair
S.5a Access to a phone, shops and facilities for obtaining meals in the canteen S.5b Access to toilet and washing machine facilities	P.5a Offer relatives directions to the shops, telephone and canteen P.5b Direct relatives to toilets and washing facilities	O.5 Relatives know the layout of the hospital and can locate: • telephone and shops • the hospital canteen • toilet and washing facilities

Continued

APPENDIX 9.2: STANDARD FOR FAMILY SUPPORT IN HOSPITAL—CONT'D

Staff–relative communication

S.6 A private area is available where members of the staff and care team can provide information/offer counselling to relatives	P.6 Relatives are made comfortable in the relatives' room prior to receiving information or having discussions with members of the care team	O.6 Relatives receive information and counselling within a private, appropriate setting
S.7 Agreed procedures exist to enable a nurse to be present when the relatives receive new information	P.7 Nursing and medical staff communicate prior to meetings to enable a nurse to be present when new information is given to relatives	O.7 Both medical and nursing staff are fully aware of relatives' current knowledge and acceptance of the prognosis and treatment
S.8 A record of multidisciplinary referrals and outcomes is available	P.8 The nurse will record multidisciplinary meetings, referrals and outcomes in the nursing notes	O.8 Staff involved in family support have access to a current record of referrals and outcomes

Social and spiritual support

S.9 A social worker is available to relatives who need specific help and advice	P.9 The nurse will, in discussions with relatives, establish their need for access to the social worker and arrange appointments as required	O.9 Relatives are able to express their socioeconomic needs and to have support and advice from a social worker
An information folder is available at the nurses' station that contains: S.10 A list of contact numbers for spiritual advisors	P.10 The nurse will maintain and update the list of spiritual advisors and will make this information available to relatives	O.10 Relatives receive spiritual support in accordance with their wishes and needs

Structure	Process	Outcome
S.11 Information about transport, i.e. bus and train timetables and taxi phone numbers	P.11 The nurse will offer information about transport times and phone numbers and will update this information as required	O.11 Relatives can travel to the hospital with the minimum delay and inconvenience

Support and information around the time of death

Structure	Process	Outcome
S.12 The information folder contains guidelines that include policy and procedures and detail the responsibilities of nursing staff around the time of death	P.12 The nurse will maintain and update the GGHB guidelines file and ensure that ward nursing staff are aware of its location	O.12 Nursing staff are aware of the policies and procedures to follow to enable them to support relatives at the time of death
S.13 An information booklet is available to newly bereaved relatives	P.13 Following the patient's death the nurse will take the family to the relatives' room and will	O.13 Newly bereaved relatives are able to express their grief within a sensitive private setting and are offered comfort, support and information
S.14 A nurse known to the family will be available to offer comfort, support and information around the time of death	• offer comfort and sympathy • provide verbal guidance about what the relatives need to do following the death • provide written guidance if needed P.14 The nurse will use sensitive questioning to check that the relatives have understood the information that has been given	O.14 Relatives are clear about what they need to do following the patient's death

EVALUATION OF CLINICAL STANDARD

Use a fresh sheet for each family   Standard applied to the family of _____

Topic: Terminal nursing care   **Subtopic:** Care of relatives

Standard statement: Relatives/significant others of terminally ill patients will be offered the maximum physical, psychological and spiritual support during the terminal stages of the patient's illness

Care group: Relatives of terminally ill patients in _____

S/P/P No.	Criterion (worded in question form)	Measured by	Achieved Yes No	Date	Signed	Comments
	Is the Unit able to offer:					
S.1	a clean private area for the use of relatives?	Observing				
S.2	facilities for rest and sleep?	Observing				
S.3	access to refreshments?	Observing				
	Is the following information available within the Unit:					
S.10	an update of religious advisors?	Asking and records				
S.11	information about transport	Asking				

		Method
S.12	a list of guidelines, including policy, detailing the responsibilities of the nurse following the patient's death?	Observing and asking
O.6	Did relatives receive information and counselling within a private, sensitive setting	Observing and records
P.7	Were nurses present at meetings when information was being relayed to relatives?	Observing and records
O.8	Does a record exist of meetings, referrals and their outcomes?	Observing and records
O.13	Were relatives able to express their grief and offered support and information within a private, non-clinical setting?	Observing and records
P.14	On sensitive questioning – were relatives clear about what they needed to do following the death of the patient?	Asking

From McIntyre 2002.

REFERENCES

Allmond B W Jr, Buckman W, Gofman H F 1979 The family is the patient. C V Mosby, St Louis, MO

Baggaley S 1997 The family. Images, definitions and development. Explorations in family nursing. Routledge, New York

Bailley R, Clarke M 1989 Stress and coping in nursing. Chapman & Hall, London

Chaplin J, McIntyre R 2001 Hope: a selected review of the literature. In: Kinghorn S, Gamlin R (eds) Palliative care: bringing comfort and hope. Harcourt Brace, Edinburgh

Department of Health 1999 Caring about carers: a national strategy for carers. HMSO, London

Eriksson E, Somer S, Lauri S 2001 How relatives adjust after the death of a patient with cancer in a hospice. Cancer Nursing 24:436–444

Folkman S 1997 Positive psychological states and coping with severe stress. Social Science and Medicine 45:1207–1221

Garry J, Arthur A 2001 Informal caring in late life: a qualitative study of the experiences of older carers. Journal of Advanced Nursing 33:182–189

Glaser B, Strauss A 1965 Awareness of dying. Aldine Press, Chicago, IL

Grant G, Ramcharan P, McGrath M et al 1998 Rewards and gratification amongst caregivers: towards a defined model of caring and coping. Journal of Intellectual Disability Research 42:58–71

Hull M M 1989 Family needs and supportive nursing behaviours during terminal cancer: a review. Oncology Nurses Forum 16:787–792

Kissane W, Bloch S 2002 Family focused grief therapy: a model of family centred care during palliative care and bereavement. Open University Press, Buckingham

Kristjanson L, Ashcroft T 1994 The family's cancer journey: a literature review. Cancer Nursing 17:1–17

Lazarus R, Folkman S 1984 Stress, appraisal and coping. Springer, New York

Lugton J 1997 The nature of social support as experienced by women treated for breast cancer. Journal of Advanced Nursing 25:1184–1191

McCormack P 1997 Families in transition: a community nursing perspective. Routledge, London, p 191–203

McIntyre R 2000 Diabetes. In: Alexander M, Fawcet J, Runcimaan P (eds) Nursing practice, hospital and home: the adult. Churchill Livingstone, Edinburgh

McIntyre R 2002 Nursing support for families of dying patients. Whurr, London

McIntyre R, Chapman J 2001 Hope: the heart of palliative care. In: Kinghorn S, Gamlin R (eds) Palliative care: bringing comfort and hope. Harcourt Brace, Edinburgh

Magni G, Silvestro A, Tamiello M et al 1988 An integrated approach to the assessment of family adjustment to acute lymphocytic leukemia in children. Acta Psychiatrica Scandinavica 78:639–642

Nolan M, Keady J, Grant G 1995 Developing a typology of family care: implications for nurses and other service providers. Journal of Advanced Nursing 21:256–265

Parkes C M 2002 Grief: lessons from the past, visions for the future. Death Studies 26:367–385

Pearlin L, Schooler C 1978 The structure of coping. Journal of Health and Social Behaviour 19:2–21

Pittman F 1988 Family crises: expectable and unexpectable. Family transitions: continuity and change over the life cycle. Guilford Press London

Ramirez A, Addington-Hall J, Richards M 1998 ABC of palliative care: the carers. British Medical Journal 316:208–211

Robinson S 1992 The family with cancer. European Journal of Cancer Care 1:29–33

Seale C 1993 Changes in death and dying: the past 25 years. Critical Public Health 4:4–11

Shea T, Kendrick K 1995 With velvet gloves: the ethics of collusion. Palliative Care Today 4:9–10

Shyu Y I L 2000 Patterns of care-giving when family caregivers face competing needs. Journal of Advanced Nursing 31:35–43

Skynner R (1976) One flesh, separate person. Constable, London

Smith N A, Ley P, Seale J P, Shaw J 1987 Health beliefs, satisfaction, and compliance. Patient Education and Counseling 10:279–286

Steptoe A, Sutcliffe I, Allen B, Coombes C 1991 Satisfaction with communication, medical knowledge, and coping style in patients with metastatic cancer. Social Science and Medicine 32:627–632

Thoits P A 1987 Gender and marital status differences in control and distress: common stress versus unique stress explanations. Journal of Health and Social Behaviour 28:7–22

Thomas C, Morris S M, Harman J C 2002 Companions through cancer: the care given by informal carers in cancer contexts. Social Science and Medicine 54:529–544

Twigg J, Atkin K 1994 Carers perceived: policy and practice in informal care. Open University Press, Buckingham

Whyte D 1997 Explorations in family nursing. Routledge, London

Wilhelm K, Parker G, Hadzi-Pavlovic D 1997 Fifteen years on: evolving ideas in researching sex differences in depression. Psychological Medicine 27:875–883

Wright L, Leahey M 2000 Nurses and families. F A Davis, Philadelphia, PA

Yates P 1999 Family coping: issues and challenges for cancer nursing. Cancer Nursing 22:63–71

Yeh C H 2002 Gender differences of parental distress in children with cancer. Journal of Advanced Nursing 38:598–606

CHAPTER TEN

Living with loss

Shaun Kinghorn, Fran Duncan

CONTENTS

INTRODUCTION

Contemporary palliative care includes the total care of patients and families confronted by disease that is no longer responsive to curative treatments, and bereavement support following the patient's death. Loss is an integral component of the human experience. Living with loss is therefore a constant companion for those patients and carers confronted by a life-threatening illness. Ellershaw & Ward (2003) remind us that the impact of death is often underestimated. Living with loss is of course not limited to the time beyond the death of a patient but is a journey that starts at diagnosis. The disease process is often accompanied by a range of losses, which can include loss of mobility, loss of self-esteem, loss of hope and loss of a sense of future to name but a few. The impact of these losses is exacerbated by the anticipation of future losses and ultimately death itself.

Developing the skills to help patients and carers to live with loss is fundamental to palliative care and requires the sensitive support of the multiprofessional team (Payne 2001). As palliative care has moved into a new millennium, public expectations have risen and it is now expected that health-care professionals will provide support during bereavement. This need is also underscored in palliative care strategy (National Institute for Clinical Excellence 2004) and includes helping patients deal with incremental loss prior to their death.

To meet these needs, health professionals working within the statutory and voluntary sectors are increasingly being encouraged to pool their resources and skills to provide services that respond to the needs of our multicultural society. Today, palliative care professionals need the skills to demonstrate empathic understanding of the needs of those who are experiencing loss. They must also be able to integrate knowledge and understanding of loss and grief theories and models and the best available evidence in this area.

Health professionals are not immune from the impact of loss and those who support patients and carers may themselves require supportive care. Providing staff support represents best practice in palliative care. It should be remembered that caring for those experiencing loss is not the sole domain of qualified health professionals. Indeed the London Bereavement Network standards for bereavement care in the UK (London Bereavement Network 2001) report that 80% of bereavement support is provided by the voluntary sector and 90% by volunteers.

AIMS OF THE CHAPTER

The aims of this chapter are to:

- Reaffirm the importance of looking after yourself while engaged in supporting those experiencing loss and grief
- Explore the nature of loss and grief within a palliative care context
- Debate the factors that influence the intensity of the grief response
- Discuss the supportive care needs of those who face bereavement.

A significant proportion of this chapter is devoted to assessment of need in those experiencing loss; this is an intentional focus. An understanding of this is fundamental to ensuring that the right care is given to the right person at the right time and also allows us to appraise whether the individual/family will need additional professional and or volunteer support.

The chapter is framed around the following themes:

- Working with loss – looking after ourselves and supporting each other
- The nature of loss, grief and bereavement
- Making sense of the loss journey
- Working alongside those living with loss
- Supporting those living with loss; some pointers to guide practice.

WORKING WITH LOSS – LOOKING AFTER OURSELVES AND SUPPORTING EACH OTHER

Looking after ourselves and other members of the team underpins the maintenance and development of our psychospiritual health. It is also an essential component of high-quality supportive care of those facing loss. Setch (2001) emphasises the fact that organisations and individuals have a joint responsibility to help develop effective coping strategies. Bereavement care involves caring for others but it also demands personal vigilance as to our own skills and emotional/spiritual capacity to deal with patients' and carers' losses. Our capacity to develop a helping relationship with patients and carers demands self-awareness and a continual investment in our own physical, psychological, social and spiritual wellbeing. This self-awareness needs to give due consideration to:

- Recognising our personal boundaries
- Recognising our own experience and limitations in managing difficult situations
- Providing support/supervision to multidisciplinary staff involved in working with those experiencing loss.

Wakefield (2000) conducted a study within the context of residential care where it was noted that the death of a patient arouses feelings of loss in the nurses. Such reactions are of course not unique to the residential care settings and such feelings of loss may be repressed or muted. Boyle & Carter (1998) also suggest that nurses working with dying patients and the bereaved may experience a variety of feelings, including unease, discomfort and lack of control. In the drive to deliver personalised care nurses are encouraged to get to know patients and relatives from a holistic point of view. It is therefore inevitable that we get to know them and all their hopes and fears.

Costello (1999), reporting on a study of anticipatory grief, suggests that listening is central to our understanding of what the patient and family are experiencing. However, this is not always easy. In a paper focusing on a critical incident involving a difficult relationship with the patient's wife, Pullen (2002, p. 488) concluded that 'it is not surprising that many nurses feel physically and emotionally drained at the end of a span of duty'. Pullen suggest that the steep learning curve that occurs in such situations offers both a daunting challenge to the nurse and the potential to enrich personal and professional wellbeing.

Saunderson & Ridsdale (1999) studied 25 GPs' beliefs and attitudes and how they had responded to death and bereavement. Almost all the doctors reported that they had felt guilty about issues relating to the death of particular patients because of their expectations of themselves in terms of not making mistakes and in diagnostic precision. The GPs also reported that they had felt bereaved by the death of well-known patients and in some instances felt the need to grieve and express emotion.

The notion that nurses 'grieve too' is highlighted in an illuminating study by McIntyre (2002) that examined nursing support for families of dying patients. The study involved interviews with relatives of dying patients and further interviews with 16 nursing staff from eight wards. The impact of caring for the dying and their relatives is graphically illustrated by the following quotes:

You get involved with the patient and involved with their relatives and you start getting to know them. . . . And they get to know you. . . . And it all becomes so painful and hard.

McIntyre 2002, p. 113

A few weeks ago we had a young 24-year-old die in the ward. That was the most difficult thing I have ever had to deal with in my whole career. It was hard watching her mother and her two brothers suffer. I couldn't switch myself from that.

McIntyre 2002, p. 113

I couldn't even speak to my husband about it because I was so upset. And he hadn't a clue what was wrong with me. He kept saying you'll have to tell me. . . so he could help me. I was like this [weeping]. The worst part of it was I was going on holiday the next day. She died the next morning. . . and I was going on holiday.

McIntyre 2002, p. 114

Such powerful experiences may resonate with your own experiences in caring for the dying, so it is important that, when engaged in delivering palliative care, 'looking after yourself' is a prerequisite of good practice and is enabling in sustaining your capacity to support those living with loss. Reflecting on the following questions with a colleague may help develop your approach to support.

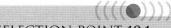

REFLECTION POINT 10.1

Supporting the bereaved – looking after yourself

Reflect on your past experience of caring for someone experiencing loss and use the following questions to guide your reflection. It might help to discuss the questions and your responses with a trusted colleague.

- How do I feel and react with people who are displaying very strong emotions as a result of bereavement?

- Is handling loss, grief and bereavement an everyday occurrence in my work?

- What are my spiritual beliefs around life and death?

- How do I show my feelings following the death of a patient?

- Who do I share my feelings with following the death of patients?

- Do I always know when I need support?

- Do I know where in my workplace to seek effective support?

- Do I know when to refer problems on to another member of the multidisciplinary team?

There are no right or wrong answers to these questions but they will help to nurture self-awareness, which is key to being able to cope with the very real stresses of working in this field. Improving your communication and listening skills will also ensure your efficacy in this work.

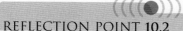

REFLECTION POINT 10.2

Organisational support

Think about your work setting and consider the following questions:

- Is there a system of clinical supervision or support in the place where you work?

- Can staff be referred on to agencies outside the organisation for additional support if required?

- Are there opportunities to review critical incidents that might arise when working with those who face loss and bereavement?

- Are ongoing programmes of education and training available?

- Are mechanisms in place to allow the referral of complex situations?

Multidisciplinary teamworking is fundamental to providing holistic palliative care. As a nurse in this team you are the one providing continuity for the patient, the family and the professional team. It is therefore crucial to understand the roles of each team member so that their skills can be utilised for the optimum benefit of the patient, family and carers. When a team works well together team members will share relevant information, problem solve, make decisions and debrief about challenging situations. Reflection and evaluation will ensure good practice and will nurture and sustain a supportive climate. It is also important to share successes within the team and have a sense of humour, as this can discharge tension, allow expression of feelings and ease pressure. The patient and family are living with their unique loss but the multidisciplinary team are living with and working with many losses. Looking after each other and ourselves is therefore a central plank of high-quality bereavement care.

THE NATURE OF LOSS, GRIEF AND BEREAVEMENT

A wide range of theories and perspectives will confront those studying loss, grief and bereavement. The terms loss, grief and bereavement are often used synonymously. According to Ringdal et al (2001) *grief* is a normal affective response to an overwhelming loss, whether in the form of a child, parent or spouse, and does not always require a therapeutic intervention if it runs an uncomplicated course. Grief is characterised by a wide range of reactions, which are manifest by alterations in thought processes, behaviour and emotions. The problem for practitioners is that not all people express every aspect of grief and individual expressions of grief are dependent on personality, cultural background, previous experience of loss and support network.

Reimers (2001) describes *bereavement* as the objective state of loss and *grief* as the emotions that accompany this loss. Factors that affect the process of grieving have been described as (1) the urge to look back, (2) the urge to cry and search for what is lost and (3) the conflicting urge to look forward and discover what can be carried forward from the past. Overlying these are social and cultural pressures that influence how the urges are expressed or inhibited. The strength of these urges can vary and change over time, giving rise to constantly changing reactions (Parkes 1998).

As patients are put in the picture regarding their illness and prognosis, anticipatory grief becomes prominent and they may experience loss arising from visualising their husband or wife coping with out them. Costello (1999) confirms that, in advance of the bereavement itself, loved ones may also experience premature grief.

Walter (1999) suggests that bereavement care is an umbrella term that covers the services to support the bereaved and the philosophy of care that underpins how those services operate. Those engaged in bereavement care need a fundamental understanding of the interrelationship between loss, grief and bereavement in order to deliver empathic and effective bereavement care. Wendell-Moller (1996) sheds some light on the relationship between grief and bereavement, suggesting that bereavement is an essential component of grief and that grief is an intense emotional response to bereavement that involves sorrow and suffering.

Mourning is yet another term; it includes the rituals and practices that help us grieve and represent observable expressions of grief. Kalish (1985, cited in Anstey & Lewis 2001) reminds us of the inevitability of bereavement by suggesting that 'Anything you can have you can lose; anything you are attached to you can be separated from; anything you can love can be taken away from you; yet if you really have nothing to lose, you have nothing' (Anstey & Lewis 2001, p. 147).

Those patients who are confronted by a life-threatening illness may experience a myriad forms of loss, resulting from the disease, treatment process and life events, which simultaneously occur throughout their illness journey.

MODELS OF LOSS AND GRIEF

The last 60 years have seen a proliferation of theories designed to make sense of the complex processes of loss and grief through the development of models of loss and grief. Greenstreet (2004) argues that a critical appreciation of theory can promote confidence in providing bereavement support. Hale (1996) also suggests that many models can provide guidelines for practice. It is beyond the scope of this chapter to provide a detailed review of all of the available models, but an overview of the key elements of a selection of models is offered in Box 10.1.

Box 10.1

Brief summary of models of grief and bereavement

Kubler-Ross (1969)

- Anger

- Denial

- Bargaining

- Acceptance

Worden (1991)

- Accept the reality of the loss

- Work through the pain of grief

- Adjust to life without the deceased

- Emotionally re-locate the deceased and move on with life

Stroebe (1998)

- Dual process model of coping with grief

- Bereaved people oscillate between *loss-oriented* and *restoration-oriented* ways of coping – a person who swings from one to the other would be deemed to be coping 'normally'

- **Loss-orientation** dominates the initial phase of grieving and incorporates traditional theories of grief with breaking bonds/ties, intrusion of grief, denial/avoidance of restoration changes

- **Restoration-orientation** is when the bereaved attend to life changes; adapting to new situations; distraction is acceptable as is denial/avoidance of grief at times; take on new roles; identities and relationships

- **Oscillation** – key construct of this model – the bereaved move between loss and restoration orientations, starting initially in loss orientation and swinging gradually into the restoration mode: key triggers initiating a swing back into loss may be anniversaries or sensory triggers, e.g. smells; music

Continued

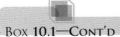

Box 10.1—Cont'd

- No time scale to this model
- Difference between the grieving of men and women – women confront their emotions more, whereas men attend to the practical tasks of bereavement

Bowlby (1980)
- Numbness
- Yearning and searching
- Disorganisation and support
- Reorganisation

Parkes (1986)
- Shock and alarm
- Searching
- Anger and guilt
- Gaining a new identity

Klass & Silverman (Klass et al 1997)
- Understanding of grief covers losses other than death, e.g. infertility, divorce
- It is normal for the bereaved to maintain a connection with the deceased that is not static
- The bereaved construct an inner representation of the deceased; the relationship diminishes but does not disappear
- Emphasis is on negotiating and renegotiating the measuring of loss over time
- Accommodation occurs rather than recovery, closure or resolution, i.e. the continual activity of seeking the meaning of the place of the deceased in the survivor's life and sense of self.

This application of guidelines and models may be taken to extremes by suggesting that care should be delivered in a prescriptive manner. Nevertheless, these models do provide a dynamic picture, charting the evolution of stage-based models which suggest that the individual will systematically work through tasks and stages in order to arrive at a state of reorganisation. More recent models, such as that of Stroebe (1998), suggest that there are gender differences in the way we grieve and that bereaved individuals can be engaged in oscillation between the 'new' post-death lifestyle and being reimmersed in the experience of grief in its many guises. These models offer frameworks to guide how we interact with patients and families. However, as practitioners we don't have to stick to one model. In practice we draw upon different elements of each model to guide our practice. Box 10.1 represents the evolution of stage-based models, for example that of Kubler-Ross (1969), through to more dynamic approaches, such as that of Stroebe (1998).

MAKING SENSE OF THE LOSS JOURNEY

Sherwood et al (2004), in a qualitative study of 43 caregivers of patients with brain tumours, provided some moving insights into the loss journey. As one participant explained, the grieving process started while the patient was alive – 'I lost him in stages, so our grief was in stages'; another noted looking back on the experience of care giving – 'I had all these empty hours that used to be spent caring for him'. Another caregiver spoke of entering the grieving process as the hardest period of your life, totally exhausted, suffering from flashbacks and still having to make decisions. The following case will illustrate that the web of grief extends beyond the immediate family.

CASE STUDY 10.1
Helen and her family

Helen, aged 35, was diagnosed with breast cancer 6 months ago. She had noticed a lump before Christmas but had delayed seeking medical help because she was so busy with her family's catering business over the festive season. Her GP immediately referred Helen to the hospital, where she had a mastectomy followed by chemotherapy. There was also evidence of spread in her lymph glands. There is a family history of breast cancer and Helen's aunt and grandmother have both died in the last 5 years with the same diagnosis.

Helen is married to Dave, aged 39, and lives with her three children – Peter (14), Joanne (11) and Gemma (7) – in a three-bedroomed semi-detached house in a small town in the north-east of England where she has lived all her life. Helen's parents, Jean and Jim, live nearby and she is particularly close to her 30-year-old brother John, who has learning difficulties. Her in-laws also live nearby but Helen has a fraught relationship with her mother-in-law Mary, whom she sees as interfering. At times this causes stress within the marital relationship. Helen works part-time as the bookkeeper in her husband's catering business, which he runs with his father, Tom, and 37-year-old brother, Bill.

Figure 10.1 is a genogram representing Helen's immediate family members, all of whom are alive.

The couple were shocked by the diagnosis and Helen's initial reaction was one of being practical and of organising her family while she was to be in hospital. She was keen to be told all the details of her diagnosis and treatment, while Dave shied away from this. He wanted to be there practically for his wife and family but found it difficult to talk about what was happening. There was also a difference of opinion about what the children

Continued

should be told. Helen believed in being open with them about her illness while Dave and his mother wanted to shield them from the exact nature and implications of it. Helen's parents have been very supportive, as has her close friend, Sarah. All are frequent visitors and offer Dave and the children practical support.

Now Helen is struggling to cope both physically and emotionally with the changes that her deteriorating condition have wrought in her. She is constantly fatigued and nauseated and trying to cope with the day-to-day demands of running a home is too much for her. She has not worked in the family business for some time and is worried about 'the books'. Dave is trying to run the business and look after Helen and the children but he finds that his relationship with Helen is becoming increasingly strained. She is shutting him out and appears depressed when she cannot do even the simplest of household tasks. She is short-tempered with the children, whose understanding of her illness varies.

The situation with their mother is starting to impact on the children. Peter is staying out with his friends more and more and is at times rude and verbally abusive to Helen; Joanne is constantly hanging around her mother wanting to help as much as she can; and Gemma has started to misbehave at school, in that she has been fighting in the playground.

Helen's prognosis is poor, as the cancer has metastasised to her brain, and she is aware of this. Her initial, practical open style of coping has been replaced by a withdrawn, frightened response as she struggles to cope with the increasing uncertainty and gravity of her illness. She knows that she is going to die but is uncertain of the timescale.

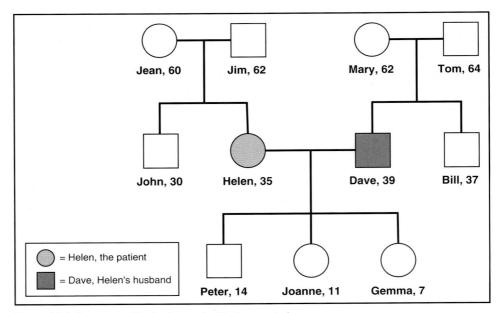

Figure 10.1 Genogram of the family described in the case study.

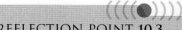

REFLECTION POINT 10.3

Supporting Helen and her family

- As the nurse working with Helen where would you start?

- What losses would Helen and her family have had to cope with?

- Whose needs and what would have to take priority?

- Who else might be involved to support Helen and her family?

- What coping strategies might Helen and her family use as they attempt to cope with the prospect of Helen dying in the near future?

BRIEF ANALYSIS OF THE CASE STUDY

The following résumé sets out the loss journey from the perspectives of various family members. These losses may be social, physical, spiritual and psychological. At first glance the unravelling of this case study may be overwhelming but by taking a careful look at the situation from the varying perspectives the cumulative life effects of living with loss should emerge.

HELEN'S LOSSES

There are a number of concurrent interrelated losses that Helen will be trying to process and make sense of. There may also be previous losses that will be reawakened in this situation. The most likely to affect her at this time are the deaths of her grandmother and aunt. She knows that they both died of the same disease that she now has. What does this mean for her?

How did they die? Is Helen aware of the details of their dying process and, if so, is this affecting her ability to cope now? If Helen has not dealt with past losses, they may add significantly to the load that she has to deal with now.

Social losses

From the initial diagnosis Helen will have experienced a sense of loss, not only of her health and physical capacity but also of her ability to function socially in the many roles that she had – as a wife, mother, daughter, daughter-in-law, book-keeper, sister and friend. How do these changes affect her now that she cannot perform as she has been used to doing? What is the impact on Helen and her family?

Physical losses

As she coped with her surgery and subsequent chemotherapy, Helen experienced physical losses, including hair loss and the loss of a breast. These losses would be cumulative the further the disease progressed. Those caring for Helen need to know how she coped with the loss of her breast. What did this do to her sense of her body image? Has it affected her intimate relationship with Dave? What are her feelings about this and about the side effects of the chemotherapy – hair loss, nausea and fatigue?

Psychological losses

In serious illness people experience debilitating symptoms and, as the illness progresses, it reduces horizons; it also reduces independence, choices and control. These are areas in our lives that we tend to take for granted but the impact of their loss can be significant to an individual's sense of wellbeing, self-worth, self-esteem and identity. Helen is also facing the loss of her future. She will not be around for her son's wedding or her daughter's graduation and other significant life events. The plans that she and Dave have made cannot come to fruition.

The psychological changes that occur when living with a range of losses and facing further uncertainties are many. The coping strategies adopted previously may or may not be effective when facing the dying process – something that is a new and lonely experience.

It may be useful to stop at this point to consider:

• How is Helen feeling about the situation she now faces?
• What are her key concerns?
• When she is having difficulty coping with things, how does it show?
• How does she cope on a day-to-day basis?
• Does she seem to have questions that need answering?

In the last 6 months Helen has initially been shocked at the diagnosis; she then took control of the situation and 'got on with it' practically until the illness started to affect her physically. Her existing coping strategies no longer sustain her in the face of worsening symptoms. Now losing control of her choices and with her social roles altering, Helen has coped by withdrawing and becoming depressed and irritable. She is aware that her cancer has spread. She feels that she has no control over her illness or her body's reaction to it. Houghton (2001) suggests that dying patients have an increased awareness of the imminence of death as their condition worsens. It may be difficult for Helen to conceive of what death or the final days of life will be like.

Spiritual losses

We are uncertain from the information we have whether Helen has any specific spiritual beliefs. McNamara (2001) suggests that those who have a strong religious commitment also have more clearly defined beliefs about the meaning of life and death than those without a strong faith. In a similar vein, Neuberger (1999) argues that dying people often have a heightened spiritual awareness. You may have access to other professionals, such as a chaplain or a social worker, who have the necessary skills to assess the patient and her family. Some of Helen's spiritual concerns might cause her to raise the following questions around spiritual issues:

- Why me? Why my family?
- Is our family being punished? (Helen has already had two female members of her family die with the same diagnosis – she may feel 'let down' by any beliefs she has)
- What does this knowledge do to my sense of hope?
- What will happen to my family in the future?
- Will Joanne and Gemma be affected?

As Helen draws close to dying there may be issues she needs to resolve privately or with family members – unfinished business that she needs to attend to.

The difficulty is that the more her condition deteriorates the more challenging it will prove for her to achieve this. There can be no 'action replay' for the dying process and for families the experience can become imprinted in their memories, with the exact details crystallising in their consciousness and informing any future similar experiences.

THE FAMILY/CARERS

In palliative care the responsibility to care for the family and carers is integral to good practice. Often their needs can be more complex than those of the patient, and managing to meet the needs of a diverse family group can prove challenging to the care team. In relation to our case study, what may Helen's family needs involve?

Helen's husband

What are Dave's losses? He faces the ultimate loss of losing his wife. In the last 6 months his losses have been similar to Helen's although he is experiencing them more indirectly than Helen. Duke (1998) identifies the multiple role loss and impact of the diagnosis on partners. Dave has lost his book-keeper for the business, his partner and the practical side of her motherly role. He has gained extra roles through child-care responsibilities, a physically dependent wife and an emotionally distant and troubled partner. Initially, Dave found it difficult to cope with the diagnosis: he used denial and being busy as his coping mechanisms. What are his coping strategies now when the situation is looking rather bleak? Who is going to support him and meet his needs?

Helen's son and eldest child

At 14, Peter has experienced the loss of two close family members through cancer since he was 9. He is also experiencing adolescence, a time of natural turbulence when his body is changing physically and he is trying to work out his identity. For children at this stage it is a time of confusion and rebellion. Peter appears to be dealing with this current crisis by absorbing himself in his peer group, as well as taking out his feelings on his mother. Does he understand what is going on, and that his mother is going to die? Has he had the relevant information he needs?

How does he feel? Does he have anyone to listen to him and give him support?

Helen's older daughter and middle child

Joanne is 11 years old and has lost two relatives since she was 6. She appears to be feeling the need to care for her mother, whose role she seems to be assuming in the household. Why? What does she understand of her mother's situation? What information has she had? How does she get on with her siblings? Who listens to her and gives her support?

Helen's younger daughter

Gemma is 7 years old and the impact of the deaths of her aunt and grandmother since she was 2 may not be so major as with her older brother and sister. However, she is clearly reacting emotionally to the situation as her behaviour at school has deteriorated. Do the school know about Helen's illness? What has Gemma been told? Are the adults protecting her because she is the youngest? Does anyone in the family take the time to talk to her and listen to her concerns?

Helen's parents

Jean and Jim face losing their daughter. This is not the natural order of life. How do they feel? Helpless? Hopeless? How do they cope? Will Helen's mother develop breast cancer too? Are they able to support one another or is the immensity of what is happening causing a rift, as it is with Helen and Dave?

Helen's brother

John is going to lose his sister but what does he understand of her illness? What have his parents and Helen told him? Who does he have to offer him appropriate support?

Helen's parents-in-law

Tom and Mary care deeply for their daughter-in-law but are very worried about Dave's reaction and his ability to cope with her death and afterwards. They want to help but Helen seems to not want them around. How do they feel? How can they support Dave and their grandchildren? What do they do?

Helen's best friend

Sarah has been a close friend of Helen's since primary school and she just wants to stop what is happening. She feels so guilty that she is well and has a future when Helen has a limited one. Sarah is there for her friend and supports Dave with the children. What is your role with Sarah? Can you share information with Sarah as you might with other family members?

SUMMARY

This case study represents one patient and the many people who are close to her, all of different ages and needs, who require support. The interaction and dynamics will vary from day to day and their level of need will also vary. As they face the ultimate loss of Helen through her death, the professionals need to assess the possible vulnerability of the key members and arrange for professional support if it is required. As you can see from the above, the more you consider the patient and their family the more questions present themselves.

Experiencing loss is a normal, natural occurrence that we all face. Living with serious loss affects each individual slightly differently. Many will cope by themselves or with the support of family and friends and without professional intervention. However, for some the sheer 'awfulness' of losing a loved one through death catapults them into an experience that is frightening, painful and lonely, seemingly without end. Some will need professional support and to identify those most vulnerable it is necessary to assess those who are most at risk.

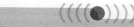

REFLECTION POINT 10.4

Responses to loss

Read the summary of psychological responses (Payne et al 2000) in Box 10.2.

Reflecting on the issues raised in Case study 10.1, which of the responses might apply to Helen's situation?

Considering Helen's case study alongside the model of psychological responses set out in Box 10.2 highlights the significant life changes that occur

Box 10.2

Psychological responses to loss and bereavement (Payne et al 2000)

Emotional

- Depression – loss of pleasure response, low mood, intense distress

- Anxiety – fearfulness, separation anxiety

- Hyper-vigilance – inability to relax

- Anger – may be expressed as hostility to friends, family, health workers or God

- Guilt – feelings of self-blame for some aspect of the deceased's death or care during dying

- Loneliness – feeling of being alone even with others

Continued

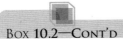

BOX 10.2—CONT'D

Cognitive

- Lack of concentration and attention – memory loss for specific events or general problems in recalling information or attending to new information
- Pre-occupation – repetitive thoughts especially about the deceased, sometimes needing to talk constantly about certain events such as a traumatic loss
- Helplessness/hopelessness – coping response which is characterised by pessimism about the future
- Feeling of distance/detachment – experience a sense of unreality

Behavioural

- Irritability – expression of anger, hospitality, suspiciousness, distrust
- Restlessness – inability to settle to specific tasks or feeling relaxed
- Searching – pacing, looking for the deceased
- Crying – tears, sighing
- Social withdrawal – remaining isolated, rejecting social groups and friendship

as a result of bereavement. These affect not only the ability of the individual to function on a day-to-day basis but also the social networks that are fundamental to high-quality bereavement care.

WORKING ALONGSIDE THOSE LIVING WITH LOSS

Supporting those who face loss or have experienced loss presents one of the most challenging dimensions of palliative care. According to Anstey & Lewis (2001), supporting the bereaved encompasses enabling them to be able to cope with emotions, thoughts and feelings associated with their loss.

According to Anstey & Lewis (2001) bereavement care involves:

- Care of the family
- Information giving and receiving
- Care of the deceased
- Supporting ritual and mourning customs
- Legal and medical interventions
- Future care and support.

The case study of Helen and her family illustrates the complexity of the loss journey and the challenges of supporting the bereaved. We must be acutely aware that the way in which death and the process of dying are perceived varies significantly from culture to culture. The diverse ways in which patients respond to the loss journey is also mediated by individual differences and gender. We believe that it is not appropriate to be prescriptive in this section. Nevertheless, as a general rule bereavement services need to consider the following questions:

- What are the information needs of those living with loss?
- How will the coping abilities of the individual be assessed and documented?
- How can we create a safe environment in which the bereaved can work through their loss?
- In what ways, if any, will the support network of the individual and the family need to be supplemented?
- How should we respond to the difficult and diverse questions posed by the bereaved?
- What are the support and training needs of staff engaged in working with those confronted with loss?
- How will the quality of bereavement services be monitored, evaluated and refined?

While specific principles will underpin how we can support those experiencing loss, a prescriptive approach towards handling loss is counter-productive. Working with loss is not totally congruent with a protocol-driven approach. Therefore, assessing risk, detailed case study review and highlighting the principles of best practice will frame this aspect of the chapter.

ASSESSING BEREAVEMENT

A key task of the team involved in caring for Helen and her family is determining how they are coping at different points in the journey. Assessing those who may be at risk from developing a difficult bereavement experience has been informed by extensive debate and research. The underlying assumption of assessing risk is that it helps us identify those individuals who may not be able to cope in the short, medium and long term following bereavement. Such assessments have become commonplace within a specialist palliative care context and may pre-empt the need for specialist help. Identifying risk is significant for a number of reasons:

- It helps us focus scarce resources on those who may need the help of health-care professionals
- Assessment may help prevent a plethora of physical, psychological, spiritual and social problems, which may persist well beyond the initial bereavement.

Bereavement services are an integral part of palliative care and are accessed by a wide spectrum of individuals who have differing levels of need. Evidence suggests that early intervention can prevent difficult and enduring reactions in bereavement, particularly when targeted towards those deemed more vulnerable or more at risk (Walshe 1997).

Family carers of patients facing a life-threatening illness can often recall experiences when a mother, grandmother, auntie or uncle, neighbour or friend died from a similar illness, and therefore they assume that the illness journey and bereavement experience will be similar. In most instances, individuals are resilient enough to 'get through', while others struggle. What are the factors that help or hinder the person's journey through grief?

The vulnerability of any individual dealing with serious losses can be identified through assessing these factors. Awareness of risk factors is essential if we are to offer focused bereavement interventions to those most in need, who themselves may not ask for help. The needs of both the dying patient and the family should be assessed holistically, taking into account the individual's societal, cultural and spiritual context, personality, age, sexuality and gender. For the patient this may be an ongoing process as they face new losses experienced in the dying process. For the family the risk assessment is often done immediately after the death. By considering the following contextual factors a tentative picture can be formed.

Societal and cultural context

Awareness of societal norms surrounding death will inform any assessment we make. We also need to assess this against the backdrop of the individual's culture and their experience of possible inequality, for instance through being disabled. Diversity occurs in different ethnic groups but also in more subtle ways in different geographical areas. People experiencing multiple social problems (e.g. poverty, poor housing) or who are coping with concurrent social losses (e.g. redundancy, divorce) will be more likely to be at risk. The grief of those living with loss may not be recognised or legitimised by society because of other presenting difficulties and stereotyping.

Personality

Coping strategies, maturity and life experience may all contribute to shaping the individual's ability to cope with bereavement. Poor self-esteem and strong self-blame would predispose someone to risk.

Sexuality

If there is openness, awareness and acceptance of the individual's sexuality then they are more likely to receive support when facing loss. However, if this is not the case there may be extra stress in living with the loss of a close sexual partner that those around them are unaware of.

Gender differences

The gender of the person will contribute to how they cope. Society promotes particular images of men as not openly expressing feelings of distress, whereas it appears to be more acceptable for women to cry and discuss their feelings. Stroebe (1998) discovered that men and women react differently in bereavement. Men tend not to express their feelings, whereas women, who generally have larger social circles, are more likely to. Men may approach their bereavement more practically than women. Statistically, in the first year of their bereavement men are more likely than women to become physically ill, suffer from depression or die.

Age

Death seems to be more normal and acceptable once we have achieved our natural life span of three score years and ten. The impact may still be great but not as universally disruptive as death occurring at a more unnatural, younger age. Parents losing an adult child find it strange that the child will die before them. The loss of a young child may produce an emotional scar that never fully heals. Losing a lifelong partner can be devastating and being older does not necessarily correlate with being accepting and philosophical about death. The important thing to remember is not to make assumptions about people's possible reactions because of their age.

Lack of social support

Does the individual have an effective means of social support? This relates to the availability of a supportive family and community network. You may discover that there are family and friends but you need to check the effectiveness of the support. In 'Helen's situation', Helen apparently has a large social network, but how does it operate? She has in fact isolated herself from her partner. She may be getting emotional support from Sarah or her parents but this is not clear at this stage. Dave, on the other hand has his parents, Sarah and his in-laws for practical support but emotionally he is isolated, as his coping strategy is not to acknowledge his feelings or talk about them. The conflict that exists between Helen and his mother may add to his stress. After Helen's death, will his coping strategies work? He will have family around but they may not be effective in supporting him emotionally. What about the children?

Family conflict is also a risk factor for a negative bereavement outcome. Concurrent social responsibilities add to the risk, as do concurrent social crises such as divorce, redundancy and moving house.

Nature of the relationship

There are likely to be difficulties in the bereavement if:

- The patient and their relative/carer/friend had an ambivalent relationship. If it was a love–hate relationship the bereaved person may experience a confusion of feelings – relief, guilt, anger, resentment – that adds to the grief already being experienced
- There was overdependency on the patient physically, financially or emotionally. The impact of the loss is heightened in this situation, as the bereaved may have no other means of support. Trying to face up to and live with the loss may seem unbearable

- There was an abusive relationship with the deceased – old wounds may be reawakened and add to the risk.

Financial

Financially, are there any major financial stressors such as loss of income or debts? Sometimes the benefits that people are eligible for before death significantly increase their income and their loss after death adds to the stress of managing.

Psychological factors

As noted earlier in this chapter, there are a range of natural expressions of grief. Immediately after the death people may feel numb and shocked. Some have described 'feeling as if they are trapped inside a bubble', with the outside world seeming remote and distant. Some people who have been coping with the dying process over a prolonged period may have experienced anticipatory grief. This is when the grieving process starts before death and the reality of the loss is absorbed over a period of time. The bereaved person will start to 'let go' of the dying person and look to a future without them. In this situation the death itself may be an actual relief and a release. A range of confusing and conflicting feelings may be felt. People may be tearful, anxious, distressed, angry, depressed, guilty, resentful, relieved – some or all of these at some time in the following months after a major loss.

Each day may be different – 'good days and bad days' – with no particular reason for this. Life can assume the pattern of being on a rollercoaster, with the highs and lows that that brings. However, if the person is displaying extreme reactions, for instance if they cannot stop crying, and are unable to function in their daily tasks, they are deemed to be at risk. The key is whether their behaviour is so extreme that it is affecting their ability to function 'normally'. Each person's 'normal' may be different, so it is crucial to assess each individual's social and emotional context objectively and not to make subjective assumptions.

You need to be aware that someone who is not reacting at all may also be at risk. It could be that they are in denial about the loss, for example if a person is carrying on with their life as if their loved one is still alive. If you cannot introduce reality gently into the consciousness of such people, then they need professional help.

It is quite common for bereaved relatives to express suicidal thoughts – 'All I want is to be with him', a wife may say after her husband's death. As a nurse in this situation it is worth checking the level of intent. You can ask: 'Have you ever thought of doing anything about being with him?' If the answer shows detailed, clear intent and planning of the method of suicide, it is important to be concerned and it's important that you get appropriate and urgent psychological and medical help for the bereaved person.

Coexisting mental illness

A history of present or past mental ill health also predisposes an individual to be at risk. The display of serious mental health symptoms such as extreme anxiety/agitation or depression is also a reason to refer to the GP for urgent psychological/psychiatric help.

Alcohol/drug dependence

Overdependence on alcohol or drugs to cope with the loss may be a cause for concern and this is a difficult one to assess as many of us drink socially and may use alcohol as a way to relax. There may be a timescale to this: many people use alcohol in the initial stages of a bereavement, for example to help them to get to sleep or to block out the pain of the loss. You need to assess whether the use of alcohol is affecting the person's 'normal' functioning. However, if this continues over a prolonged period it may be necessary to refer for medical help.

Physical factors

If bereaved people are suffering from a serious illness then they are more likely to be at risk. It is also useful to check the bereaved's level of self-care and sleep pattern. Generally these will be disturbed but if the situation appears to be chronic and disruptive there may be cause for concern; for example they may be suffering from clinical depression, which needs medical intervention.

Spiritual factors

A complete sense of hopelessness and an acute loss of faith may combine to cause a serious depression that could result in a suicide risk. If the relevant rituals and religious practices have not been observed after the death, this may put the bereaved at further risk.

Nature of dying and process of death

Circumstances surrounding the dying process and death may not happen as the family/carers have been lead to expect – for example, it may be a traumatic happening (a sudden bleed). Their hopes around the dying process may not have been fulfilled – they may have wanted to be with the dying person but were unable to be there. Often it is something that has either been done or not done that in retrospect causes distress. People use hindsight a great deal when they are mourning and talk over again and again the circumstances of what has happened – 'If only' and 'I should have' are commonly heard. People often have irrational expectations of themselves in their bereavement, which are unrealistic. Irrational feelings, for instance guilt, can become overwhelming in the bereavement. People feel responsible and blame themselves for things that they consider contributed to the death when in reality nothing would have made any difference. This may be an unconscious way of trying to undo what has happened, as the reality of accepting the finality of death is too much. In assessing a person's vulnerability it is always worth talking through their expectations, experiences and feelings about the dying process and death itself.

HOW DO WE ASSESS BEREAVEMENT?

A number of bereavement assessment tools have been developed from research to help practitioners discern the degree of risk facing an individual. Melliar-Smith (2002) mentions that the aim of risk assessment is to lessen the possible long-term effects of unresolved grief for families and carers through using a systematic assessment. Such frameworks can also act as an educational framework for the multidisciplinary team. Some tools measure vulnerability with a score, others rate it as high, medium or low. Such tools are useful as they are an aide-mémoire when considering the needs of the bereaved and can be a focus for multidisciplinary education and discussion.

Assessing the vulnerability of a bereaved individual is a complex task. Using a tool may help as it will cover the significant areas of risk. One needs to be careful not to pathologise what can be a normal, albeit painful, disruptive and distressing individual experience.

The role of the nurse is twofold. First, there needs to be an ongoing assessment of the patient and how they are dealing with increasing loss and uncertainty. In our case study, Helen's reaction and method of coping varied as she became sicker and more dependent. This in turn affected the dynamics of the family and strained her relationship with her husband. Your role in this situation might be to discuss this with Helen and possibly to refer on to the relevant team member, for example the social worker or counselling or the chaplain for spiritual support. Dave may also value input from the nursing staff as Helen continues to reject him.

There are other family members whose need for support will also need to be assessed throughout the period of Helen's dying. The children may need specialist intervention but any contact with them would have to be agreed with Helen or Dave.

Second, following the death of the patient you need to ensure that the risk assessment has been done and that the information is passed on to the bereavement service or the worker in the team who provides bereavement support.

BEREAVEMENT ASSESSMENT: AN EXAMPLE
OF PRACTICE DEVELOPMENT

As has already been suggested, efforts to assess bereavement have resulted in a plethora of assessment tools. The following offers an example of the work of St Ann's Hospice (UK) to develop a bereavement assessment tool. This gives insight into ways in which the process and outcomes of developing a bereavement assessment tool have influenced the practice of bereavement care in the hospice. The bereavement assessment document has now been used within St Ann's Hospice for 6 years. Within this time it has had two reviews and is shortly coming up for its third. There have been changes and the document has been developed to suit the needs of different bereavement care needs within the organisation. The development of improved services and the consideration of new avenues for approaching bereavement support have evolved from the original bereavement assessment documentation.

The main outcomes of this initiative were as follows.

- As a result of increased social work referrals, a bereavement helpline was set up to respond to carers whose bereavement was initially assessed as low or medium risk. This helpline has continued to grow and thrive, being run by bereavement support volunteers. This bereavement helpline itself brought bereavement volunteers together in a different way and the initial training by the Samaritans training team proved invaluable.

- A staff induction programme was implemented to raise bereavement assessment awareness, together with an extended programme of training for bereavement support volunteers. The bereavement assessment document has proved an invaluable training tool for sessions on bereavement assessment, both for trained staff and for volunteers.

- Supervised bereavement counselling services were developed and have now moved on and extended, including more work with families and children. The Neil Cliffe Cancer Care Centre, now part of the St Ann's Hospice organisation, has adapted the bereavement assessment document for community bereavement work.

- The bereavement service was extended through the launch of the community bereavement programme, offering general bereavement support for those within the South Manchester area and, again, the original bereavement assessment document has been adapted to serve this service.

- As a result of the formation of a review team for the bereavement assessment documentation, a cross-site bereavement providers group now meets quarterly to discuss issues around bereavement support services both within the organisation and nationally.

- An integrated care pathway (ICP) covering care for the last 24 hours of life triggered bereavement assessment and support. This was added to the new ICP documentation implemented in 2002 and was recently audited positively by the organisation.

- The organisation is now a member of the Bereavement Research Forum, a national bereavement coordinators' group run through the Association of Hospice and Palliative Care Social Workers, and contributes also to the Manchester Bereavement Forum.

- Ongoing development of bereavement assessment continues following the initiation of this project.

Other policies, guidelines and developments within the organisation have also touched on the bereavement services. The lone worker policy, for example, integrated the bereavement support volunteers for the community bereavement service and general bereavement support services. The training and support of bereavement support working in-house with bereavement follow-up of patients' families and running the bereavement line[119]. This has proved very successful and created new incentives and motivation within this training programme.

The conclusion is that bereavement assessment documentation like this can have surprising potential to develop practice and, if the initial difficulties during implementation are handled positively, these guidelines can provide a sound base for future adaptation as the organisation develops.

((((●))))

REFLECTION POINT 10.5
Use of a bereavement assessment protocol

Think about your own area of practice. What benefits or difficulties might you expect if a bereavement assessment protocol was to be implemented into your area of practice?

WORKING WITH THE BEREAVED

CASE STUDY 10.2
Peter's experience

Peter, aged 45 years, married Julie when he was 23 years old and was diagnosed with multiple sclerosis when he was 25. Peter and Julie's son, Joe, was born at the time when Peter was diagnosed. Initially, Peter could cope with his symptoms, which consisted of numbness and fatigue. However, as his condition worsened he was unable to continue working as a window cleaner because of his poor mobility and he became depressed. His relationship with Julie deteriorated and she left him 5 years ago, taking Joe with her. Peter returned to his parents and now lives with his mother, Mary, who is in her early seventies. She suffers from anxiety, arthritis and chronic obstructive airways disease. Peter's father died of a stroke 6 months ago. Peter has one brother, Bill, who is 3 years older than him, and a younger sister, Marilyn. They are both married and live in the same village as Peter and Mary, whom they support as best as they can – they both have full-time jobs and families.

Peter sees Joe when he is on leave from the army. Their relationship is strained at times, as Joe has never had a father who was well and could do the normal fatherly activities with him.

Continued

CASE STUDY 10.2—CONT'D

Peter's multiple sclerosis has developed to the extent that his limbs are now in spasm and he spends long periods of the day in bed. Peter insists on staying at home and resisted accepting care until after his father's death. His father had been providing a lot of the care until his sudden stroke. At this point it was clear that Mary would not be able to provide the necessary physical care to maintain Peter at home. Peter reluctantly agreed to a home care package. He also accepted periods of respite care in the local hospice, which gave him and Mary a break from one another. He has stoutly refused day care, seeing it as 'just for old folk'. Now his symptoms have worsened and he has a serious chest infection as well as being incontinent. He is likely to die in the next few weeks.

Throughout his illness Peter has not wanted to acknowledge his diagnosis or prognosis. He has had periods of depression when his condition relapsed and when his illness forced him to lose yet another vital role or function (e.g. stopping work, needing a wheelchair). Mary has tried to support him but she is unwell herself and she is struggling to cope with the death of her husband. Marilyn and Bill are concerned about how Mary will cope in the future. They also express concern for Joe, who is unaware of how seriously ill his father is. Peter has insisted that Joe should not be told about his current condition. This is partly because Peter is in denial and unable to cope with hearing about his prognosis.

When assessing the needs of Mary and Joe, with Peter's death being imminent:

- What are the risks for Mary and Joe?

- Complete the bereavement risk assessment tools for both Mary and Joe.

- What sort of help may they require – as Peter is dying; immediately after his death and in the longer term?

SUPPORTING THOSE LIVING WITH LOSS

Supporting those living with loss is one of the most daunting challenges within palliative care. The lack of rigorous evidence-based recommendations has led to a lack of consensus on what is the most helpful package of care for the bereaved (Forte et al 2004). Bereavement is an area where a rigid set of guidelines is neither appropriate nor practical. Nevertheless we need to consider a selection of principles that can inform practice. The whole area of bereavement support is vast and it is beyond the scope of this chapter to cover it all. Therefore the remainder of this chapter will consider some aspects of supporting those living with loss.

When the bereaved person is facing life without their loved one a constellation of painful experiences, feelings and thoughts will unfold. This emotional/spiritual/physical pain may surface at times that are inconvenient and when the person is least expecting it. Support throughout the loss journey is critical to the person adjusting to life without a loved one. Generally only a small number of individuals need professional help, the majority of people requiring sustained support from people who are supportive, understanding and good listeners. What people need is to have their expression of feeling accepted, affirmed and validated.

Social support is critical but not always readily available to all. Payne et al (2000) note that there are a number of factors – such as geographical mobility, loss of support provided by the deceased, impact of bereavement on social network, changes in role and status, anxiety faced by others when interacting with the bereaved, and personality factors – that all influence the support experience. Therefore we need to assess risk but also to anticipate and give some thought to the scope of social support that is likely to be available to the bereaved person. This should ideally take place before the death of a loved one.

Good practice in supporting the bereaved includes:

- Looking after yourself as you look after the needs of the bereaved
- High-quality pain and symptom control in the run-up to the patient's death
- Assessing risk and identifying current and future social support networks
- Referring on to other members of the multiprofessional team for more specialist support
- Good-quality information and communication at all points in the bereavement journey.

It doesn't always go to plan. Review Case study 10.3 and consider what went well and what could have been done to improve the care. Following your review of this scenario, consider how immediate and long-term support of the bereaved is addressed in your area of practice.

CASE STUDY **10.3**
Jean's experience

Jean is 42 years old and is married to Keith. They have been married for 16 years and have two children, Stephen aged 12 and Amanda aged 7. Jean developed breast cancer 5 years ago. Following 12 months of treatment, including a lumpectomy, radiotherapy and chemotherapy Jean was able to resume her work as a primary school teacher. Unfortunately, 3½ years after the completion of her initial treatment it was discovered that Jean had developed bone secondaries in her right hip, two ribs and her left humerus. Pain, nausea and increasing disability have become a problem over the last 3 months. Within the last year Jean has been cared for at home with the support of the district nurse, the GP, the Marie Curie Nursing Service and a Macmillan nurse. Jean is aware of her diagnosis and prognosis and has, along with her husband, expressed a desire to die at home.

Over the last month Jean has become increasingly immobile, has become confused and has developed right-sided weaknesses. It is decided that she should be admitted to an emergency admissions ward within the local district general hospital for investigations and further treatment. Within 24 hours, Jean has been transferred to a four-bedded room within a 30-bedded acute medical ward. The team focuses on treating symptoms and active treatment to arrest any further deterioration. Jean has never been admitted to the hospital before and doesn't really know the staff. At no time during her 3 days in hospital do Jean and Keith's children visit their mum. Their grandmother, who lost her husband to cancer 3 years ago, cares for them for while Jean is in hospital. Visiting is difficult for Keith, who is a self-employed plumber and has to meet the requirements of a sizeable contract.

Following a computed tomography scan it is confirmed that secondary deposits in Jean's brain indicate that the disease has progressed further than anticipated. The ward is really busy, with five admissions over a 5-hour period. The registrar plans to see Keith that evening to put him in the picture on the results of the scan and the planned regime of treatment. In the evening, prior to visiting, one of the health-care assistants goes to check that Jean is comfortable prior to her husband coming to visit her, but unfortunately Jean has died. No one was with her at the time of her death.

Keith arrives on the ward alone and is briefed by the doctor and Jean's named nurse. He is devastated, extremely upset, and angry. Keith contacts Jean's brother and within half an hour there are seven relatives in the four bedded ward to say their goodbyes to Jean. There are no private areas or offices available on the unit or the adjacent ward.

- As the nurse responsible for Jean's care how would you handle this situation?
- What is undesirable about this situation so far as the bereavement care of Jean and her family is concerned?
- What are the support needs of other patients in the four-bedded ward?
- What are the support needs of staff on the ward?
- Are such situations avoidable?
- How would you prevent such a situations arising in the future?
- What are the support needs of the family?

Situations in which bereavement has not been handled well need to be considered alongside situations where bereavement has been handled well.

REFLECTION POINT 10.6
Handling bereavement situations

Think back and try to recall a bereavement situation which you think was handled well. Using the headings below, try to summarise what it was that contributed to the positive outcome for the patient and family (or staff) concerned:

- What was the age of the patient?
- What was the diagnosis?

Continued

- What gender was the patient?

- Who were the main sources of support for the patient and family?

- What was the quality of the relationship between staff and patient/carers?

- Were there any specific bereavement risk factors that suggested future difficulties?

- What did you do as an individual to help prepare the patient and their family?

- What did you do as a team to help ease the situation and prepare the patient and family for the bereavement?

- How did you feel about the situation? How did you cope?

- Any other comments?

SOME SUGGESTIONS TO HELP SUPPORT THE BEREAVED

THE EARLY DAYS

Immediately after the death the nurse plays a central role in supporting the family. The family should be given as much time as they require with the deceased to disengage and to say their final goodbyes. At this point they may be unable to absorb information, so written information is useful as well as checking through their understanding of what has happened. Families need time; bereavement support is time-consuming. Listening and just being there is what people need. Be alongside their grief and pain. You may need to communicate through touch and you may find that the distress you are witnessing causes you to cry. Shared tears demonstrate genuine care. Bereavement assessment should be completed and, if any serious risk factors are identified, referral should be made to the appropriate support services, assuming that the family agree to this.

Do not attempt to offer solutions or answer questions where no solutions or answers exist. In addition to practical help in the early stages, do not underestimate the value of just being there and just listening – this includes listening in a genuine manner to stories and conversations concerning the qualities of the person who has died.

- **Listen and accept the person in a non-judgemental way**. Allow people to grieve in a way that suits them. There is no right or wrong way to grieve. Part of this involves giving the person permission to express the unhappiness they are feeling at that moment in time.

- **Demonstrate empathy with the person's position and challenges**. Use good listening skills.

- **Tolerate and stay with the silences**. Silence is often a productive time during which the bereaved may experience new insights about themselves and the situation they now find themselves in.

- **Stay in touch with your own feelings about death and dying**. In order that the bereaved can make sense of what they are experiencing, you need to maintain an awareness of your own reactions to death, personal experiences and vulnerabilities and stay focused on addressing their experience, needs, and challenges. If the situation has made you feel angry, helpless or sad it is worth checking out with the individual how they feel. That way you will ensure that you are working with their feelings and not yours.

- **Offer assurances based on the person's actions in the run-up to the death** – 'You did everything you could'

- **Encourage the person to be patient with themselves**, especially in the months ahead, when they will be confronted with the gaps left by their loved one.

- **Don't take anger personally**. This and other emotions are likely to be part of the grief process. It is important to keep calm and to try and understand the cause, always ensuring that you are safe in the situation. If there is an escalation then you should remove yourself and seek help.

- **Consider diversity/cultural differences**. Different cultures, religions and ethnic groups may have different views, values, rites and rituals around the dying process and death. As a nurse it is imperative that you find out what these are to ensure the appropriate care. It will also help you to understand the patient's and family's reactions to their situation. You may need to seek an interpreter to aid with communication but you must ensure that (except in an emergency) the interpreter is not a family member but a properly qualified, external interpreter who is acceptable to the patient.

- **Allow for coping strategies**. These will vary from day to day and depend on what the person is facing, their personality, belief system, cultural background, age, life experience and loss history. The reaction may vary from tearful distress to philosophical stoicism to acceptance. Each reaction is equally valid but some may be more difficult for the helping professional to deal with, e.g. anger or giving up.

INFORMATION

When people are bereaved they become more dependent and may feel disempowered. As professionals we can seek to redress this imbalance by ensuring that the bereaved person and family have all the information they want and need to make the necessary choices and decisions. This will increase their sense of control in a world where they may feel they are increasingly losing it. Information needs to be given sensitively and at a pace that the patient and family can cope with. This takes skill, time, privacy and patience. The language used needs to be free of jargon and appropriate to the listener. The professional needs to be open and willing to answer questions and go over topics again and again to ensure understanding. Never assume, always check out how the person has processed the information.

Remember, nobody grieves in exactly the same way. Each individual is different and reacts differently; nevertheless experience suggests that some of the following emotions and thoughts are commonplace. Such an array of suggestions provides a framework for the informational needs of the bereaved.

- It may be difficult to accept the loss and at times you may deny what has happened
- At times it may seem as if there is no point in going on and the intensity of your grief is overwhelming and difficult to get away from
- You might experience sleep disturbances or periods when you feel very tearful and exhausted
- You may experience feelings that are foreign to you such as anger or guilt
- As time progresses you might find that you are able to look back on events and memories without the same level of distress
- You may feel that people are avoiding you – in some instances this is understandable when they themselves are not sure what to say or do to help you
- Don't be afraid to share your feelings with a sympathetic listener.

LONGER-TERM BEREAVEMENT SUPPORT

Anyone living with a loss through death will cope in the first year with all the changes without requiring professional intervention. Accepting the reality of the permanency of death can take some time. Generally people will acknowledge the death intellectually but emotionally the permanency can be too distressing to accept. Stroebe's (1998) model, in which the bereaved swing from expressing their feelings of distress and grief to a more practical way of coping, is in fact what often happens. The more recent theorists have produced concepts that illustrate the experiences of many bereaved. Klass et al (1997) describe the ongoing relationship with the deceased in a different way, more as an inner representation. This allows the bereaved to continue to have a relationship with the dead person and not to have to let them go, resolve their grief or readjust, as orthodox theories would suggest. If this was not achieved in a specific time scale, they would be deemed to be pathological in their grief reaction. Now there is much more individuality to grieving, with no clear time scale.

Questions to consider at a later stage in the bereavement include:

- Are suicidal or extreme emotional reactions to the death being displayed regularly?

- Is the bereaved person 'stuck' in their grief, for example going to the cemetery every day after a year?
- Has the bereaved sought to deny the death; for example, have they kept all the dead person's possessions, created a shrine to them, made radical changes to their lifestyle, actually denying that the death has occurred?
- Is the bereaved displaying similar symptoms to the deceased and is phobic about their illness?
- Has the bereaved person's level of functioning broken down completely?

If the answer to any of these questions is yes, the person is struggling to cope and may not be able to deal with their losses. Bereavement counselling might help and you should consider referral on to an appropriate service.

CONCLUSIONS

Supporting the bereaved is a vast topic and has been the subject of wide-ranging research by nurses, psychologists, social workers, medical staff and voluntary agencies, to name but a few. The nurse working alongside the multiprofessional team can play a significant role in helping prepare those who are dying and also to help bereaved relatives navigate the difficult days ahead. The emphasis of this chapter has been on an orthodox picture of grief, where pain and sadness are constant companions. However, Kissane (2004) provides a timely reminder that hope can exist in the knowledge that creativity and new beginnings may be an emerging feature of life if the person is able to successfully pass through the mourning process.

ACKNOWLEDGEMENTS

We are grateful to the many patients, carers and families from whom we have learnt so much, and to Caroline Melliar-Smith and the team at St Ann's Hospice for sharing the work they have undertaken on bereavement assessment.

REFERENCES

Anstey S, Lewis M 2001 Bereavement, grief, and mourning. In: Kinghorn S, Gamlin R (eds) Palliative nursing: bringing comfort and hope. Baillière Tindall, Edinburgh

Bowlby J 1980 Attachment, loss, sadness and depression, vol. 3. Penguin, Harmondsworth

Boyle M, Carter D 1998 Death anxiety amongst nurses. International Journal of Palliative Nursing 4:37–43

Costello J 1999 Anticipatory grief: coping with the impending death of a partner. International Journal of Palliative Nursing 5:223–231

Duke S 1998 An exploration of anticipatory grief: the lived experience of people during their spouses' terminal illness and in bereavement. Journal of Advanced Nursing 28:829–839

Ellershaw J, Ward C 2003 Care of the dying patient: the last hours or days of life. British Medical Journal 326:30–34

Forte A, Hill M, Pazder R, Feudtner C 2004 Bereavement care interventions: a systematic review. Biomedcentral 3. Available on line at: www.biomedcentral.com/1472-684X/3/3

Greenstreet W 2004 Why nurses need to understand the principles of bereavement theory. British Journal of Nursing 9:590–593

Hale G 1996 The social construction of grief. In: Cooper N, Stevenson C, Hale G (eds) Integrating perspectives on health. Open University Press, Buckingham

Houghton P 2001 On death, dying and not dying. Jessica Kingsley, London

Kalish R A 1985 cited in Anstey S, Lewis M 2001 Bereavement, grief, and mourning. In: Kinghorn S, Gamlin R (eds) Palliative nursing: bringing comfort and hope. Baillière Tindall, Edinburgh

Kissane D 2004 Bereavement. In: Doyle D, Hanks G, Cherney N, Calman K (eds) Oxford textbook of palliative medicine, 3rd edn. Oxford University Press, Oxford

Klass D, Silverman P R, Nickman S L 1997 Continuing bonds: new understandings of grief. Taylor & Francis, Washington, DC

Kubler-Ross E 1969 On death and dying. Tavistock, London

London Bereavement Network 2001 Standards for bereavement care in the UK. London Bereavement Network, London. Available on line at: www.bereavement.org.uk/standards/index.asp

McIntyre R 2002 Nursing support for families of dying patients. Whurr, London

McNamara B 2001 Fragile lives. Open University Press, Buckingham

Melliar-Smith C 2002 The risk assessment of bereavement in a palliative care setting. International Journal of Palliative Nursing 8:281–288

National Institute for Clinical Excellence 2004 Improving supportive and palliative care for adults with cancer – the Manual. NICE, London. Available on line at: www.nice.org.uk/page.aspx?o=110007

Neuberger J 1999 Dying well: a guide to enabling a good death. Hochland & Hochland, Hale

Parkes C M 1986 Bereavement. Penguin, Harmondsworth

Parkes C M 1998 Coping with loss. British Medical Journal 316:856–859

Payne S 2001 Bereavement support: something for everyone. International Journal of Palliative Nursing 7:108

Payne S, Horn S, Relf M 2000 Loss and bereavement. Open University Press, Buckingham

Pullen M L 2002 Joe's story: reflections on a difficult interaction between nurse and patient's wife. International Journal of Palliative Nursing 8:481–489

Reimers E 2001 Bereavement – a social phenomenon? European Journal of Palliative Care 8:242–244

Ringdal G I, Jordhoy M S, Ringdal K, Kaasa S 2001 The first year of grief and bereavement in close family members to individuals who have died of cancer. Palliative Medicine 15:91–105

Saunderson E M, Ridsdale L 1999 General practitioners' beliefs and attitudes about how to respond to death and bereavement: qualitative study. British Medical Journal 319:293–296

Setch F 2001 Looking after yourself. In: Kinghorn S, Gamlin R (eds) Palliative nursing: bringing comfort and hope. Baillière Tindall, Edinburgh

Sherwood P R, Given B A, Doorenbos A Z, Goven C W 2004 Forgotten voices: lessons from bereaved carers of persons with a brain tumour. International Journal of Palliative Nursing 10:67–75

Stroebe M S 1998 New directions in bereavement research: exploration of gender differences. Palliative Medicine 12:5–12

Wakefield A 2000 Nurse responses to death and dying: a need for relentless self-care. International Journal of Palliative Nursing 6:245–255

Walshe C 1997 Whom to help? An exploration of the assessment of grief. International Journal of Palliative Nursing 3:132–138

Walter T 1999 On bereavement: the culture of grief. Open University Press, Buckingham

Wendell-Moller D 1996 Confronting death: values, institutions and human mortality. Oxford University Press, Oxford

Worden J W 1991 Grief counselling and grief therapy, 2nd edn. Routledge, London

USEFUL WEBSITES

Growth House: www.growthhouse.org/

AARP: www.aarp.org/griefandloss/coping.html

Hospice net: www.hospicenet.org/

Grief and bereavement: www.psycom.net/depression.central.grief.html

CHAPTER ELEVEN

Ethical issues in palliative care

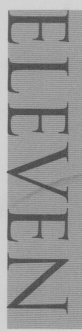

Kate Jones, Jacqueline Husband

This chapter will focus on everyday ethical issues and some potential dilemmas that arise in palliative care nursing. Ethical theories and ethical principles will be outlined and explored, applying these to the analysis of case studies that contain ethically challenging situations. We hope to provide readers with opportunities to develop the knowledge, skills and attitudes required to contribute to ethical decision-making and the competence to apply these within palliative care practice.

AIMS OF THE CHAPTER

- Define ethics and its relevance to progressive palliative care development
- Identify some moral and ethical approaches to decision-making
- Analyse some common ethical dilemmas, which may arise in palliative care.

INTRODUCTION

The moral demands of care require radical responses and moral courage, as well as political astuteness.

Cooper 1991

There are no easy solutions to ethical problems faced by health-care professionals in contemporary palliative care. Society today is pluralistic and recognises and respects claims of different groups to maintain their own customs, moral values and rules. This makes a moral and political consensus difficult within society, and has major implications for palliative nursing, especially around issues of life and death (Webber 1996).

There are many tragic dilemmas to be faced by nurses in the palliative care setting. Because of this, the moral and ethical choice between actions to be taken and what is considered reasonable, practical and right is complex. Right answers are few, wrong answers can be devastating. That is the challenge! However, it is right that nurses examine their actions in terms of acceptability and they should continually question their practice within a supportive and interdisciplinary team environment.

DEFINING ETHICS IN PALLIATIVE NURSING

What is it about contemporary palliative care that brings ethical issues more into focus? Beauchamp & Childress (1994) define ethics as the systematic examination of the moral life, which seeks to provide sound justification for moral decisions and actions of people. However, 'ethical' might mean:

- Having to do with the study of morality (an ethical question)
- Conforming to recognised standards of practice (ethical conduct) (Boyd et al 1997).

Anyone can be immoral but only those who fail to live up to publicly professed obligations tend to be called unethical.

While there is a widespread consensus on the moral values that influence decision-making in health-care settings (Downie & Calman 1995), deciding what is right or wrong is not quite as simple in palliative care. We may question whether the issue of right or wrong is helpful in palliative care. In difficult situations the parallels of right and wrong can be difficult to tease apart and we often make decisions within a complex tangle of emotions, options and possible outcomes. Decision-making in terms of interventions and treatments can involve deciding what ought to be provided, what is optional and what ought not to be provided (Randall & Downie 2001). This is supported by Johnston (1999, p. 14) who states that: 'Ethics is a form of philosophical enquiry and generally understood to be a system of action guided principles and rules which function by specifying the type of conduct permitted (allowed), required (obligatory) and forbidden (never allowed).'

The aim of palliative care is to relieve suffering and to improve quality of life (World Health Organization 2003), but it is more than that! It is about last chances, the meaning and value of life, endings and making the situation better or right (ultimately dying). This philosophy was well grounded by Cecily Saunders, pioneer of the modern hospice movement in the 1960s. Her statement of intention of care, 'To help you live until you die', has become more complex in modern-day palliative care. However, there was excellence in its simplicity in those beginnings when the distinction between living and dying was less blurred than it is today.

Medical consideration is one among many considerations related to health and quality of life (Lloyd 1997), and ethical dilemmas often stem from problems of communication within the health-care team (Scott 1995). Although it is nurses who spend the greatest amount of time with a patient, all team members involved in caring for the patient should contribute to the decision-making process. Care will only be ethical if we offer practical, physical, psychosocial and spiritual help. This involves holistic care within the context of a patient's life history, character, values and culture.

Today, responding to the unmet needs for palliative care for people earlier in their diagnosis, and for those with advanced and progressive non-malignant illness, makes the division between acute care and palliative care less clear (NCHSPCS 1998).

ETHICAL DILEMMAS AND DECISION MAKING

An ethical dilemma is a difficult problem for which there is no totally satisfactory solution, or which involves a choice between equally unsatisfactory alternatives. The most difficult moral decisions lie in the 'grey areas' where the choices made may not result in the ideal or personally desired outcomes. Johns (1999) describes the use of structured reflection, whereby the key ethical principles of autonomy, justice, beneficence and non-maleficence are applied to the analysis of a complex problem in the practice situation. He suggests that this approach will enable practitioners to become more ethically sensitive in responding to similar situations they may encounter in the future. His description of ethical mapping highlights important questions a nurse may reflect upon when faced with ethical dilemmas in the palliative care setting (Fig. 11.1). This reflective approach to decision-making is also supported by Doane (2002), who suggests that nurses should step back from themselves to think more objectively about the challenging situation.

In Figure 11.1, each of the boxes represents a different perspective from which to consider the particular dilemma. This allows a more balanced view to be taken when seeking the right solution for a given dilemma. The analysis should be patient-focused and should be considered at a team level before a decision is reached.

Factors that may influence the decision-making process may include the prognosis of the patient, the relationships between the health professionals,

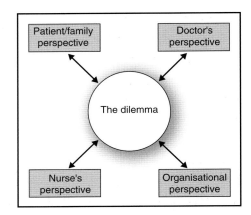

Figure 11.1 A framework for approaching an ethical dilemma (adapted from Johns 1997).

the patient and the family, and the expectations and wishes of the patient. Additionally, the professional's own values and morals may impact on the approach to the dilemma. Influences from both society and the health-care organisation will affect the outcome. It is for this reason that all perspectives must be considered when responding to a situation or dilemma.

Johns asserts that ethical theories and principles, like all extant sources of knowledge, exist only to inform the practitioner. They cannot prescribe what is best within an individual situation. By definition, ethical dilemmas are often conflicting – for example, truth telling may be harmful; respecting the autonomy of one person may conflict with the rights of another, making it difficult to know what is the right decision to make. The practitioner needs to consider issues such as:

- Who has the authority to make the decisions?
- Who has the power and position to act within the particular situation?
- Is there a clear understanding of how and why these decisions were made?

Nurses may therefore benefit from using a framework such as the one described above to enable them to reach a balanced view and to enable them to apply ethical decision-making in practice.

REFLECTION AS A FRAMEWORK FOR ETHICAL REASONING

Ferrell (1998) offered an alternative model of ethical reasoning based on reflection for nurses who are facing a moral or ethical dilemma. This uses relevant questions at each point of the reflective cycle. Like similar models, it helps the nurse explore and analyse the context within which the dilemma is occurring. The main elements of this model include:

1. Reflection or analysis
2. Judgement and action
3. Justification and reflection.

The questions below are based on Ferrell's model of ethical decision-making and will be applied later in the chapter when analysing specific scenarios within a palliative nursing context.

1. Reflection or analysis
   • What is the nature of the dilemma – what is really happening?
   • What are the ethical principles involved?
   • What are the moral/legal rights of everyone involved?
   • What are the professional's responsibilities?
   • Whose decision is it and who will be affected?
   • What are the likely outcomes in terms of burdens, risks and benefits?
2. Judgement and action
   • Making the decision and acting upon it.
3. Justification and reflection
   • Evaluating the decision – was it the right option to take?
   • Use personal reflection to consider the results of the action and how it may affect your future practice.

Nurses should remember that no one single approach works best in all situations. It is likely that differences in care settings and situations will require different approaches to addressing potential ethical problems and will be dependent on the values of the decision maker, the nurse and other parties involved (Fry & Johnstone 2002). At an everyday level, the nurse working with patients in the palliative care setting, where death and dying are regarded as normal processes, may still be faced with difficult ethical dilemmas in end of life care (Box 11.1).

BOX 11.1

Examples of ethical problems in end-of-life care

• Withdrawing or withholding treatment

• Unintended but foreseen consequences, e.g. sedating a patient

• Conflicts of interest – involving dying patients in research

• Extraordinary versus futile treatments

THEORETICAL APPROACHES

Before considering the main ethical principles it is important that we draw attention to the underlying theories that inform ethical decision-making. These theories may be interpreted through a number of different approaches. However, adopting an ethical approach is not always about having a set of rules to obey but is rather about transforming oneself into someone for whom the duty of care for the individual is inherent (Lloyd 1997).

For the purpose of this chapter, we will be considering three ethical theories offering a mixture of classical and modern thinking. No one theory can be right for every situation – but some contemplation of the meaning and understanding of each can support decision-making. Ethics is concerned with value judgements (Box 11.2) and in particular with value judgements about right and wrong, good and bad behaviour. However, another role of ethical theory is to support the judgements that are made (Fry & Johnstone 2002). Beauchamp & Childress (1994) and Johns (1997) also argue that, when dealing with ethical and moral dilemmas in practice, it is crucial that we understand why decisions were made and how the actions can be justified. This underscores the importance of communication and interdisciplinary decision-making.

ETHICAL THEORIES

The ethical theories that will be discussed are:

- **Deontology** – a theory based on obligations and duty
- **Utilitarianism** (consequentialism) – this theory considers what actions achieve the greatest good
- **Virtue ethics** – considers particular character qualities, e.g. courage, wisdom and justice, and what is a right and virtuous way to act.
  Each of these theories will be considered separately. Their application to the analysis of practice-based dilemmas will be addressed later in the chapter.

Deontological ethics

Central to deontology is the notion of duty – doing what is right. Modern deontology is based on unconditional respect for persons and in doing what is

Box **11.2**

Definition

Value judgement

A judgement that, in the broadest sense, is made on behalf of someone else but may not necessarily reflect the right decision for the individual patient and family.

right regardless of the consequences. What is right, however, may not necessarily always be good; therefore the theoretical approach does separate 'good' from 'right', in that a good action can have a bad outcome (the end does not justify the means).

In Kantian ethics (named after Immanuel Kant, 1724–1804, the originator of the theory), duty is central and universal. The difficulty with universalising a moral maxim (rule) is that the principle of moral equality in caring can conflict with the duty of delivering care. This can present challenges for nurses in the palliative care setting, where situations can change quickly and where decisions and actions have to balance the principles of beneficence (doing good) and with non-maleficence (not causing harm). In palliative care there is often a tension between these principles. Randall & Downie (2001) argue that in palliative care actions are judged to be either appropriate or inappropriate depending upon the individual situation and that no single rule can be applied generally to all patients.

An example in practice is that deontologists would view truth-telling as always 'right' regardless of the situation. They would argue that one should always tell the truth. In modern nursing, the traditional duty of the nurse as a protector and truth-teller could be challenged. In palliative care, nurses may face a conflict of what rule to obey to satisfy their duty of care, for instance whether to keep a confidence or to protect someone who is vulnerable by breaking that confidence. The deontological approach does have a place in palliative care particularly if we use it as a basis for individualised interaction in practice settings.

Utilitarian ethics (consequentialism)

Utilitarian theory considers the value or merit of an outcome of an action rather than the action itself. This theory evaluates the ends produced by an action to determine its goodness or rightness. In its broadest interpretation, utilitarianism should strive to maximise happiness (or benefit) and minimise misery for the greatest possible number. The difficulty is that one person's happiness can be another person's misery. For example, take the case of an elderly lady with a slow-growing head and neck tumour, admitted to hospital having had a 'stroke' associated with the progression of the tumour. Further active treatment is not indicated and she wants to be admitted to the local hospice. She states: 'This is the type of care I want and need at this stage of my illness.' Her prognosis, however, is indeterminate: clinically she could deteriorate quickly and equally she could deteriorate over many months. A decision is made that hospice care, although appropriate, has to be denied her because of pressure on hospice beds for others, defined as more urgent, waiting for admission. For the length of time that this lady might occupy a bed, many others could benefit for shorter periods, until they died.

The lady is distraught. She cries out that nobody wants her and she is dying. A health-care professional who believes that hospice care should be available for all the dying will have difficulties accepting this decision. From a utilitarian perspective, it is justifiable to deny this lady hospice care, when so many others could use the bed she might occupy for months. A lack of local resources can make policy makers look at actions and outcomes in terms of a long-term perspective – extremely valid when you are trying to be fair to the greatest number but often difficult and stressful for nurses in the front line of care.

Virtue-based ethics

Virtue-based ethics dates right back to Plato and Aristotle in the 5th century BC but has had a recent revival within contemporary moral theory and has been held up as the ultimate essence of care and compassion (Hursthouse 1999).

Virtue ethics could be described as 'person-centred' rather than 'practitioner-centred', in that it focuses on what is a right and virtuous action as opposed to what guides actions in terms of rules and obligations. Historically, human virtues (character) and responsibilities, in terms of the duty of care, were paramount in nursing. Duty was seen as a sacred obligation, a loyal service and a professional religion. Contemporary virtue ethics looks more deeply into the 'ethic of caring', being guided by a moral view of a person and the relationship and strength of caring (Gilligan 1982). Macedo (1992) describes these characteristics in terms of tolerance, empathy, willingness to dare, receptiveness to new ideas, active involvement, fairness, impartiality, the pursuit of excellence, respect for others and the willingness to enter a public debate.

In palliative care nursing, principle- or rule-based ethics cannot fully encompass the human interaction that takes place between a nurse, a dying patient and distressed family. Arguably the virtues of moral courage, wisdom and justice are needed far more today in the context of decision-making because of the developing scope of palliative care (Thompson et al 2000).

For example, a distressed, dying patient asking to be released from their suffering may challenge the very basis of professional codes and conduct. It may take a degree of moral courage to change the process of care at that stage and not to abandon human dignity, autonomy and justice for the fear of being seen as not acting in a virtuous way in trying to save a life at all cost.

Grayling (2001, p. 72), considering Aristotle's statement that 'A life truly worth living is being watched over by a good angel', argues that the meaning behind 'being virtuous' is complex and multiple in character. Being virtuous involves respect and concern for others, and a duty to improve oneself and to use one's gifts for the sake not only of others but also for the quality of one's own experience. This concurs with Randall & Downie (2001), who argue that the virtues and dispositions of health-care professionals are important to patients and families when difficult decisions have to be made.

It must be appreciated that the theories described above may, and can, overlap in most discussions around ethical dilemmas in practice.

You may wish to read further in this area (Thompson et al 2000) to help clarify and supplement this topic.

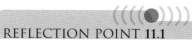

REFLECTION POINT 11.1
Ethical theories

Drawing on your past experiences, reflect on two examples of difficult situations in practice. Apply the framework suggested by Johns or Ferrell. Identify possible alternative outcomes to the situations when applying the ethical theories.

ETHICAL PRINCIPLES

Ethical theory, as defined by early philosophers, cannot always be easily transferred to contemporary health-care situations, as the theories were built upon the value systems of earlier times. The underpinning ethical principles, however, do still provide a sound foundation for our own personal beliefs, morality and actions when applied to modern-day living. Moral and ethical judgements are intrinsic to our daily practice in palliative care. We use them in almost every interaction with our patients but often do not recognise that we are doing so. The central focus of ethical decision-making and its links to caring confirm the need to develop understanding of the connections between caring and ethics.

To be credible, ethical behaviour must be based not only on our shared values but also on universally recognised principles. Writers such as Beauchamp & Childress (1994) and Randall & Downie (2001) classify ethical principles as:

- Respect for the individual
- Autonomy
- Justice and utility
- Beneficence
- Non-maleficence.

While such principles provide the foundation of nursing and personal moral guidelines, they do not provide answers in individual situations. An understanding of the ethical principles will support the nurse involved in decision-making within the clinical setting. Each of the ethical principles will be explored separately, but it must be remembered that, within the clinical setting, consideration of more than one principle may be required. Application to analysis of professional dilemmas will be addressed later in the chapter.

RESPECT FOR THE INDIVIDUAL

What do we mean by respect? Due regard for the feelings or rights of others, avoiding harm or interference is the definition provided in the *Concise Oxford Dictionary* (1999). These concepts mirror and provide the foundation of all the ethical principles, suggesting that respect for the individual encircles any ethical approach. The overarching principle of respect forms the basis of the code of professional conduct (Nursing and Midwifery Council 2004). Accountability for our own practice is determined by the demonstration of respect for the patient or client as an individual.

As nurses we have a duty to respect the rights, autonomy and dignity of our patients, to be truthful and honest and to promote their wellbeing (Thompson et al 2000). Unrestricted respect for the dignity, worth and uniqueness of the individual should envelop all provisions of care. In modern multicultural society, we are taught that everyone is entitled to hold their own beliefs and opinions. Patients and professionals alike should not be prevented from expressing these views and should not be discriminated against because of them (Thompson et al 2000). However, this can create an environment for many potential ethical dilemmas.

Respect and caring are vital components of the role of the nurse, particularly when practising within the palliative care setting. These elements reflect the central role of the patient and the importance of a person-focused approach to care. At a simple level, respect for persons includes considering the manner we use to discuss our patients. To describe patients as 'the lung cancer in bed 3' implies that the patient is no longer a unique individual with a distressing life-threatening illness but only a cancerous tumour to be managed and eliminated if possible. If we consider the vulnerability of patients in our care, any sense of identity is lost in this one statement.

However, the goal of valuing the patient as an individual is often compromised by the superficial knowledge we obtain from patients and upon which we base our judgements. The necessity of taking time to elicit information from the patient and having regard for their needs and wishes acknowledges the principle of respect and the uniqueness of the person.

Issues that should not affect respect for patients are their 'likeability' or their attributed responsibility for their illness. Did the patient bring their circumstances on by their lifestyle? Personal opinions are subjective, open to interpretation and contravene the ethical principles mentioned above.

Another dimension of respect is confidentiality and privacy. This can create dilemmas within health-care provision. It is easy to be drawn unwittingly into conversation about a patient when faced by obviously concerned friends and relatives. In the community setting, your arrival at the home may be seen by concerned neighbours, who can place you in a difficult position by enquiring after their friend. This can create a tricky situation for a nurse who is trying to maintain confidentiality but provide reassurance. Similarly, in the hospital setting, discussion of sensitive and confidential information often takes place behind curtains, which are not soundproof. Is this a breach of privacy or a necessity arising from limited resources?

Nurses do not work in isolation but are part of a wider professional team. Mutual respect for one another's roles and opinions is integral to providing effective palliative care. The benefit of multidisciplinary team working is the combination of a variety of skills striving to improve the quality of patient care. But with many different viewpoints on offer, decision-making can become a challenge. Differences in opinion are common within a team but, if the opportunity to air these differences is missed, conflict will arise and resolution will not be reached. Consider the situation where the care environment is focused on cure and survival but the patient is not responding to treatment. The staff may feel guilty, a failure, for not preventing the death of the patient, creating additional stresses within the team. Decisions regarding the direction of treatment strategies may exacerbate this tension.

Arguably, we ought to allow everyone the right to express their views on ethical matters on the basis of the overarching ethical principle of respect for the individual. However, role conflicts can occur, as nurses have many roles in life, for example team member, manager and member of society as well as nurse. The stance nurses take up in their personal life may differ from their role as a nurse. The application of the ethical principles to a dilemma offers the opportunity to use reasoned thinking to provide a number of possible solutions (Webb 2000).

By acknowledging the importance of our own moral and ethical stance, it will be easier to respect the importance of others. This will ease the decision-making process, reducing the opportunities for conflict within the team and with the patient. Nouwen (1976, p. 36), supporting this, writes: 'When we have seen and acknowledged our own hostilities and fears without hesitation, it is more likely that we will also be able to sense from within the other pole towards which we want to lead not just ourselves but our patients as well.'

AUTONOMY

Respect for autonomy underpins several important foundations of ethical practice such as confidentiality, consent and effective communication (Have & Clark 2002). But what exactly does 'respecting autonomy' mean? The notion is partially understood as respecting the unique individual and the way they define themselves through the way they live and the values and beliefs they hold. Respecting autonomy means respecting choices. This should be done in a non-judgemental manner, without inflicting our own beliefs on the person. Making choices and deciding one's goals is what makes the person individual (Beauchamp & Childress 1994).

In palliative care, the dilemma arises when the person's choices make demands on other individuals or society (Have & Clark 2002). No one lives in a vacuum, which renders it unacceptable to demand unlimited respect for autonomy when choices will impinge on others who have an equal right to their own life and choices. Autonomy is further restricted by other factors, such as the law, social tradition and the prevailing circumstances of a person's life. There are a number of questions we must ask ourselves in order to establish autonomy's place in health-care ethics:

- Are all individuals equally autonomous?
- Are different decisions made by the same individual equally autonomous?
- To what extent are we obliged to respect these autonomous decisions?

Individuals live within a network of relationships and choices may be influenced by consideration for others (Have & Clark 2002).

Consider the 'rights' of the patient who chooses to die at home. The nurse may feel that the home circumstances are not suitable for the patient's needs but, if this is the patient's wish, can the nurse deny it? In another situation, carers may want to keep the patient at home, not fully understanding the implications of this decision and the demands it will make. Additional stress and tension among family members may be exacerbated, raising the question: Does this decision respect the autonomy of all concerned? The application of the principle of autonomy requires that the person has sufficient knowledge to exercise control. This may not resolve the initial dilemma involving allocation of resources but will undoubtedly allow the relatives to make informed choices, within their own limitations.

Respecting autonomy requires that care provision be directed to the needs of the individual (Thompson et al 2000) but nurses also have a duty of universal fairness (equal opportunity) and equity (equity of outcomes). This can create dilemmas around individuals' rights and fairness and justice for all.

JUSTICE

What is meant by justice in palliative care ethics? A focus on partnership between the patient and the care providers has been highlighted in recent policy documents (Department of Health 2001, NHS Scotland 2003). Tensions can and do exist between just and equitable care for the individual and the equitable allocation of resources to meet the needs of the majority. In current palliative care provision, there are limited resources, raising the question of fair distribution of these scarce resources. Conflicts exist between justice, fairness, equality and utility – utility being the principle of providing the greatest good for the greatest number of people (Randall & Downie 2001).

Consider the Calman–Hine report (Department of Health 1995) proposing centralisation of specialist cancer services. By applying the principle of utility, concentrating the largest amount of resources where the largest population is sounds ethically supportable. But this has implications for those patients living in rural areas, who would be obliged to travel great distances for the same level of care. Does this seem just and fair? Justice requires of us that any personal rule of action should in principle be capable of being universalised for all people.

Difficult decisions must also be made around the provision of specific services. A great deal of the money available goes towards funding research, and much of the media attention focuses on the 'high-tech', highly emotive spectrum of health care. It could be argued that investment in less attractive aspects of health care such as health promotion would provide greater utility of resources. This point was raised in 1995, in the case of 'Child B', who had a complicated form of leukaemia and who was denied treatment by the local health authority (Economics of Health Care 2004). The case was taken to court on the grounds that the decision was made on economic rather than clinical grounds. It was settled privately out of court but highlighted public opinion about their right to the best treatment available. The principle of justice encompasses equal respect for a person's rights for fair and equal access to treatment, as well as being aware of the legal implications. According to the Human Rights Act (Department of Health 1998), people have the right to choose, the right to equity of service and the right not to be discriminated against.

Nurses who are committed to the principle of equity and justice have a duty to campaign for further resources to improve services and to maintain standards of care. Nurses also have an obligation to remain competent, recognise their own limitations and acknowledge areas for further learning (Nursing and Midwifery Council 2004). The ethical principle of justice demands that care provision is based on current evidence and best practice. The provision of quantifiable evidence of quality raises problems in palliative care. Does this mean that the care provided is unimportant? Does this create an injustice in the evaluation of palliative care services? (Randall & Downie 2001). The ethos of palliative care is the provision of high-quality care for each individual patient. This raises the question: 'What is quality?' There is a moral obligation on health professionals to improve the quality of care and to demonstrate this in quantifiable and qualitative terms.

BENEFICENCE AND NON-MALEFICENCE

The principle of beneficence (doing good) underpins the duty to care. Conversely, whenever nurses are committed to helping others, they may in turn risk doing harm. We must consider the principles of beneficence and non-maleficence together, as the balance of burdens and risks must not outweigh the benefits of any choices or decisions. Beneficence rises from a relationship of trust between the patient and nurse. If the main focus is to benefit the patient, then telling them the truth is often ethically correct. This will enhance the trust and honesty in the therapeutic relationship.

The Nursing and Midwifery Council (2004) state that nurses must recognise and respect the role of patients as partners in their care. This involves identifying their preferences regarding care and respecting these within the limits of professional practice. In simplistic terms, if a patient refuses a specific course of treatment, with the view that it won't benefit their quality of life, the nurse is obliged to respect this decision unless it may cause them additional harm. The subsequent dilemma that arises is between respecting the patient's autonomy and not causing harm (non-maleficence).

In practice, however, patients may choose to do things their way, reflecting values different from those held by the nurse. The skills of communication, listening and maintaining confidentiality are paramount in respecting autonomy. However, for patients to make critical choices they also require to be provided with complete and accurate information (Browne 1998).

Dilemmas surrounding truth-telling in palliative care often arise not from the rights of patients but from the internal conflict between the nurse's own rights and duty to care. The desire to protect vulnerable patients from the painful realisation of their deteriorating condition may affect the nurse's ability to share accurate information. By protecting patients from harm the nurse is in fact preventing them from making their own choices. The modern concept of patient empowerment through information-giving is essentially a combination of the principles of respect for autonomy and beneficence (Gillon 1994). This not only respects patients' choice but also enhances their autonomy.

The issue of informed consent is crucial in maintaining a patient's autonomy (Scott et al 2003). According to Vincent (1998, p. 1253), the doctor–patient relationship changed from: '[t]he traditional, paternalistic doctor-guided care, to a much more shared approach, with increased public awareness of and openness to discuss disease and death.' This shift has occurred at the same time as an increased emphasis on the nurse–patient relationship and the patient advocacy role of nurses (Nursing and Midwifery Council 2004, Scott et al 2003). The necessity for information, in order to inform the patient, requires truthfulness and honesty. For patients to give their informed consent for a procedure implies that they have sufficient information and understanding of it. Habiba (2000, p. 184) describes informed consent as: 'a voluntary, un-coerced decision, made by a competent autonomous person, to accept rather than reject some proposed course of action'. This would suggest that informed consent is ideally mutually participative, involving shared decision-making between the patient and the health-care team.

Some patients may choose not to be given the full details of the risks or benefits of a procedure or treatment. This is their autonomous decision but it is not informed consent. However, if the nurse reveals information to the patient against their wishes, suffering could result. It is commonly argued within palliative care that most patients do not wish to know the full truth about their prognosis, as they will lose hope. However, there is little evidence to support this (Fallowfield et al 2002). Establishing where patients are in their understanding, providing the necessary information and then revisiting their understanding is a good way to support decision-making, and thus patient autonomy, without causing harm.

REFLECTION POINT 11.2
Truth-telling in the workplace

Reflecting on previous experience, describe a situation where you did or did not withhold information from a patient or family and consider whether this was ethically sound. What ethical principles were at work here, and in what way?

APPLYING REFLECTION TO DECISION-MAKING

The focus will now be on four case studies in which ethical and moral dilemmas have arisen. An ethical reasoning model approach, based on Ferrell (1998), will be applied, using reflection, analysis and discussion in each situation, to enable readers to identify how they might develop their own moral reasoning in the practice setting. Nurses working with patients and relatives in any palliative care setting may recognise situations such as these, where decisions have to be made under difficult circumstances and also where there may be conflict between the personal beliefs and values of all those involved.

Within each of these case scenarios, we will apply the ethical principles of respect for the individual, autonomy, justice, beneficence and non-maleficence to our analysis. These principles guide moral action and are the centre of moral and ethical judgements in professional practice. They generally confirm that actions 'ought' or 'ought not' to be taken, and they can serve as a justification for the process of decision-making and the outcomes in patient care.

CASE STUDY 11.1
Michael

Michael is a 50-year-old single man who has been admitted to the oncology unit with an advanced cancer of the head and neck.

Michael is self-employed and lives alone but has many friends whom he sees at his local social club. Over the last 2 years, he has had surgery to remove the tumour bulk, radiotherapy and chemotherapy. He has now developed more local recurrence and lung metastases and is very frail and unable to work. On admission to the unit he has dysphagia, dyspnoea and is very weak. Michael has refused a gastrostomy to enable feeding to be commenced and has stated that he wants no further active treatment but only to be looked after.

REFLECTIVE ANALYSIS OF MICHAEL'S SITUATION

Michael has refused a treatment that ultimately might prolong his life and possibly make him feel stronger. However, his illness is so advanced it is uncertain what overall good it would do and it might only serve to prescribe a lingering death. The nurse and other team members are concerned that he is starving himself. Nutrition is a basic human need and requirement for life. Failure to commence a method of feeding could hasten Michael's death. His refusal to agree to be fed places a burden on the health-care professionals, who may feel they are failing in their duty of care.

The central ethical principles in this situation are the right to refuse treatment, respect for the individual's choice and personal autonomy. Respect for the individual, compassion and care are the overarching elements in the role of the nurse in the palliative care setting. To have respect for the individual is to value their personal liberty to determine their own actions and make a choice. Respecting a person as an autonomous individual is to acknowledge that their choices stem from their own personal values and beliefs. Michael may want full participation in decisions about his care and health-care professionals should respect this situation for this particular individual.

An autonomous, fully informed patient makes a decision about care based on their own values and priorities. Michael may have decided that artificial feeding, given the advanced stage of his disease, offers no future benefit for his view of the quality of his life. However, it is important and wise to revisit these decisions throughout his care.

The role of the nurse in Michael's situation is to support his right to the decision he has made, in terms of his treatment and care, and to respect his reasons for the decision. The care of any patient is a collaborative and collective one and, although it is the patient who has refused feeding, all professionals should be involved in supporting him at times of vulnerability and offer alternative approaches to alleviate any suffering.

Decisions such as these are often challenging and difficult to make in palliative care. Deontologists, for whom the principle of respect is morally supreme, argue that there are many circumstances in which a person's autonomy must be respected even if to do so will result in a foreseen worse outcome for the patient. For Michael, not to be fed will probably hasten his death but to override his decision might ultimately cause him more harm and distress. This could be difficult for staff to accept when his choice is different from what they feel should be done on ethical grounds.

If Michael is fully aware of the consequences of refusing to be fed, and he has sufficient information and time to make a choice, then the role of the professional is to support this. Gillon (1986) describes rejection as an acceptance of the human condition and, if Michael understands the benefit, risk and burdens, then his decision should be respected.

Tumour of the head and neck can cause distress and suffering either by a sudden acute event or in a protracted terminal phase of the illness. Tube feeding allows Michael to live longer but may cause more harm through the possibility of resulting in a final event of tracheal obstruction or haemorrhage. Not feeding may hasten the process of dying by causing Michael just to fade away.

This is a complex situation. There are times when death appears to be a benefit from both the patient's and the professional's perspective. The distinction between active and passive euthanasia (Box 11.3) is problematic, especially if the action has the consequence of hastening Michael's death without the intention that a supposed bad consequence may follow. In ethical terms, this is known as the 'doctrine of double effect' (Box 11.3; attributed to the theologian Thomas Aquinas) and describes the situation where an individual performs an act that may have two effects, one of which is good (Michael's autonomy and choices respected) and the other which is bad and not desired

---

Box 11.3

Definitions

Euthanasia

The act of killing someone painlessly, especially to relieve suffering, from an incurable disease.

Doctrine of double effect

The doctrine of double effect permits an act, which has the potential to have both good and bad effects. The act itself is good and the good effect is the reason for acting. For example, sedation for distress may shorten life but the intent is good although the result is a possible shortening of life.

(hastening his death). This is said to be morally permissible if the agent did not *intend* the bad consequence to happen. To take such a decision takes moral courage (virtue ethics) and there must be a reason for the action – it must be worthwhile (for Michael) to be able to justify the outcome. Gillon (1986) reminds us that actions cannot only be judged ethically in terms of their consequences. In the practice situation, the conditions under which the actions are carried out, and why they are carried out, are a vital aspect of the moral assessment.

In this case, Michael's refusal to be fed artificially relieves the possibility of prolonging his suffering (as he sees it) and gives the team the opportunity to manage and plan his care in the terminal phase of his illness. Michael's reasons come from his personal values. However, such decisions need to be revisited regularly with Michael throughout his care. Although the decision may remain the same, the priorities of care offered should be continually assessed and evaluated as his condition deteriorates, and Michael should still be part of this. Randall & Downie (2001) suggest that effective relief of prolonged suffering in palliative care may sometimes justify the use of measures that entail a risk of shortening life.

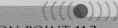

REFLECTION POINT 11.3

Patient autonomy

If you were a nurse caring for Michael, how comfortable would you feel with the level of control that he has taken over his situation? Can you suggest any reasons for your answers?

CASE STUDY 11.2
Emily

Emily is 75 years old and has advanced lung cancer; she also has significant chronic obstructive airways disease and is now confined to bed. Emily is keen to remain at home and is being cared for by her 80-year-old husband, Joe, with the help of the primary health-care team and specialist palliative care service. Over the last few days, her condition has deteriorated, her pain and dyspnoea have not been well controlled and she is becoming increasingly distressed and exhausted. Previous increases in her dosage of opioid have not improved her pain but have only made her drowsy and confused.

Emily is asking to be eased of her suffering and has previously expressed her wish to be allowed to 'slip away' when death is imminent. Joe is exhausted and distressed by the situation but wants to continue to look after Emily at home. Their only son lives in the USA and visited a few months ago. He is constantly in touch and has asked to be informed of any planned changes to Emily's management.

The multidisciplinary teams are meeting to discuss three possible options:

- Increase or change Emily's opioid therapy
- Use sedation to relieve her distress
- Admit her to the hospice.

REFLECTION AND DISCUSSION

There are a number of sensitive issues to address in this situation and some difficult decisions to make. Emily is distressed and is asking for an end to her suffering. She has previously expressed a wish that her life should not be prolonged if her death is imminent. Her elderly husband is her main carer and is exhausted and overwhelmed by her distress.

The multidisciplinary teams are meeting to discuss the best solution for both the patient and her family. We bring in the principles of autonomy (of patient, carers and professionals), beneficence and non-maleficence, and consider what is necessary to reach an acceptable outcome by collective team working.

Randall & Downie (2001) remind us that decision-making involves the team understanding the patient's problems and using the options of treatment approach. The team already knows that increasing Emily's opioids has not always improved her pain and they must consider the fact that her dyspnoea may be more of a problem, making her frightened and thus exacerbating her pain.

Emily is exhausted and relieving her distress is paramount. This would also ease her husband's suffering and it is necessary in the first instance to decide whether her continuing care should be at home or in the hospice. This would also allow the opportunity for Emily's son to be made aware of and involved in the decision process.

In palliative care, the practice of sedating a patient who is imminently dying is sometimes defined within the parameters of 'killing and letting die'. Health-care professionals have a moral obligation to use every reasonable means available to free patients from symptoms that cause them to suffer. This has nothing to do with euthanasia, its purpose and intent being to relieve the patient from the intense discomfort that dominates their consciousness and leaves no space available for the important things they want to think and say before they die (Roy & Rapin 1994).

Sedation of the imminently dying in palliative care practice means that:

- The patient is close to death (hours or days)
- The patient has one or two severe symptoms that are proving refractory to standard palliative care
- The physician treats these symptoms with an effective therapy
- The therapy has a dose-dependent effect of sedation that is a foreseen but unintended consequence of trying to relieve the symptom of distress (Jansen & Sulmasy 2002).

In Emily's case, there is a significant risk that her death may be hastened. Nevertheless, the team may offer this option for the benefit of alleviating her suffering, which, for the patient and family, may outweigh the harm in shortening her life. Emily has made her wishes known and her values and priorities should have been documented in her records and therefore could be used when discussing the treatment approach with the family. They also help to justify the course that has been chosen and explain why.

Advanced directives/statements (Box 11.4) can assist health-care professionals in making decisions for patients, particularly if the patient's autonomy is impaired. This requires practical wisdom and moral courage and there is no moral absolute in these situations. The team can only reasonably expect to provide a balance between 'doing good' and causing the least harm to Emily and her family. Although Emily has made no formalised advanced directive, it is important that nurses should be reminded of their relevance, particularly to patients who have a life-threatening illness.

An advanced directive is a statement about future medical treatment, to take effect if:

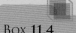

Box 11.4

Definition

Advanced directive (living will)

A formal written advanced statement by a patient refusing treatments in specific stated situations that may occur in a future illness.

- The maker of the advanced directive should become unable to communicate at some future time
- The circumstances specified in the advanced directive arise.

Moral dilemmas in the health-care setting can be eased by the existence of a 'living will' and the use of such documents may increase as medicine advances its technical possibilities (Downie & Calman 1995).

In this case, the primary health-care team and specialist palliative care team have a collective responsibility to the way decisions are made and the outcomes resulting from those decisions. Each team member will have differing moral values and should listen carefully to all the arguments to be able to modify their views accordingly. The professionals, the patient and the family will all contribute to the decisions, with the patient remaining the central focus (Randall & Downie 2001).

In Emily's case, it is important that the teams have decided to meet together and discuss the options of care. Ultimately, the quality of care of Emily and her family is paramount. The moral and ethical content of the decisions made are dependent on the process of how and why the decisions are reached, not only on the outcome.

REFLECTION POINT 11.4

Dying with dignity

The doctrine of double effect relies on a moral distinction between intended and foreseen outcomes. Consider a patient where a difficult decision regarding sedation has to be made.

- How and why did your team arrive at a solution?
- How can advanced statements benefit health-care professionals in making difficult decisions?

CASE STUDY 11.3

Elizabeth

Elizabeth is a 60-year-old widow and has advanced cancer of the breast, with lung and cerebral metastases. She was previously a very independent person who, although she lived alone, had a large extended family in regular contact with her. Her condition has quickly deteriorated at home and the GP feels that specialist intervention is now necessary.

Elizabeth has been admitted to an acute medical ward in the local general hospital with increasing confusion, poor pain control and dysphagia. Her large family is constantly on the ward and is extremely anxious about her current condition. Following assessment by the hospital palliative care team, a syringe driver has been commenced, administering analgesia and a sedative. The intravenous infusion to administer fluids that was commenced on initial admission is still in progress.

The team feels that Elizabeth is dying and recommend an increase in her sedation to alleviate her agitation. It is also felt appropriate to discontinue the intravenous fluids at this point, as there is evidence of her chest becoming increasingly moist.

REFLECTIVE ANALYSIS AND DISCUSSION I

There are a number of issues in this scenario but what is essentially happening in Elizabeth's situation is the withdrawing of futile and non-beneficial treatment that may potentially be causing her harm. Consequently, this causes some alarm among her family, raising the dilemma of who should be making decisions about care plans. Elizabeth's condition is so advanced that she can no longer voice her wishes and it is the health-care team who must decide the best course of treatment in her last few days. This, however, may cause tension with her family if they do not fully understand what is happening and why.

The ethical and moral principles to consider in this case are beneficence and non-maleficence. Would keeping the intravenous fluids running improve the patient's quality of life and dignity in these last few days and would withdrawing the intravenous fluids at this stage cause her more harm than good? Within palliative care, we have a duty to care but not to prolong the process of dying. Withdrawal of treatment when it is no longer possible to restore health or reverse the dying process is perfectly acceptable, but this can create problems for health-care professionals when relatives equate continuing treatment with maintaining hope (Webb 2000). Death is a normal part of living but in modern society it is often perceived as frightening and unfamiliar. The unrealistic expectation of society today is that the medical profession can cure everything and prevent death, which often leads to a difficult situation when dealing with grieving relatives.

Quality of life in the last few days of life is generally a subjective experience (Edwards 2002). This suggests that treatment choices should be made with the best interests of the patient at the centre of the decision. Consider the patient's wishes if they are known, in order to respect the individual's choices, but, if this isn't possible, an alternative strategy must be considered. The aim of alleviating distress and suffering without causing harm or hastening death is central to the palliative approach. Which course of action would be in Elizabeth's best interests?

Research evidence about the effect of providing hydration in palliative care is inconclusive. Some say that it may even be detrimental (Twycross & Wilcock 2001). It can be argued that dehydration might improve the analgesic effect of medication, diminish the risk of incontinence and reduce pulmonary secretions, thus relieving the patient from requiring nasopharyngeal suctioning in the end stage of life. Alternatively, the use of parenteral fluids may make the patient more comfortable at the moment of death. However, Jeffery (1998) proposes that intravenous fluids have little effect unless the patient is complaining of thirst. But either way, for many families, the withdrawal of fluids can be associated with feelings of guilt and abandonment. Everyone is aware of the need for fluids to maintain life. By refusing to provide the patient with fluids, professionals can be accused of incompetence, neglect and hastening death.

By improving communication between professionals and families, a better understanding of the patient's wishes may be reached. Sensitivity to cultural and religious beliefs is paramount at this stage. Culture shapes fundamentally how individuals make meaning out of living and dying. Studies have shown cultural differences in attitudes towards decision-making in the end stage of life (Kagawa-Singer & Blackhall 2001). Thus the risk of cultural misunderstanding surrounding care is increased.

Regardless of cultural background we should ensure family involvement in decision-making. In every case, frank and open discussion with the family is crucial. Decisions might not rest with the family, but proper information and good communication can lead to them supporting the medical decision taken. In Elizabeth's case, the additional fluids appear to be causing more harm than good. Her chest is becoming increasingly moist and may even be adding to her agitated state. The risks outweigh the benefits, suggesting that ethically the health-care team is obligated to withdraw this treatment. If this is explained to the family, they will feel included in the care but will not have the burden of making the difficult decision to stop treatment.

Nurses working in any palliative care setting will have had to face situations where decisions had to be made under difficult circumstances. Collaborative decision-making will assist in most situations but ethical dilemmas continue to arise. The application of the ethical principles to the situation may help guide you to an answer but will not provide the answer when used alone.

REFLECTION POINT 11.5
Decision-making

Can you think of a situation in your own workplace where treatment was withdrawn from a patient? Who was involved in the decision-making process?

CASE STUDY 11.4
Jack

Jack is a 66-year-old man with chronic congestive cardiac failure. His main carer is his wife, Mary, also 66 years old. They have no children but have had a very close marriage of 41 years.

Recent admissions to hospital for acute episodes of breathlessness have become more frequent and Jack's responses to treatment less efficient. He can no longer be left alone at home without his anxiety levels rising and consequent episodes of breathlessness occurring. Mary is exhausted, sleeps little at night and has no free time for herself during the day.

Currently, the district nurse visits twice a week but there is no social service support involved. The GP has requested a 'respite' admission to the local hospice but Jack wishes to remain at home. In spite of his deteriorating condition, Jack's prognosis is indeterminate and the hospice is reluctant to offer more than 1 week respite care.

REFLECTIVE ANALYSIS AND DISCUSSION 2

Within this scenario there are two key dilemmas arising; respect for the individual's right to choose their place of care and the equity of access to palliative care services for patients with an indeterminate prognosis. In Jack's situation, his autonomous wish to remain at home has an impact on his wife and on the resources available within the community setting. The current limitations on palliative care funding raise the question 'Can palliative care provisions be a right for all, irrelevant of diagnosis?'

The current strategy for allocation of resources is inextricably linked with the ethical principle of justice (Hunt 1996). This is a complex issue but generally involves a careful balancing of the benefits and burdens for the individual with the benefit for society as a whole. It is widely accepted that palliative care should be available at a basic level for everyone but how can we support the autonomous rights of the individual to access any service appropriate to their needs? Current services are stretched thinly even when only attempting to meet the needs of patients with cancer.

The utilitarian approach would suggest the use of outcome measures to identify areas deserving of resources. An example of a validated palliative care outcome measure is the Palliative Care Outcome Scale (Hearn & Higginson 1999). It is based on symptom assessment and quality of life issues, measuring issues important to patients where the more traditional mortality outcome measures are not important. By using such a tool, Jack's GP may be in a better position to justify the individual's right to access hospice care for longer than 2 weeks. However, this may be disputed, as it contravenes the principle of utility. By admitting Jack to the hospice for an indeterminate period, access to palliative care services will be denied for a greater number of patients.

The other key issue is around Jack's wish to remain at home. 'Autonomy' is the ability to make decisions independently based on honest information. If Jack wishes to remain at home, and is in possession of all the facts, this decision should be respected by the nurse and supported by any accessible resources. But if this decision is based on lack of knowledge and fear of hospice care, the nurse has an obligation to explore things further and provide information as desired by Jack. People must be free to make choices even if we don't agree with them but we can ensure that choices are based on accurate information.

If, however, Mary states she is no longer willing to care for Jack at home, and the resources to support his needs are not available, a further dilemma will arise. Unless Jack is deemed incompetent, he cannot be removed from his home even if the professionals feel he is not receiving the care he requires. Interestingly, the opposite is the case if Jack was in hospital and wished to die at home. According to the Community Care Act (Department of Health 1990), if Mary refused to take Jack home after his stay in the hospice and a sufficient care package was not demonstrated to be in place, the palliative care team would be obliged to keep Jack in their care. This causes problems when the patient's choice about place of care is considered to be paramount.

Beyond the consideration of the principle of respect for the individual's autonomy are the principles of beneficence and non-maleficence. By removing Jack from his own home, where he feels safe, will we be causing more harm than good? But by keeping him at home, what harm are we causing his wife? The World Health Organization (2003) identifies the fact that responsibility often falls upon the shoulders of the family and suggests that, if a society encourages home care, it also has an ethical responsibility to look after both the patient and family caregivers. But, in an environment where investment in palliative care services is scarce and often supplemented by charitable donations (NCHSPCS 1997), we must be certain that resources are used in the best way. Ultimately, the patient should be able to choose where to be cared for, even if the circumstances are far from ideal. The decision would be best made in partnership with both the patient and family, with the ability and willingness of the family to participate in the care clearly identified.

Jack's story highlights the type of situation in which many nurses working in the community setting may find themselves. The apparent inequity of access to resources for patients with a non-malignant condition can cause frustration and often a sense of being unable to fulfil our duty to care for our patients. The conflict between respect for the patient's wishes and respect for one's professional responsibility in providing the best possible care reflects many of the day-to-day concerns facing nurses.

REFLECTION POINT 11.6
Palliative care services

Do you know what palliative care services are available in your local area? If not, seek out the nearest palliative care service and find out what might be offered should a patient in your care require more help than your professional team can supply. How accessible are these resources and services to patients with non-malignant disease?

IMPLICATIONS FOR NURSING PRACTICE

Nurses working with patients and relatives in any palliative care setting may face similar situations to those described in these case scenarios. In this chapter we have chosen to focus on the ethical principles – respect for the individual, autonomy, justice, beneficence and non-maleficence – applying the underpinning of some ethical theory to each case.

Professional nursing is all about having the knowledge and skills to do things, and an awareness of the relationship between how you act and about the potential outcome (end) result of those actions. Nursing practice is not an end in itself but a means to achieve positive outcomes and experiences for the patient, family or community. It depends upon the interactions between people being patient focused rather than practitioner focused (Wainwright 1999).

Through reflection, analysis of the ethical dilemmas in nursing practice, and discussion around these, the nurse can become more ethically sensitive in responding to future situations (Johns 1999).

Nurses have always been seen as the care protectors and advocates for the patient and this is even more important today due to advances in medical care, technology and the growing possibilities of palliative care patients being included in research trials. These developments require the nurse to be more ethically aware of the moral and legal implications of the care they deliver. In palliative care, patients and families are at their most vulnerable (Box 11.5) and need to be safeguarded and informed of their rights. Nurses must be aware of issues of care and justice that might arise and that might need to be addressed.

The adoption of reflection and an interpretive approach such as the 'ethical reasoning model' (Ferrell 1998) may help practitioners develop intuitive skills alongside ethically based reflection, based on previous experiences. One of the critical roles of ethics is to provide sound justification for the decisions and judgements that are made in ethically challenging situations.

Box 11.5

Definition

Vulnerable patient
Someone capable of being emotionally wounded or hurt – for example a patient with end-stage disease who is fragile and dependent and may be easily coerced or manipulated because of this.

CONCLUSION

In this chapter we have highlighted some common dilemmas that nurses may have to face in the palliative setting to help the reader to develop 'ethical insight' into these situations.

Palliative care has developed steadily over the last 20 years, its widening scope resulting in more complex issues to unravel, particularly in decisions at the end of life. Technological interventions can prolong life and this has blurred the distinction between acute care and end-of-life care, and indeed between life and death. Moreover, patients and families are now able to access information from many sources and can influence choices about their care.

Nurses are in the front line of caring and should have a voice in the discussions and decision-making around these issues. This is why we chose to focus on case scenarios that present ethical dilemmas. Some of the questions these raised may be able to be answered, but perhaps many more questions will be raised as you reflect on your own experiences.

A structured reflective approach was used in the concept of 'ethical mapping', where the various contextual factors within the decision-making environment are viewed – for example the position of the patient and family and who has the authority to take action. We also applied an approach using an ethical reasoning model, based on reflection, to identify and understand what might be occurring in each situation.

Johns (1999) defines reflection as a window for practitioners to look inside themselves and know who they are as they try to understand their work in everyday practice. This exemplifies the challenge that ethical dilemmas present in palliative care nursing and enables us to develop our own understanding and knowledge. It is the contradictions within some of the decisions that must be made that create the challenge in palliative care nursing.

You may recognise this in the case scenarios we have discussed. A major concern in palliative care settings is the vulnerability of patients who are in the final stages of illness. The fear of pain and dying, as well as the fear of death, may add to the burden of decision-making. In addition, there may be uncertainty and confusion about the options of future care. Recognising the closeness of ethical principles to the practice of nursing dying patients may enable the study of ethics and of ethical problems to be related directly to the practice of palliative care.

Nurses face situations with ethical implications on a daily basis, but these become problems only when no solution is to be found. However, it is important to remember that nurses do not work in isolation: they are part of a multiprofessional team and participate in prescribed treatments, and must acknowledge their personal and professional accountability for this. If an ethical question arises, then the nurse should voice any concerns there may be in a climate of mutual support and respect within the team. Debate and dissension, however, are integral to the ethical decision-making process, and having different perspectives, and alternative views and outcomes for consideration is crucial in decision-making (Botes 2000).

'No man is an island' and ethical decisions made without interaction between the various members of a multidisciplinary team could be deemed ineffective.

The idea of collaborative interprofessional working is to reach some sort of consensus on issues that can be challenging. In doing this, the team can then support their decisions and reasoning, thus completing the reflective cycle.

For nurses, ethics is not so much about theoretical arguments as about practical activities and attitudes that influence care. Palliative care should ultimately strive for excellence in the terms of a holistic approach to every patient as a unique individual. The value of considering ethical issues in some detail is that it can assist in adopting a framework for problem-solving in situations where there appears to be no easy answer.

The application of ethical principles to practice often demonstrates different potential outcomes, sometimes resulting in tensions. For example, the principles of beneficence and non-maleficence may conflict with an individual's right to autonomy. Applying an ethical model or framework to complex health-care issues may help reconcile these tensions.

Perhaps it is right to end by completing Cooper's quote (1991, cited in Chinn and Kramer 1999), with which we began:

Ethical choices should be guided not only by roles and principles but also by thoughtful analysis of feelings, intuitions and experiences.

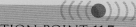

REFLECTION POINT 11.7

Ethics and the practice of nursing

We leave you to consider the following question:

- How does your knowledge of ethics enable you to reflect on and develop your practice?

REFERENCES

Beauchamp T, Childress J 1994 Principles of biomedical ethics, 4th edn. Oxford University Press, New York

Botes A 2000 An integrated approach to ethical decision making in the healthcare team. Journal of Advanced Nursing 32:1–10

Boyd K, Higgs R, Pinching A 1997 New dictionary of medical ethics. BMJ Publications, London

Browne N 1998 Truth-telling in palliative care. European Journal of Oncology Nursing 2:218–224

Chinn P, Kramer M 1999 Theory and nursing: integrated knowledge development, 5th edn. Mosby, St Louis

Concise Oxford Dictionary 1999 Concise Oxford Dictionary, 10th edn. Oxford University Press, Oxford

Cooper M C 1991 Principle-orientated ethics and the ethic of care: a creative tension. Advances in Nursing Science 14:22–31

Department of Health 1990 The NHS and Community Care Act 1990. HMSO, London, c. 19

Department of Health 1995 A policy framework for commissioning cancer services (Calman K, Hine D). HMSO, London

Department of Health 1998 The Human Rights Act. TSO, London

Department of Health 2001 Quality and fairness – a health system for you. TSO, London

Doane J 2002 In the spirit of creativity: the learning and teaching of ethics in nursing. Journal of Advanced Nursing 39:521–525

Downie R, Calman K 1995 Healthy respect: ethics and healthcare, 2nd edn. Oxford University Press, Buckingham

Economics of Health Care 2002 Case study – Child B. OHE. Office of Health Economics. Available on line from: www.oheschools.org/ohech1pg8.html

Edwards D 2002 A philosophical discussion of end-of-life decision-making methods for incompetent patients. International Journal of Palliative Nursing 8:146–151

Fallowfield L, Jenkins V A, Beveridge H A 2002 Truth may hurt but deceit hurts more: communication in palliative care. Palliative Medicine 16:297–303

Ferrell L 1998 Doing the right thing: customary vs reflective morality in nursing practice. In: Johns C, Freshwater D (eds) Transforming nursing through reflective practice. Blackwell Science, Oxford, ch 3

Fry S, Johnstone M 2002 Ethics in nursing practice, 2nd edn. Blackwell Science, Oxford

Gilligan C 1982 In a different voice: psychological theory and women's development. Harvard University Press, Boston, MA

Gillon R 1986 Philosophical medical ethics. John Wiley, Chichester

Gillon R 1994 Medical ethics: four principles plus attention to scope. British Medical Journal 309:184–188

Grayling A 2001 The meaning of things. Weidenfeld & Nicholson, London

Habiba M A 2000 Examining consent within the doctor–patient relationship. Journal of Medical Ethics 26:183–187

Have H T, Clark D 2002 The ethics of palliative care: European perspectives. Open University Press, Buckingham

Hearn J, Higginson I 1999 Development and validation of a core outcome measure for palliative care: the palliative care outcome scale. Quality in Health Care 8:219–227

Hunt S 1996 Ethics of resource distribution: implications for palliative care services. International Journal of Palliative Care Nursing 2:222–226

Hursthouse R 1999 On virtue ethics. Open University Press, Buckingham

Jansen L, Sulmasy D 2002 Sedation, alimentation, hydration, and equivocation: careful conversations about care at the end of life. Annals of Internal Medicine 136:845–849

Jeffery D 1998 Ethical issues in palliative care. In: Faull C, Carter Y, Woof R (eds) Handbook of palliative care. Blackwell Science, Oxford

Johns C 1997 Commentary on reflection – 'reflections on reflection'. Nursing in Critical Care 2:144–145

Johns C 1999 Unraveling the dilemmas within everyday nursing practice. Nursing Ethics 6:287–298

Johnston M 1999 Bioethics: a nursing perspective, 3rd edn. Harcourt Saunders, Sydney

Kagawa-Singer M, Blackhall L 2001 Negotiating cross-cultural issues at the end of life: 'You got to go where he lives'. Journal of the American Medical Association 286:2993–3001

Lloyd D 1997 Revision notes in diploma of healthcare ethics. Centre of Law and Ethics, King's College, London

Macedo S 1992 Liberal virtues: citizenship, virtue and community in liberal constitutionalism. Clarendon Press, Oxford.

NCHSPCS 1997 Making palliative care better. National Council for Hospice and Specialist Palliative Care Services, London

NCHSPCS 1998 Reaching out. National Council for Hospice and Specialist Palliative Care Services, London

NHS Scotland 2003 Partnership for care – Scotland's health. White Paper. Scottish Executive, Edinburgh

Nouwen H 1976 Reaching out. Collins, London

Nursing and Midwifery Council 2004 The NMC code of professional conduct. NMC, London

Randall F, Downie R 2001 Palliative care ethics: a companion for all specialties, 2nd edn. Oxford University Press, Oxford

Roy D, Rapin C 1994 Regarding euthanasia. European Journal of Palliative Care 1:57–59

Scott A 1995 Moral obligation. Nursing Times 91(5):50–51

Scott P A, Taylor A, Valimaki M et al 2003 Autonomy, privacy and informed consent 4: surgical perspective. British Journal of Nursing 12:311–320

Thompson I, Melia K, Boyd K 2000 Nursing ethics, 4th edn. Churchill Livingstone, Edinburgh

Twycross R, Wilcock A 2001 Symptom management in advanced cancer, 3rd edn. Radcliffe Medical, Oxford

Vincent J 1998 Information in the ICU: are we being honest with our patients? The results of a European questionnaire. Intensive Care Medicine 24:1251–1256

Wainwright P 1999 The art of nursing. International Journal of Nursing Studies 36:379–385

Webb P 2000 Ethical issues in palliative care. Hochland & Hochland, Manchester

Webber J 1996 Ethical dimensions in palliative nursing. International Journal of Palliative Nursing 2:61

World Health Organization 2003 Cancer pain relief and palliative care. WHO, Geneva

CHAPTER TWELVE

Evidence-based palliative care

Catriona M Kennedy, Karen Lockhart-Wood

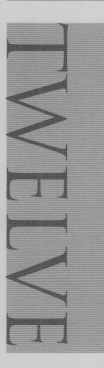

CONTENTS

Caring for patients and families who have palliative care needs requires a knowledge base that encompasses the physical, psychosocial and spiritual aspects of care and a range of interpersonal skills. Increasingly, nurses are required to explain and justify their actions and identify the evidence on which their practice is based. This is not a new requirement, as over 30 years ago the Briggs Report stated that nursing should become a research-based profession (Department of Health and Social Security 1972). Furthermore the quest for excellent, effective and appropriate clinical care for patients and families has been identified in an increasing number of policy and strategy documents (Department of Health 1993, 1996, 1998, Royal College of Nursing 1996).

Nurses working in palliative care require knowledge drawn from the physical sciences, social sciences, arts and humanities to provide holistic, patient and family focused care.

> [K]nowledge underlying nursing grows like a spiral. There can be no end point as the universe will never be totally mastered. It is this continuous never ending potential to create and use further knowledge, the opportunity for ongoing learning, that not only enables nursing to develop its all important body of knowledge but also makes life exciting and worthwhile for us all.
>
> Hockey 1996, p. 5

If palliative nursing care is to be based on the best available evidence there are three key questions that, individually and collectively, nurses need to consider:

- Where do you look for the evidence on which to base decisions and subsequent actions?
- When you find suitable evidence, how do you evaluate it – what counts as evidence?
- How can 'good evidence' be applied to practice in a usable form?

This chapter seeks to provide you with information to help develop these essential skills to ensure excellent, effective and appropriate palliative care for patients and families.

AIMS OF THE CHAPTER

The aims of this chapter are to enable the reader to:

- Critically appraise the sources of evidence available to inform palliative care nursing practice
- Evaluate the application of evidence to the practice of palliative care
- Evaluate quality of care within the context of clinical governance
- Explore the ethical issues relevant to palliative care research.

WHY SEEK TO CHANGE PRACTICE?

There is a saying 'If it ain't broke, don't fix it', so why seek to change practice? Nurses are, quite reasonably, expected to know what they are doing. It is expected that the basis of what they do or say is judged to be appropriate and based on an appraisal of the range of alternatives for action. Traditionally, some aspects of nursing practice have been based on ritual and routine. In some respects this is not surprising, as people required care long before the existence of nursing research. However, explaining the evidence base on which decision-making and subsequent actions are based is impossible if the profession depends on ritual and routine as the basis of practice.

The growth in nursing research in the UK since the 1960s can be attributed to the development in undergraduate and postgraduate programmes of education and in nursing research. Forty years is a relatively short period of time for the development of an evidence base for a profession and the evidence base for nursing is at an early stage of development. Therefore we do not always know whether our decisions and subsequent interventions are effective and appropriate. In the absence of evidence, who chooses what to do? What are decisions based on if evidence does not exist for a particular clinical issue or available evidence is not accessed and appraised by us as practitioners?

The exploration of the knowledge underpinning nursing practice can largely be attributed to the seminal work of Carper (1978), who examined early nursing literature and named four fundamental ways of knowing in nursing (Box 12.1):

- Empirics, the science of nursing
- Ethics, the component of moral knowledge in nursing
- Aesthetics, the art of nursing
- Personal knowing in nursing.

These have remained the fundamental ways of knowing reflected in current literature (Jacobs-Kramer & Chinn 1988, Rolfe 1998, White 1995). Traditionally, nursing has followed the positivist research paradigm in the pursuit of academic credibility (Rolfe 1998). However, it could be argued that focusing on knowledge derived from empirical, quantitative research has limited the development and exploration of knowledge in use within nursing. Randomised controlled trials (RCTs) may offer the right basis for

---

Box 12.1

Ways of knowing in nursing (adapted from Carper 1978)

Empirics: Scientific or propositional knowledge consisting of theories and models that can be tested empirically

Aesthetics: The artistic component of nursing, including the expressive and technical skills of nursing – based on the actions, conduct and interaction of the nurse with others

Personal knowledge: 'Know-how' in everyday practice

Ethical knowledge: Moral knowledge of what is good and right, based on beliefs and values.

judging the merit of certain treatments in both medicine and nursing. However, the espousal of holistic nursing care, with its recognition of the key psychosocial and spiritual aspects of health, suggests that alternative ways of gathering evidence will be necessary. This is especially true in relation to palliative care, which holds quality of life to be an underpinning philosophy of care.

Carper's (1978) work has drawn attention to the fact that, currently, nurses and nursing need and depend upon knowledge additional to that provided by empirical science, and this recognition has been crucial to the development of nursing knowledge.

Nursing is a practice-based discipline and it is expected that knowledge will be gained through experience in practice. Clearly, nurses working in palliative care require a broad knowledge base derived from a range of disciplines. Much of the knowledge of experienced palliative care nurses is personal and not easily explained or transferred to others. It involves knowing what to do with a particular patient and/or relative at a particular moment in time.

In recognition that scientific enquiry alone cannot account for the evidence base of nursing practice, nursing scholars have attempted to legitimise the knowledge that is derived from experience and practice rather than scientific enquiry alone (Kennedy 1998, Luker & Kenrick 1992, Macleod 1996, Meerabeau 1995).

It would appear, then, that practitioners' knowledge is based on an amalgam of theoretical (knowing that) and practical (knowing how) knowledge. Practitioners themselves may not be able to easily identify the knowledge on which they base practice. Research has identified that practitioners may be unable to articulate the sources of their knowledge and that a large proportion of their practice is based on experiential knowledge (Kennedy 2002, Luker & Kenrick 1992, Macleod 1996). This may be because experienced practitioners have developed an integrated knowledge base that does not differentiate between knowledge, experience and science. A significant proportion of nursing practice is therefore likely to be based on a mix of public (in the public domain) and private (known to the individual) theories.

A BASIS FOR DECISION-MAKING

Deciding how to act (or deciding that no action is necessary) has an enormous impact on quality of care and subsequent outcomes for the patient and family. Therefore, the knowledge base of the nurse and its impact on decision-making about whether and how to act are important. Decision-making work relevant to nursing mainly focuses on information-processing theory such as the nursing process and the hypothetico-deductive approach. These are descriptive models of decision-making that suggest discrete stages on the decision-making process (Box 12.2). There is in nursing practice, however, intense interest in intuition either as a form of knowledge or as a mode of cognition. The reality may lie somewhere between these two positions, as practitioners'

Box 12.2

Stages in decision-making: the hypothetico-deductive approach (Elstein & Bordage 1979)

- **Data collection** – the process of gathering and collecting information

- **Hypothesis generation** – the process of generating alternative formulations of the problem

- **Cue interpretation** – the process of interpreting the evidence in the light of these hypotheses

- **Hypothesis evaluation** – the process of combining information to reach a diagnostic decision or judgement

expertise may influence how they are able to use the appropriate mode of cognition for the decision-making tasks.

For example, if you are responsible for setting up a syringe driver and explaining the procedure to a less experienced colleague, you would probably be able to describe the procedure of setting up the syringe driver and explain how to calculate the doses of prescribed drugs. You might also be able to identify the sources of knowledge for the task as those drawn from theory about the purpose of the syringe driver and knowledge of drug doses and compatibility, and have experience in completing the task. However, deciding what information to give to the patient and appropriate family members may be rather less clear-cut and will be context-dependent. You need to judge what information is appropriate to give in each case. How well you know the patient, their expressed wishes and their condition are likely to influence your actions as a nurse. It is in a scenario such as this that we are likely to say 'Well, I just knew what to do' and attribute our actions to intuition.

Attributing aspects of nursing practice to intuition is arguably dangerous for the profession in a climate where transparency of actions and individual accountability are paramount. If nurses are unable or unwilling to articulate what they do and why, this will limit development of the evidence base of the profession.

We need to challenge current practice: Why am I doing this and how can my actions be justified? Every nurse needs the skills to critically appraise the evidence available to inform practice and many nurses need to be involved in the generation of new knowledge in order to ensure that the evidence base for practice is robust and fit for purpose. Nurses also need to ensure that any changes made to practice are likely to improve the experience and outcomes for the patient and family.

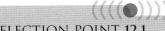

REFLECTION POINT 12.1

Identifying your own knowledge (adapted from Rolfe 1998)

Identify one aspect of your role from your day-to-day work.

- On a scale of 1–10, rate how confident you are (10 being absolutely confident) that you have the knowledge required to carry out this action?

- How did you gain the necessary knowledge, e.g. theory, reading, practice experience?

- What kind of knowledge is it?

SOURCES AND LEVELS OF EVIDENCE

Evidence-based practice is a process of systematically reviewing, appraising and using clinical research findings to inform care decisions, and is a component of clinical effectiveness. The drive towards evidence-based practice has its origins in North America and the McMaster Medical School in Canada originally coined the term 'evidence-based medicine' in the 1980s (Deighan & Boyd 1996). In the recognition that all health care needs to be evidence-based, this term has been broadened from its original medical focus. Evidence-based practice is a process that integrates the best available evidence from systematic research with clinical practice. Without evidence, clinical practice may become routine and outdated. The question is, then: Where do we look for evidence?

Evidence for practice may be drawn from two main sources: published materials and expert clinical practice. If we are to use evidence from published sources to inform our decision-making and subsequent actions, we need to determine the quality of the evidence available and be able to distinguish research from other forms of reporting. For example, research articles are usually published in an academic journal, typically with the word 'journal' or 'studies' in its title. Similarly, review articles are usually published in academic journals and may be identified as a 'review' to distinguish them from the other contents, but may also be published in a professional journal.

Professional journalism, which focuses on current professional issues, is usually published on a monthly or weekly basis. This type of publication is generally not considered to be a reliable source of evidence for practice, as it may be opinion-based or biased towards the views of the author. The important point to remember is that not everything that is published is good-quality research, so nurses need to be able to discern what is or is not sound and reliable evidence.

Research evidence is presented in many forms, and its value can be ranked according to its level of credibility. However there appears to be a lack of consensus over the exact classification of different levels of evidence, but these can be divided into six broad areas with the 'best' level of evidence at level 1 (Table 12.1). Such grading of evidence into different levels is used to inform the production of clinical guidelines, where recommendations for practice are made and the level of evidence used to inform this recommendation is made explicit (SIGN 2000, Wiffen 1998).

USING EVIDENCE TO SUPPORT RECOMMENDATIONS FOR PRACTICE

The best level of evidence available is the systematic review or meta-analysis of RCTs. Systematic reviews follow a clear protocol that sets out the review methodology from the outset and are more comprehensive and inclusive in their search than the traditional literature review (Hearn et al 1999). Efforts are also made to locate studies that have not been published, also known as 'grey literature', as well as published sources. A detailed inclusion and exclusion list of criteria is given and the justification for excluding studies from the review is made explicit.

Thus the systematic review provides clinicians with a reliable overview of all the available research evidence on a particular topic and is therefore the most rigorous approach to assessing the quality of the evidence available in a particular field or area (Hearn et al 1999). In contrast, traditional published literature reviews have been identified as subjective, as the authors may be selective about which studies they include, thus introducing a source of bias.

Meta-analysis pools together the results from a number of trials, often with different sample sizes, age ranges and contexts, thus providing a larger sample size from which to draw conclusions. Although less rigorous than the systematic review, this approach provides greater confidence than might be placed in the findings of otherwise smaller-scale studies. No matter how well they are conducted, individual studies are unlikely to provide conclusive evidence relating to a particular research question; thus, when a particular finding is

TABLE 12.1
Levels of evidence

Level	Evidence obtained from
I	A systematic review or meta-analysis of randomised controlled trials
II	At least one randomised controlled trial
III	Systematic review of non-randomised controlled study
IV	At least one other well designed quasi-experimental study
V	Well designed non-experimental descriptive studies (e.g. comparative studies, correlation studies, case studies and qualitative studies)
VI	Consensus of expert opinion (e.g. Delphi studies)

Box 12.3

Systematic review: do hospital palliative care teams improve care for patients or families at the end of life? (Higginson et al 2002)

Higginson et al (2002) conducted a systematic review of literature to determine whether hospital palliative care teams improved care for patients or families at the end of life. Using detailed search terms, the review included electronic searches of ten databases, hand searching of specialist journals, contacting authors and examining the reference lists of all papers retrieved. A detailed set of inclusion and exclusion criteria was given and all eligible studies were graded for quality and rigour. While only one randomised controlled trial was found, other studies examined the intervention of a hospital palliative care team in relation to outcomes such as symptoms, quality of life, length of time in hospital or palliative care, and changes in professional practices such as prescribing habits. The reviewers concluded that, from their findings, there was some evidence to support the belief that hospital palliative care teams offered positive benefits to patients and carers at the end of life; however, the evidence available was quite weak, which presents a challenge to palliative care practitioners.

The results of this review highlight the need for further good-quality research. Indeed, the authors called for further evaluation of the cost-effectiveness of hospital palliative care teams in meeting the needs of patients and carers.

obtained in a number of studies, there is greater confidence that this general principle is true (Burns 2000).

Systematic reviews or meta-analyses of several randomised trials have become the 'gold standard' for judging whether a treatment does more good than harm. However, some aspects of care do not lend themselves to this type of research or cannot wait for trials to be conducted. Therefore, if no randomised trial has been carried out for our patient's predicament, we look to the next best level of evidence and work from there.

THE ROLE OF CLINICAL PRACTICE GUIDELINES

Within the UK two organisations have been set up to coordinate the production of evidence-based clinical practice guidelines. In Scotland this is the Scottish Intercollegiate Guidelines Network (SIGN) and in England and Wales it is the National Institute for Clinical Excellence. The SIGN guideline on control of pain in patients with cancer (SIGN 2000) provides an example of an area of practice that draws on evidence from the various levels outlined in Table 12.1. Evidence from level 1 is available to support the recommendation of using paracetamol, aspirin and non-steroidal anti-inflammatory drugs for mild pain. However this level of evidence may also be used to cast doubt over the efficacy of interventions. For example the use of transcutaneous electrical nerve stimulation is considered by many to be useful in the management of cancer pain but evidence from level 1 suggests that there is no clear evidence of therapeutic benefit (SIGN 2000). For nurses working in palliative care this type of evidence can cause a dilemma when making decisions about interventions.

Additionally, it is widely acknowledged and supported by the available research that effective pain management requires accurate and regular assessment. The research available to support this recommendation for practice comes from comparative studies, non-experimental descriptive studies and case studies, which are grouped in level 5. SIGN also advocates the use of a standardised assessment tool when assessing patients with cancer pain; however, the level of evidence available to support the use of this recommendation is from the lowest category in Table 12.1. This does not mean that we can ignore the evidence that supports pain assessment, just that this evidence is acknowledged to be at a lower level. Given the nature of palliative care and the need for a holistic approach to symptom management, evidence will require to be drawn from a range of sources.

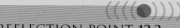

REFLECTION POINT 12.2

Levels of evidence

Consider an area of practice that you are involved in. How do the levels of evidence support your practice? It may be that the evidence to support the area is from a 'low' level. Consider the reasons for this. Is it because there has been limited research activity in this area or is the area of practice not amenable to 'scientific' research?

QUANTITATIVE AND QUALITATIVE RESEARCH APPROACHES

Research approaches can be broadly divided into quantitative (positivist) and qualitative (naturalist) methods of enquiry. Nurse researchers have expended considerable energy in debating the differences between and relative advantages of quantitative and qualitative methods.

Quantitative and qualitative research has evolved from a range of disciplines and each approach has rich and varied traditions. Both approaches have been employed to address a range of research topics and the choice of research approach should be driven by the research question/s – different questions have different emphasis. While it is important to understand the principles underpinning these two research approaches we should avoid driving a wedge between them as many studies use a 'mixed methods' approach.

For example the work of Herth (1990), which explored the meaning of hope and identified strategies that foster hope in terminally ill patients, used qualitative and quantitative methods. This study used semi-structured interviews to collect qualitative data and self-report instruments to collect quantitative data. Herth's work is important for palliative nursing as it provides a framework for practice that can help nurses to identify strategies and interventions that are likely to foster hope in terminally ill people throughout their illness.

Quantitative methods are based on the scientific method and modelled on the processes used in the natural sciences. They involve measurement, deductive reasoning, causality and hypothesis testing (MacKenzie 1994). Quantitative studies tend to have a clearly defined focus, large sample sizes and data that can be tested by using a set of procedures and rules. The drive for nursing to contribute to the establishment of a sound body of evidence for practice may be seen as an incentive for nurse researchers to adopt the positivist approach (NHS Management Executive 1994, Wilson-Barnett 1998).

In qualitative (naturalist) methods, the social researcher studies phenomena within the natural setting in order to understand human behaviour. This approach allows the researcher to interpret people's worlds and understand behaviours, opinions and interactions using real examples (Hammersley & Atkinson 1995). The sample sizes in qualitative studies are generally smaller than those used in quantitative ones and purposive or convenience-sampling strategies are normally employed.

The remainder of this section will explore the contribution and use of quantitative and qualitative research in palliative nursing care.

QUANTITATIVE RESEARCH IN PALLIATIVE CARE

Quantitative research is considered to be the science of discovering how the world works with the aim of creating laws and determining predictability of actions. Quantitative research is based on the belief that causal relationships can be proved in a systematic and objective manner. Characteristics of quantitative research are that it is objective, systematic, rigorous and concerned with measurement and the statistical representation of findings. The aim of this type of research is for the findings to be generalisable to a wider population.

Quantitative research is therefore reductionist, as it breaks down the phenomenon under study into its component parts, which are then described and termed 'variables'. Variables may be related to the characteristics and attributes of the participants in the study, to interventions or events and to the outcomes measures that are to be examined. Effects are then observed, measured and described. In palliative care, however, description of variables is often not an easy task as the outcome measure can be abstract in nature – for example quality of life, comfort or distress. In such instances an operational definition will usually be given to guide the research project and aid a common understanding of the concept.

A useful definition of quantitative research is offered by Porter & Carter (2000, p. 19) who state that: 'Quantitative research is a formal, objective, systematic process for obtaining quantifiable information about the world, presented in numerical form and analysed through the use of statistics. It is used to describe and test relationships and to examine cause-and-effect relationships.'

The philosophical underpinnings of quantitative research come from the traditional sciences. Because of this influence it is often termed 'positivist' or 'empirical' research. Quantitative research has traditionally been held in high regard, with proponents of this approach asserting that it provides a more objective and thus more reliable source of knowledge for practice. Evidence from funding bodies would support this, as historically quantitative research studies have received significantly more funding than qualitative studies (Carr 1994). However, it is now recognised that both quantitative and qualitative research methods provide valuable contributions to knowledge.

TYPES OF QUANTITATIVE RESEARCH

The term 'quantitative research' relates to a variety of research designs, including surveys, descriptive research, correlational research, experimental and quasi-experimental research, as well as the controlled trial, which may or may not be randomised. There are many comprehensive texts that give fuller explanations of quantitative research methods but for the purpose of this section the relevance of these research methods in palliative care will be explored.

Surveys

Surveys are a common approach to quantitative research and are usually in the form of a questionnaire. Many of us are familiar with this type of research through responding to different types of survey in our day-to-day life. Surveys have the advantage of being able to reach a large number of potential participants, are relatively cheap and easy to administer. One of the main disadvantages, however, is that surveys often have a poor response rate (Polit & Hungler 1995).

Surveys can be descriptive or explanatory. Descriptive surveys seek to describe the characteristics or variables under study, whereas exploratory surveys aim to explore areas of practice where there is little information.

Surveys into palliative care such as Linklater et al's study (Box 12.4) have mainly been at the descriptive level, with some of these using very large samples to gain a national representation of palliative care provision (Copp et al 1998) or to research care provision in a particular setting (Froggatt et al 2002).

Another common type of survey conducted in palliative care is the patient or carer satisfaction survey. This type of survey seeks to elicit the views of those using the services provided and to quantify the responses with a view to producing a meaningful report. Such a report can influence the provision and

BOX 12.4

An exploratory study: pain management services in palliative care (Linklater et al 2002)

A recent exploratory survey by Linklater et al (2002) used a postal questionnaire to explore the experiences and views of palliative care physicians with regard to input from anaesthetists in the management of complex pain. The researchers concluded that the majority of consultants were satisfied with the level of input from anaesthetists but felt that their role could extend to include advice on prescribing drugs. The survey also identified a lack of formal arrangement between palliative care units and anaesthetic departments as problematic.

This type of study provides practitioners in palliative care with information regarding service provision, from which recommendations may be made.

focus of service provision. However satisfaction surveys are fraught with difficulty because of the abstract nature of the concept of satisfaction. Other variables such pain and symptom distress, as well as depression, may significantly influence the respondent's perception of satisfaction. Tools used to measure such factors are described more fully under data collection methods.

DESCRIPTIVE RESEARCH

Descriptive research may be used to describe the characteristics of a certain population. Further research would be required to find out why this is the case and to help health-care professionals target this service more effectively to other groups of the population.

CORRELATIONAL RESEARCH

Correlational research is concerned with the systematic investigation of the relationships between two variables. For example, in testing the relationship between two variables we examine the strength of correlation between two characteristics. Burns (2000) uses the example of the correlation between locus of control and self-esteem. The usefulness of this sort of research in palliative care is that it may help practitioners to identify patients who might benefit from interventions designed to promote a stronger internal locus of control, thus promoting self-esteem, which may improve perceived quality of life. Obviously, this is an assumption that would require further research to substantiate it.

EXPERIMENTAL AND QUASI-EXPERIMENTAL RESEARCH AND THE RANDOMISED CONTROLLED TRIAL

The experiment is considered to be the most powerful type of quantitative research as it tests cause and effect in order to demonstrate whether a treatment or intervention is effective. It involves comparing one group who are receiving active treatment or an intervention against a control or placebo group. The characteristics of both groups must be similar. This can be achieved through randomisation of the participants to either group, thus eliminating any source of selection bias.

Control groups are used to compare the effectiveness of the treatment or intervention under scrutiny. Ideally, participants and researchers should not know whether they are receiving 'active' treatment. This is a process called 'double-blinding'. However it is not always possible for the participant and/or the researcher to be blinded. Hodgson (2000) conducted a RCT of reflexology to determine the impact on patients' quality of life. During the pilot it became apparent that patients who had previous experience of reflexology were able to determine whether or not they were in the active treatment group or the placebo group, thus becoming unblinded. This led to patients with previous experience of this therapy being excluded from the main study.

The RCT is considered to be the gold standard of experimental design, as it has been argued that it provides the most rigorous method of determining whether or not a cause and effect relationship exists between a treatment or intervention and an outcome (Sibbald & Roland 1998). In the table of levels of evidence, the RCT is ranked as the second best level of evidence, with only the systematic review of RCTs being considered better. However, for practical reasons, as illustrated above, or for ethical reasons it is not always possible to meet the rigorous standards required for a RCT. A quasi-experimental design study (Box 12.5) would then be an appropriate design. This term relates to experimental design studies in which either there is no control group or participants have not been randomly allocated to the treatment or intervention group.

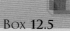

Box 12.5

Quasi-experimental study: the essence of cancer care: the impact of training on nurses' ability to communicate effectively (Wilkinson et al 2002)

A good example of such a study is that of Wilkinson et al (2002), who conducted a quasi-experimental study to evaluate the effectiveness of a communication skills training programme delivered to cancer and palliative care nurses. In this study it was hypothesised that a statistically significant improvement between pre- and postintervention scores would be observed.

The findings supported the positive effect of communication skills training on the participants' ability to communicate with patients, particularly in situations that were emotionally charged.

SAMPLING

Careful consideration is given to selecting participants for quantitative studies as one of the aims of quantitative research is that the results can be generalised to a wider population than the study sample. This means that participants must be representative of the wider population to whom the results will relate. To achieve this a detailed list of inclusion and exclusion criteria is normally drawn up prior to the study commencing.

DATA COLLECTION METHODS IN QUANTITATIVE RESEARCH

There are a number of data collection methods used in quantitative research but the concepts that are being researched must ultimately be able to be quantified in some way. The process of selecting and/or developing a data collection instrument or tool can be a very challenging aspect of the research project. The key principle of data collection in quantitative research is that of measurement to allow comparison between variables and statistical analysis. Polit & Hungler (1995) categorise data collection methods into three broad categories: self-reports, observation and biophysiological measurement.

Self-reports

If we are to investigate what people think, feel or believe the easiest and most reliable way of doing this is by asking them directly. Self-reporting is a common method of data collection used in quantitative research. Varieties of self-report include questionnaires, rating scales and attitude scales. Demographic data can also be gathered in this way and can be coded to allow for quantification.

There are many tools that have been designed for assessing the distress and quality of life of people with different illnesses. However it is important, when choosing a tool, that it meets the criteria of being valid, reliable, sensitive to changes over time and appropriate for the purpose for which it is being used (Box 12.6).

There is a plethora of measurement tools available but not all will meet the criteria set out in Box 12.6. Therefore, selection of a tool for research purposes needs careful consideration. Table 12.2 presents some of the more common tools used in palliative care research.

Observation

Both quantitative and qualitative researchers may use observation; however, the way observation is conducted differs. Quantitative researchers conduct observation in a structured manner. For example they may observe interaction between patients and health-care professionals and have predetermined categories that help to break down the phenomena under study. This differs greatly from the qualitative approach to observation, where it is likely that extensive field notes will be written following observation.

Box 12.6

Criteria for measurement tools

Validity – is the term used to describe whether the tool measures what it is intended to measure (Polit & Hungler 1995). For example, a valid depression measurement tool, for palliative care, needs to differentiate between normal sadness and grief associated with dying and clinically significant depression.

Reliability – is the term used to describe whether the tool consistently measures the same concept, when applied in different settings by different people. One would expect a reliable tool to yield the same results when measuring the same concept at different times (test–retest reliability) and when employed by different users (interrater reliability).

Sensitivity – is concerned with the ability of the measurement tool to detect clinically significant changes over a period of time. Visual analogue scales are considered to be the most sensitive scales, while simple verbal descriptive scales are usually less sensitive.

Appropriateness – is concerned with the ability of the measure to be used in the intended setting. Is it short enough for ill patients to complete? If it was designed in a different country, is it culturally appropriate?

Table 12.2

Evaluation tools to support palliative care practice

Name and author	Areas measured	Comments
Symptom distress scales		
Rotterdam symptom checklist (De Haes et al 1990)	34 symptoms, including physical and psychological problems. Each problem assessed on a Likert scale	The scale was developed in patients with different stages of cancer, either disease-free or undergoing chemotherapy. There is evidence of validity and reliability but its length makes it inappropriate for use with those who are very ill
Edmonton symptom assessment system (Bruera et al 1991)	Nine physical and psychological symptoms measured on visual analogue scales	The scale was developed for use in hospices but may equally be of value in a hospital setting. It is designed so that the scores are 'charted', making the tool a good ongoing clinical assessment and audit tool. Evidence of validity and reliability is limited to the North American population

Continued

Table 12.2—Cont'd

Name and author	Areas measured	Comments
Symptom distress scale (Holmes 1989)	Ten physical and psychological symptoms measured on a numerical scale	This tool was developed from McCorkle & Young's (1978) tool in the USA. It has been extensively used in the UK and is the most commonly used scale in cancer research nursing. Although simple to use, very ill patients may find it difficult
Wisconsin brief pain inventory (Daut et al 1983)	Measures pain and its impact on the psychological and social wellbeing of the patient on 12 scales. Items are measured on a 0–10 scale	This tool is particularly useful in palliative care as it considers pain as a multifaceted concept. It is well validated in patients with chronic pain. An abbreviated version has been used to study the incidence of pain in patients with cancer in different settings in Scotland (J Welsh, personal communication)
Hospital Anxiety and Depression Scale (HADS) (Zigmund & Snaith 1983)	Two subscales, consisting of 14 items, measuring anxiety and depression	Designed for use in patients with a physical illness. Easy and quick for patients to complete. Its use has been validated in the palliative care setting (Le Fevre et al 1999)
Quality of life (QOL) tools Spitzer quality of life index (Spitzer et al 1981)	Measures five domains of QOL: physical activity, daily living, perception of own health, support from family and friends and outlook on life. Within each area there are three statements, which are scored 0, 1 or 2	Developed as a brief and simple measurement of QOL. Shown to be valid and reliable in oncology patients. However, there is little evidence of testing in patients with advanced cancer. Designed to be completed 'by proxy' by the patient's physician, and therefore the validity of the results may be questionable
The functional living index (cancer) (FLIC) (Schipper et al 1984)	22 items covering physical, functional, psychological and social areas. Each question is measured on a seven-point numerical scale	Although quite long, patients can complete it in 10 minutes. It was tested on ambulatory oncology patients but has since been widely validated for use within palliative care settings

TABLE 12.2—CONT'D

Name and author	Areas measured	Comments
European organisation for research and treatment of cancer – QLQ-C30 (EORTC QLQ-C30) (Aaronson et al 1993)	30 questions and a global QOL core covering the physical, functional, psychological and social domains of QOL. Also has a number of tumour-specific modules developed to be used in conjunction with the core questionnaire	Internationally tested, demonstrating good validity and reliability among cancer patients with early and advanced stages of disease. It is sensitive to changes in QOL over time. Its length may make it difficult for some patients to complete
Global QOL Score	May be administered as a single visual analogue score or a numerical scale (as found in the EORTC QLQ-C30)	Most patients could rate their QOL on a single scale. Donnelly & Walsh (1996) report that this is the QOL assessment tool of choice for seriously ill patients. A major disadvantage is that it does not give information on what component of QOL, e.g. physical or social, is good or poor
Specific palliative care evaluation tools		
Support team assessment tool (STAS) (Higginson 1993)	17 items assessing areas of importance to patients with palliative care needs, including: communication, planning family affairs and home support	Designed for use by community specialist palliative care services. Widely used and well validated. It relies on being completed by the professional and is therefore only as valid as the person who is able to make accurate judgements on behalf of the patient. Also limited on the assessment of the patient's symptoms
Patient-evaluated problem score (PEPS) (Rathbone et al 1994)	Patients are asked to list problems 'impairing their quality of life – whether physical, emotional, social, or spiritual'. These problems are then rated by the patients, as mild, moderate or severe	This is a patient-centred approach (rather than a tool) for evaluating patient problems, which, when combined with, for instance, a global QOL score, provides a useful clinical assessment and audit tool. Can be used on first assessment visits and repeated, e.g. at weekly intervals, to provide information on effectiveness in helping patient problems. Little information is available regarding the validity and reliability of this approach

Continued

TABLE 12.2—CONT'D

Name and author	Areas measured	Comments
Palliative care assessment tool (PACA) (Ellershaw et al 1995)	Measures symptom control (eight core symptoms plus patient-reported symptoms), patients' and relatives' insight, and facilitation of patient placement	Specifically designed to assess the impact of hospital palliative care teams, in the areas measured, over a time period. Initial tests of reliability are good but more evidence of validity is required to be confident of its usefulness
Palliative care outcome scale (POS) (Hearn & Higginson 1999)	The POS consists of two almost identical measures, one of which is completed by staff, the other by patients. Agreement between staff and patient ratings was found to be acceptable	Developed as an outcome measure for patients with advanced cancer and their families, which would cover more than either physical symptoms or QOL-related questions. Validated for use in a variety of palliative care settings, including inpatient care, outpatient care, day care, home care and primary care. The questionnaire takes approximately 10 minutes to complete by staff or patients. Has acceptable validity and reliability. Can be used to assess palliative care prospectively for patients with advanced cancer

Biophysiological measurement

This term covers the data collection methods associated with quantitative research that collect numerical data through measurement. For example a study researching cachectic patients' response to nutritional supplements would be likely to include measurement of the patient's weight, and possibly determination of body muscle mass. When using instruments of measurement, reliability is of great importance to ensure that confidence can be upheld.

DATA ANALYSIS IN QUANTITATIVE RESEARCH

Data analysis in quantitative research takes place once all the data have been collected. If quantitative research is concerned with measurement then it follows that the data collected will be numerical. However Parahoo (1997) suggest that not all phenomena under study can be measured with the same degree of precision, as some phenomena cannot be easily transformed into numbers. For example, temperature can readily be measured but perception of quality of life is not so easily defined. Numerical data can therefore be classified in four levels. Like the levels of evidence, the levels of measurement of numerical data are ranked hierarchically (Parahoo 1997).

Nominal-level data

This level of data is ranked lowest on the hierarchy as it pertains to phenomena that cannot be measured against each other. Such data are usually collected for descriptive purposes only. Examples of this level of data include gender and marital status. Such factors are assigned a numerical code for identification purposes.

Ordinal-level data

This level of data is produced by ordering or ranking numbers, for example on a satisfaction scale:

Very satisfied	1
Satisfied	2
Unsatisfied	3
Very unsatisfied	4

Here the numbers signify the ranking of the phenomenon but the scale is not specific in that the difference between being satisfied and unsatisfied is not absolute.

Interval-level data

In contrast to the ordinal-level data, interval-level data are precise, as the difference between the numbers is specific. However there is no absolute zero in this level of measurement. For example a thermometer measuring temperature measures the precise temperature and the difference between two temperatures is specific, but 0° does not mean no temperature.

Ratio-level data

This level of data has an absolute zero point. Examples might be income, number of drugs taken or a measurement on a ruler.

STATISTICAL ANALYSIS

Statistical analysis is a process whereby a large amount of numerical data can be handled in an objective and unbiased way. The use of statistics allows the presentation of a set of data allowing the main characteristics of the study to be identified, allows summarisation of the main features and helps to identify any relationships between variables. While it is beyond the scope of this chapter to discuss statistical analysis in great depth, a brief summary is provided. For a more detailed description of this subject consultation of a specialist statistical text book such as *Statistics at Square One* (Swinscow & Campbell 2002) is recommended.

There are two types of statistics, descriptive and inferential. Descriptive statistical analysis is used mainly in descriptive research studies where the purpose of the study is to summarise the frequency of a particular characteristic or variable. For example, Linklater et al (2002) used descriptive statistics to report that 72% of the respondents in their survey believed that the frequency of anaesthetic consultations for patients with complex cancer pain was adequate. However descriptive statistics may also be used in correlational or experimental studies as descriptive information to provide some background information before more sophisticated statistical techniques are used.

Inferential statistics are used to demonstrate the relationship between variables. For example, Wilkinson et al (2002) used inferential statistical analysis to demonstrate the link between communication skills training and improved skills in communicating effectively.

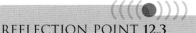

REFLECTION POINT 12.3

Quantitative research

Using an area of palliative care practice that you are familiar with, consider the strengths and weaknesses of quantitative methods as a research approach.

SUMMARY OF QUANTITATIVE RESEARCH

This section has discussed the different types of quantitative research and explored some of the data collection and analysis methods. Quantitative research is a valuable research methodology in palliative care and contributes to providing evidence for practice. There are several limitations of this type of research, the most notable being that not all phenomena lend themselves to measurement and quantification. This is where qualitative methods may be more appropriate.

THE ROLE OF QUALITATIVE RESEARCH IN THE EVALUATION OF PALLIATIVE CARE NURSING

Qualitative research plays an important part in providing evidence for practice in nursing and is gaining greater acceptance within medicine. Qualitative research is particularly suited to palliative care as both qualitative research and palliative care acknowledge the importance of the perspectives of the individuals involved and holism is viewed as an underpinning principle. Qualitative research is based on the belief that it is important to explore an individual's experiences within the context in which these experiences occur. There is more to 'knowing' than what can be seen or measured – knowing involves making settings, human actions and experiences comprehensible.

Qualitative research, as a set of interpretative practices, utilises many approaches, including phenomenology, grounded theory and ethnography. These research approaches all have potential to provide important insights and knowledge for palliative nursing care (Denzin & Lincoln 1994). These approaches share certain features, including the centrality of the subjective experience and the multiple realities that can exist within any phenomenon. Each has different traditions and philosophies and an overview of each approach follows, alongside an example of how these approaches have been used in palliative care research.

GROUNDED THEORY

Grounded theory was developed during an important period of growth in social research in the 1960s and 1970s and is often cited in research literature as the dominant framework underpinning many qualitative studies. Atkinson (1995) states that grounded theory is not a philosophical position or a theory in itself. Grounded theory has its roots in certain sociological theories and the theoretical framework is derived from symbolic interactionism. Symbolic interactionism focuses on the symbolic meanings that people attribute to events and transactions in their lives, and on the ways people interact within their social roles (Glaser & Strauss 1967, Holloway & Wheeler 1996).

Grounded theory begins with an area of study and what is relevant to that area is allowed to emerge; therefore, the research does not begin with a hypothesis to test (Box 12.7). The essence of grounded theory is that the concepts and theory that emerge are inductively derived from the phenomenon investigated. The theory is therefore grounded in the data. The research process involves formulation, testing and redevelopment of propositions until a theory develops. Central to the grounded theory approach are the principles of data saturation and theoretical sampling (Kubler-Ross 1970, Strauss & Corbin 1990) with data gathering and analysis occurring concurrently.

PHENOMENOLOGY

Phenomenology is variously interpreted as a philosophy and a research approach that focuses on the meaning of the 'lived experience' for the individual with the purpose of promoting human understanding (Cohen 1987, Morse & Field 1996). The researcher asks the question 'What is it like to have a certain experience?' It is a requisite of phenomenology that the researcher comes to the study with few preconceived notions, expectations or frameworks (Omery 1983), although the extent to which this is possible is arguable. The goal in the phenomenological method is to provide an accurate description of the phenomenon being studied (Box 12.8), unlike grounded theory, where the goal is to develop theory (Morse & Field 1996).

Box 12.7

Grounded theory: *On Death and Dying* (Kubler-Ross 1970)

The seminal work of Kubler-Ross adopted a grounded theory approach to explore the experiences of very sick and dying patients. Her 1970 work was based on interviews, which formed part of a seminar, with 200 dying patients.

Originally the researchers, who included students, encountered difficulties in accessing patients, as colleagues were resistant to 'interference'. The patients themselves, however, were relieved to share their stories and in-depth interviews were conducted. The interviews were conducted with students present and an audience behind a screen. The interviews were followed by discussions among the research team and the seminar audience. This allowed the researchers to identify emerging concepts grounded in the data as the study progressed.

Analysis of this large database revealed five coping mechanisms used by dying patients at the time of a terminal illness: denial and isolation, anger, bargaining, depression and acceptance.

Kubler-Ross's work has been influential in palliative care and has made a major contribution to helping us understand the experiences of patients who are very ill and dying.

Box 12.8

Phenomenology: 'The experience of dysphagia and its effect on the quality of life of patients with oesophageal cancer' (Watt & Whyte 2003)

Watt & Whyte (2003) used a phenomenological approach combined with the use of a validated quality of life questionnaire to explore the experience of dysphagia in patients with oesophageal cancer and how this impacted on their quality of life. As the aim of the study was to add to the knowledge and comprehension of this poorly understood symptom, the authors argue that phenomenology was an appropriate choice of method.

Using purposeful sampling, 11 patients with advanced oesophageal cancer were identified as being suitable for inclusion in the study. However, because of the progression of their illness, five participants were unable to take part, which is a commonly reported problem in palliative care research.

Although drawn from a small sample, the findings provide insight into the physical, emotional and social impact of this symptom on the patient's quality of life. Acknowledging the limitations of the study, the authors concluded that a much larger qualitative, multicentre study was required to provide a comprehensive picture of the phenomenon. They contend that the strength of this study is that it provides some insight into an area where little work has been undertaken.

ETHNOGRAPHY

Ethnography represents the third major branch of qualitative research. Ethnography has a long history with its roots in anthropology and has been described as the most basic form of social research (Hammersley & Atkinson 1995). The overall aim of ethnography is to make one culture understandable to another and may be considered to be a generalised approach to developing concepts and to understanding human behaviours from the insider's point of view (Morse & Field 1996).

Leininger (1985) defines ethnography as a systematic process that includes observing, detailing, describing, documenting and analysing what is going on in a specific situation in order to explain the culture of specific groups of people. Hammersley & Atkinson (1995) interpret ethnography in a more flexible way by viewing it as a set of methods involving the researcher participating in people's lives for a period of time and collecting data to explain the topic under study.

Ethnographic studies are conducted in the natural setting where the phenomenon under investigation actually occurs and normally involve an eclectic research style, resulting in an extensive account of the phenomenon being studied (Box 12.9). Ethnographic studies normally employ multiple methods of data collection, including participant observation, interviews and field-notes.

Box 12.9

Ethnography: 'Contemporary hospice care: the sequestration of the unbounded body and "dirty dying"' (Lawton 1998)

Lawton's ethnographic study was an exploration of inpatient hospice care. The study was conducted in a context where home care was viewed as the most appropriate form of care for dying patients and prioritising hospice care was a social and economic reality. Lawton worked alongside nursing and volunteer staff for a period of 10 months in the role of participant observer. She was therefore 'immersed' in the context in which the study was being conducted and was able to make sustained and repeated observations on patients, families and staff in all areas of the hospice.

Lawton's findings are challenging for specialist palliative care because she concludes that many patients are admitted to hospices because of the way the disease affects the physical 'boundedness' of the body through deformation and decay. She cites examples of patients who develop faecal fistulas, facial and fungating tumours, persistent and uncontrolled incontinence and vomiting. As such, the findings challenge the philosophy of specialist palliative care, which professes to accord equal importance to psychosocial aspects of care.

DATA COLLECTION METHODS IN QUALITATIVE RESEARCH

Data in qualitative research are words/textual and the following are the main research data collection methods associated with it.

Participant observation

Participant observation is one of the main methods of data collection in ethnographic research. In nursing, possible sites for nurse observers are endless and vary on a continuum from open (public) to closed (private) settings. The role undertaken by the researcher may range from complete observer through the participant as observer and the observer as participant to the complete participant (Gold 1958). While the roles of complete participant or complete observer are relatively clear, the distinctions between participant as observer and observer as participant are less clear. Field notes of the observations would normally be recorded (Kennedy 1999).

Qualitative interviewing

The qualitative interview has been described as: 'an interview whose purpose is to gather descriptions of the life-world of the interviewee with respect to interpretation of the meaning of the described phenomena. Technically the qualitative research-interview is "semi-structured" it is neither a free flow conversation nor a highly structured questionnaire' (Kvale 1983).

There are three main approaches to qualitative interviewing. The informal conversational interview is almost entirely participant-led and often occurs in participant observation. The second approach involves the compilation of a general interview guide, which outlines the issues to be addressed with each individual. The third and most structured approach, the standardised open-ended interview, consists of a set of predetermined questions and can be used to minimise variation and bias. Within each of these approaches it is essential that interviewees can respond in their own way (Bryman 2001, Patton 1980). Qualitative interviews are normally taped and then transcribed word for word, constituting the materials for subsequent analysis and interpretation.

Focus groups

An interview using predominantly open questions may be conducted to ask a group of participants questions about a specific situation or event relevant to them and of interest to the researcher.

Documents/text sources

Documents can provide useful data and these include personal documents in written forms (diaries, letters) and visual form (photographs) and also autobiographies and media materials.

DATA ANALYSIS IN QUALITATIVE RESEARCH

Once data are collected they need to be analysed. Qualitative research is normally, although not exclusively, exploratory and inductive. This means that the purpose of analysis in qualitative research is to produce a coherent and inclusive account of the phenomenon under study, resulting in rich description. Normally, the analysis aims to identify and construct themes that arise from the data.

Qualitative research does not always remain at the level of descriptive account and may result in typologies and theoretical models being developed. Davies & Oberle (1990) developed a model of supportive care in palliative care that comprises six interwoven but discrete dimensions: valuing, connecting, empowering, doing for, finding meaning and preserving own integrity. In seeking to describe the clinical component of the nurse's role in supportive or palliative care, the researchers gathered data based on one nurse's experience of caring for ten cases. The researchers suggest that the concept of supportive care is complex and that the model provides a framework for understanding the role of the nurse and provides a theoretical framework for further research in the area.

Data analysis in qualitative research commences at the very early stages of the research and continues throughout to the production of the final report. Dey (1993) describes qualitative analysis as a circular process that involves describing, classifying and connecting data. Developing thorough and broad descriptions of the phenomenon under study is the first step in qualitative analysis. This step starts with open coding, which is the process of breaking down, examining, comparing, conceptualising and categorising data (Bryman 2001, Strauss 1987, Strauss & Corbin 1990).

The next stage is to identify the concepts that facilitate understanding of the data, and the development of analytical categories evolves with this process. Once categories have been created the next stage is to organise the data around the categories generated. Tesch (1990) calls this 'recontextualisation' of the data as it allows the connections between categories to be explored and provides new insights and understanding of the phenomenon under study.

For example, one of the aims of McIntyre's (1996) study was to explore the needs of relatives of cancer patients who were dying in acute hospital wards. Thematic analysis revealed data that could be categorised as 'experiences of hospital care'. Within this category, McIntyre identified several themes, including the fact that relatives' experiences of the ward climate and facilities during their loved one's illness did not always match their needs. Similarly, within this category of relatives' experiences there were issues related to initiating contact with staff, as it was not always clear to them who they should approach and when it was appropriate to do so. Furthermore, relatives identified that often their information needs were not met. This example illustrates that under the heading of 'experiences of hospital care' the analytical process identified a wealth and complexity of detail of the lived experiences of the relatives who participated in this study.

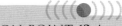

REFLECTION POINT 12.4

Qualitative research

Identify a question from practice which you could address using qualitative methods.

- Why are qualitative methods appropriate for this question?

- What practical issues would you need to consider if you were to carry out this study?

THE CONTRIBUTION OF QUALITATIVE RESEARCH TO PALLIATIVE NURSING CARE PROVISION

The focus of this chapter is to provide you with strategies to ensure that the clinical care you provide is the best possible care option for the circumstances in which it is given. This means that you need to be able to determine what is 'good evidence' on which to base interventions. Qualitative research can contribute to theory development and deepen understanding of what constitutes effective and appropriate care for patients receiving palliative care and their families. Qualitative methods can also help to bridge the gap between the evidence derived from quantitative methods and clinical practice. As such, qualitative methods have much to offer palliative care but should not be seen as a soft option (Clark 1997).

Qualitative research plays an important part in providing evidence for palliative care nursing, as the focus on the individual and holism is a shared philosophy. However, questions exist as to the most appropriate criteria for evaluating qualitative research and, to date, limited systematic evaluation of qualitative research in palliative care has been conducted. Disagreements exist about the standards by which qualitative studies should be assessed and establishing trustworthiness is a source of concern to both those conducting research and those who seek to use it. Some writers suggest that the standards applied to quantitative research of validity and reliability, which are based on clear relationships between the findings and the properties being measured, are applicable to qualitative enquiry. However, qualitative research is based on different assumptions from those of quantitative research and attempts to apply these criteria may amount to self-justification.

Ensuring trustworthiness and rigour in qualitative research should be approached using appropriate criteria such as those identified by Lincoln & Guba (1985): credibility, transferability, dependability and confirmability. A number of actions can be taken to ensure that these criteria can be met. For example, demonstrating that the analysis and interpretation are based on the accounts of the participants can enhance credibility. This involves using in-vivo quotes to support the presentation and discussion of the findings. Similarly, dependability may be illustrated by returning the data and/or findings to the participants in order to obtain their comments and subsequent validation.

For nurses, the ability to evaluate the quality of research available on which to base practice is crucial. However, as there exists an ongoing debate among researchers as to the most appropriate criteria with which to evaluate their work, the problems faced by those seeking to use research findings are apparent. Bailey et al (2002) carried out a systematic evaluation of the nursing contribution to qualitative research in palliative care between 1990 and 1999. The full study evaluated 138 research papers drawn from 50 journals using a tool developed to assess their content and quality. A subset of these data, which included 67 nursing papers together with an analysis of 29 papers from a comparison group of death studies, medical anthropology and sociology journals, was presented in order to explore the strengths and weaknesses in qualitative palliative care research.

There were some positive findings in that nearly 50% of the nursing papers were well written and nearly 33% were judged to enhance understanding or knowledge. However, the reviewers concluded that in nearly 50% of the papers in this sample, which had been published in nursing journals, the relationship between data, analysis and findings was not clearly presented. The authors did, however, caution against using a checklist approach to ensuring rigour and trustworthiness.

Qualitative research demands of the researcher a high level of self-awareness and reflective skills. The sensitive issues surrounding the care of the dying demand that anyone undertaking qualitative research in palliative care needs highly developed interpersonal skills.

ETHICAL ISSUES IN PALLIATIVE CARE RESEARCH

Readers are referred to Chapter 11 for more in-depth coverage of ethical issues in palliative care. Good clinical practice should be based on sound evidence. It is therefore not ethically acceptable to follow tradition or received wisdom without question. However all research involving humans is conducted at some cost to the participants. What must be considered is whether this cost is ethically justified or not. Biomedical ethical principles of beneficence, non-maleficence, justice and autonomy, which are discussed in more detail in the Chapter 11, are the overriding principles that guide researchers.

Following the principle of beneficence researchers must ask themselves: 'Will this research do good?' Sometimes the answer is quite simple, as the participants are indeed expected to gain from participating in the study. However more often the answer is not clear, as the findings may help patients in the future but may not necessarily benefit all the participants in the research study. An example of this would be patients participating in a placebo-controlled RCT. Some patients would be randomised to receive a placebo treatment and would therefore not be expected to gain any therapeutic benefit from participating in the research. This not only presents a dilemma for those asked to participate in the research but also for those involved in conducting the research and for other caregivers supporting participants.

Secondly the principle of non-maleficence may be considered. Those involved may consider whether participation in the study would cause undue harm to the participants. Patients participating in research studies may be exposed to side effects of treatments such as drug therapies. Participants may also be exposed to psychological harm, particularly in research studies that use interviews or questionnaires. Scott et al (2003) suggest that in such studies participants may be exposed to deep probing of personal issues, which may be psychologically damaging if not expertly executed. Therefore it is not only experimental research that requires ethical consideration.

A number of documents have been produced to guide researchers on the ethical aspects of research. The most notable of these is the Declaration of Helsinki, which quotes from the Declaration of Geneva, stating that: 'The health of my patient will be my first consideration' (Randall & Downie 1999, p. 236). In congruence with this guidance, the Nursing and Midwifery Council code of conduct (2002) states that all practitioners must 'act to identify and minimise risk to patients and clients'. Using patients or clients as research participants to explore the effectiveness of therapies or interventions may or may not have detrimental effects as well as desirable effects. The researcher must weigh up whether or not such detrimental effects outweigh the potential benefits, while maintaining that particular patient's best interests.

To achieve this, the ethical aspects of any research study must be carefully examined prior to the research study being conducted. This is usually detailed in the research protocol or proposal. Local research ethics committees (LRECs) now exist to scrutinise the ethical aspects of research projects. All research involving human participants or personal information relating to them requires the approval of the LREC. Therefore it is wise for researchers to make contact with the LREC at an early stage in the project development. There is usually a protocol to be completed and the committees meet at certain times throughout the year, so gaining ethical clearance may take some time.

Cerinus (2001) developed an ethics protocol for her action research study on the introduction of clinical supervision (Box 12.10). The protocol was developed from a principle-based framework and clarifies the rights and responsibilities of both the participant and researcher. The ethics protocol

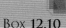

Box 12.10

The ethics of research (Cerinus 2001)

Each participant, in agreeing to participate in the planned study, has the right:

- To withdraw from participation in the research at any time

- To be fully informed of the purpose, design and dissemination of the research

- To control the disclosure of personal information within the data collection process

- Of privacy and security in data collection, storage and handling

- To be confident that data will be destroyed on completion of the study

- Of anonymity in data reporting (or to give explicit consent if anonymity is not possible)

- To expect fairness, accuracy and relevance in data reporting and dissemination

- To benefit, via participation and appropriate acknowledgement, in the research outcome(s).

contributes to research rigour by providing a set of statements that may act as a benchmark against which actions may be judged.

Inherent in this protocol are the ethical issues pertaining to informed consent, autonomy and confidentiality. When researching in palliative care these issues have special relevance.

INFORMED CONSENT

Informed consent assumes that participants are given comprehensive information to help them make an informed choice as to whether or not to participate. The researcher must ensure that participants receive adequate information, understand the information they have been given and are free to consent voluntarily. Randall & Downie (1999) question whether patients in the palliative care setting can ever give consent that is truly voluntary. They argue that patients who are in pain and discomfort, distressed or frightened are more vulnerable and dependent on carers and health-care professionals. They state that patients who do not have a terminal prognosis feel constrained and bound to participate in research and that therefore it is easy to assume that this is compounded in those who are terminally ill. They argue that such patients should be left in peace to share the time they have left with relatives and friends. However the counter-argument to this is that, in the pursuit of more effective treatments that may promote quality of life for such patients,

further research to provide an evidence base for practice is needed and therefore justified.

How much information to give participants to enable them to give informed
consent has also been the focus of some debate. Benton & Cormack (2000)
state that withholding information that might allow patients to make an
informed decision as to whether or not to participate in research studies is
indefensible and that researchers who attempt to do so should not be given
consent to conduct their study. Conversely, some researchers argue that giving too much information may jeopardise the research findings and that withholding some of what is known is warranted on these grounds.

AUTONOMY

Autonomy is closely linked with the individual's right to give informed consent, as information is an important element of autonomous control.
However in palliative care, as with many other health-care settings, many
patients are unable, through being incapacitated, to give consent. The Law
Commission report on mental incapacity (1995, cited in Randall & Downie
1999) states that research on patients who do not have the ability to consent
is illegal and amounts to unlawful battery. However the Declaration of
Helsinki states that 'where physical or mental incapacity makes it impossible
to obtain informed consent, or when the subject is a minor, permission from
the responsible relative replaces that of the subject in accordance with
national legislation' (North Glasgow University Hospitals NHS Trust 2005).
In palliative care Randall & Downie (1999) use the example of artificial
hydration at the end of life to illustrate a situation where patients may not
be able to consent to participation in research but argue that such research is
needed as there has been intense debate among practitioners as to the effectiveness of this treatment. In such cases, research can only be conducted on
patients who are in the last stages of life and as such are unable to consent to
participation.

CONFIDENTIALITY

Throughout the course of a research study the researcher may be privy to confidential information divulged to them by the participants. Such information
should be handled with respect and not divulged outwith the sphere of the
research study. As outlined in the ethical protocol in Box 12.10, the individual's right to confidentiality and anonymity must be upheld.

SUMMARY OF ETHICAL ISSUES RELATING TO RESEARCH

In conclusion, this section has explored the ethical aspects of conducting
research in the palliative care setting. The ethical principles of beneficence,
non-maleficence, justice and autonomy have been discussed in this context.
The importance of developing and adhering to an ethical protocol has also

been stressed as well as the implications for patients participating in palliative care research.

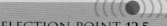

REFLECTION POINT 12.5

Ethical issues relating to research

In relation to palliative care research within your own clinical area, identify the ethical issues that you anticipate might arise in relation to:

- Potential participants

- You as the researcher.

CHANGING PRACTICE

The preceding parts of this chapter have focused on defining levels of evidence and exploring the research approaches used to build the evidence base for palliative care. There are gaps in the available evidence for palliative care nursing practice, so questions remain as to how nurses can act within the bounds of professional accountability and ensure that they are providing clinically excellent care based on best evidence rather than tradition, assumption, personal preference and/or ritual (Walsche & Ford 1995).

Focus on the quality of clinical care is not a new phenomenon in the National Health Service. Assuring quality in the NHS is currently defined in the Clinical Governance Framework (Department of Health 1999a), which ascribes a new 'duty of quality' to health-care providers and envisages a single, coherent, local programme for quality improvement. Clinical governance recognises the importance of teams, organisations and systems rather than individuals working in isolation.

The clinical governance framework combines different strands of quality. These include:

- Audit and feedback
- Clinical effectiveness
- Error reduction
- Risk management
- Evidence-based practice
- Patient involvement
- Lifelong learning.

Nurses need to ensure that they contribute to the clinical governance agenda at local and national levels and the publication of *Making a Difference*

(Department of Health 1999b) reinforces the nursing contribution to quality improvement.

The quest for excellence in the NHS is supported by a number of structures and processes and two examples are given here. A comprehensive list of clinical governance resources can be found in Royal College of Nursing (2003).

THE NATIONAL INSTITUTE FOR CLINICAL EXCELLENCE (NICE)

The National Institute for Clinical Excellence (NICE; www.nice.org.uk) is a special health authority established in 1999 in order to provide clinicians with evidence of best practice and information about the best and most cost-effective treatments. NICE was established as concerns were growing about the costs of new technology and treatments and variations in practices – so-called 'postcode rationing'.

Currently, NICE is producing a series of cancer service guidelines that aim to advise how NHS services should be configured to provide effective services. The guidelines are based on an evaluation of the available evidence and guidelines for those providing supportive and palliative care are currently under construction and consultation. The guidelines for supportive and palliative care encompass the information needs of patients and families, communication, psychological support, specialist and generalist palliative care services, and terminal care. The guidelines were constructed in recognition of a scarcity of evidence for specialist palliative care. They are derived from a systematic review of the available evidence with the level of evidence identified on which a particular guideline is based. For example, in reviewing the impact of a specialist palliative care team, evidence identified by the researchers at level 1A and below supports such teams working with patients at home, in hospitals and hospices as a means of increasing the outcomes for cancer patients in relation to pain and symptom control and overall satisfaction with the care provided.

In day-to-day practice, how then can such evidence be used? It may be used to provide the rationale for the establishment of a specialist palliative care team within a certain area or to support the strengthening of an existing team.

NATIONAL HEALTH SERVICE QUALITY IMPROVEMENT SCOTLAND

National Health Service Quality Improvement Scotland (NHS QIS; www.nhshealthquality.org) was established in Scotland on 1 January 2003 to improve the quality of health care in Scotland. Its function is to set standards, monitor performance and provide advice, guidance and support to NHS Scotland on effective clinical practice and service improvements.

NHS QIS incorporates the Clinical Standards Board for Scotland, the Clinical Research and Audit Group, the Health Technology Board for Scotland, the Nursing and Midwifery Practice Development Unit and the Scottish Health Advisory Service. Links are available through www.nhshealthquality.org.

CLINICAL EFFECTIVENESS

Clinical effectiveness is an important aspect of clinical governance and has been defined as 'the extent to which specific clinical interventions when deployed in the field for a particular patient or population do what they are intended to do, that is, maintain and improve health and secure the greatest possible health gain from the available resources' (NHS Executive 1996).

Clearly, nurses have a responsibility to ensure that they keep up to date with available evidence for practice; however, they need to evaluate the evidence before initiating any changes in practice. Similarly, if change is implemented then this must be evaluated. Change is therefore a dynamic process, which operates on a cyclical basis of obtaining, implementing and evaluating the evidence. Movement between these steps is cyclical and multidirectional.

Introducing change in clinical practice is notably difficult and requires strong leadership and probably additional resources. The next section will consider the implementation and evaluation of evidence-based practice.

EVIDENCE-BASED PRACTICE

Transferring research-based knowledge into clinical practice involves a complex change process. The utilisation of research in practice has long been acknowledged as important for improving patient outcomes, providing 'value' for money and also increasing job satisfaction for professionals. Furthermore, professional accountability and quality of care are recognised as important aspects of clinical care provision.

Research utilisation equates with evidence-based practice, which seeks to provide clinically effective care. Clinical effectiveness is linked to quality assurance so the issues involved in research utilisation are complex and multifaceted.

Evidence-based practice aims to incorporate the systematic, explicit and judicious use of best available research evidence to inform patient care. Earlier in this chapter we explored the hierarchy of evidence that seeks to classify the quality, validity and reliability of research evidence. The purpose of working with such a classification is to increase the transparency of clinical decision-making by identifying whether decisions are based on best scientific evidence, expert opinion and/or anecdotal evidence.

So, in relation to day-to-day work, how does the practising nurse incorporate research findings into clinical care? Responsibility for ensuring that practice is evidence-based carries responsibility for decision-making at individual, group and organisation levels.

Evidence-based practice involves:

• Identification of the practice problem
• Identification of research knowledge related to the problem
• Critical appraisal of the evidence

- Transfer of knowledge into clinical decisions and actions
- Evaluation of the effects of decisions and subsequent actions (Fig. 12.1).

DEVELOPING CLINICAL GUIDELINES

Clinical guidelines are one method by which evidence-based practice may be implemented. The processes involved in developing guidelines reflect the evidence-based practice (EBP) process. As many clinical guidelines are available, it is likely that local guidelines will be developed from these and a plan for local implementation agreed and implemented.

Identification of the practice problem

In many respects this should be the easiest step of the EBP process, although if ritual and routine is the basis of practice within a clinical area then people may fear and be resistant to change. Identification of an area worthy of exploration may result from a range of sources, including audit, research, critical incident reviews, identified clinical risks or following complaints.

Identifying and agreeing a problem should engage all those involved and in palliative care will often require a multiprofessional approach to change. Achieving consensus will require frank and honest discussion and identification of the issues that are driving the need for change and those that are likely to restrict the successfulness of change.

For example, pain can be controlled in the majority of patients; despite this, evidence exists to demonstrate that a significant number of patients experience unacceptable levels of pain. Assessment is the process that aims to provide the nurse with an accurate picture of the patient's condition. Evidence suggests that nurses do not assess pain well and that a number of factors contribute to this, such as patients not being asked about their pain, patients' reluctance to report pain, poor documentation and underuse of pain measurement tools (McCaffery & Ferrell 1997, SIGN 2000).

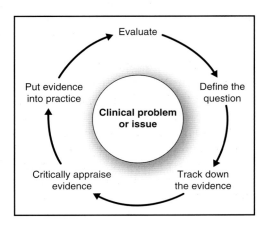

Figure 12.1 Evidence-based practice

So an area worthy of attention may be to develop guidelines for pain assessment. Guidelines should be evidence-based and provide summaries of knowledge that can be used for reference by practitioners. Guidelines can also provide standards for clinical audit. The most important reason for developing guidelines is to improve patient care. Changes in clinical behaviour will only happen if the process of development is systematic and those involved experience ownership.

Identification of research knowledge related to the problem

Once the problem has been identified the next stage of the process is to find the right evidence and knowing where to look and how to search for evidence is a skill required by all nurses.

The main library databases include MEDLINE, CINAHL, Cancerlit and PsychInfo, although there are others. The Cochrane Collaboration publishes a database of systematic reviews and can be accessed at www.cochrane.co.uk. Decisions need to be made about the depth and scope of the search and most search facilities allow you to predetermine aspects of your search, including the time span and design of studies you wish to retrieve.

Critical appraisal of the evidence

Critiquing research is a process of critical reading and thinking in order to assess the scientific merit of research studies and the validity or trustworthiness of their findings to determine their value for practice or further knowledge development.

Continuing the example of guidelines for pain assessment, guidelines already exist at local and national levels (www.sign.ac.uk). The task of a local group is to review what is available and discuss how the findings and recommendations could be applied in a particular clinical area. The validity of any guidelines should be assessed and the steps are similar to those used for evaluating research.

There are a number of frameworks to use when critiquing research; however most reflect the main stages of the research process (Table 12.3).

In reading a paper it is important for you to decide if all the categories in Table 12.3 have been addressed and to make an overall evaluation as to the reliability of the findings as a basis for changing or advancing clinical practice.

Transfer of knowledge into clinical decisions and actions

Once appropriate evidence has been retrieved and critiqued the next stage is to consider how the findings can be used to inform practice. At this stage, negotiation and discussion among group members to reach consensus are vital. Guidelines should be sent out for as wide consultation as possible as this process is likely to increase feelings of commitment and ownership and increase the success with which the change can be implemented. Education, information and feedback to those who participate are also crucial to the implementation process if newly developed guidelines are not to be cast aside.

TABLE 12.3

Critiquing research reports

The aim of the research	Is the aim clearly stated?
Literature review	Is the literature review comprehensive?
	Is the literature critically evaluated?
	Are gaps in the literature/knowledge base identified?
Data collection methods	Are the data collection methods identified and justified?
	Are sampling details supplied and consistent with aims of study?
Data analysis methods	Are the data analysis processes clearly explained?
	Does the approach to data analysis seem relevant to the aims and scope of the study?
Validity, reliability or trustworthiness	Are the processes used to ensure the credibility, dependability and transferability of the data clearly explained?
Ethical issues	Are the ethical issues identified and addressed?
Results and conclusions	Do the results answer the research questions/aims?
	Are the strengths and limitations of the study identified?
	Are the implications for future research, practice and education identified?

THE ROLE OF CLINICAL AUDIT

One of the ways in which practice can be evaluated is through the use of audit. It has to be remembered that audit is an important process in identifying areas of practice that need to be addressed – so audit can be prospective and/or retrospective to any process of clinical change.

Clinical audit is a well-established method of reviewing clinical practice against agreed standards with the aim of identifying areas for improvement in quality of care. Audit in health care has been defined as: 'A cyclic activity incorporating evaluation of the quality of clinical practice and action taken in response to the results of this evaluation' (Department of Health 1994). Audit is the process by which practice can be systematically monitored and evaluated. A programme of audit is required to monitor the achievement of standards, the implementation and effectiveness of clinical guidelines and integrated care pathways.

The quality assurance process within nursing is not new. Much of the early work focused on the framework for quality assurance proposed by Donabedian (1980). This framework breaks down services into three separate but interrelated components that continue to influence the development of best practice statements and clinical standards.

- **Structure** – the physical and organisational aspects of a service, such as staffing levels or equipment
- **Process** – the manner by which care is delivered
- **Outcome** – what is achieved from the structure and processes of care.

Clinical audit certainly has a place in palliative care and the start of most audit and quality assurance programmes necessitates the identification of a standard. Over recent years there have been significant moves to produce national standards and guidelines that can be used and adapted at a local level. For example the Clinical Standards Board for Scotland (as of 2003, now known as NHS Quality Improvement Scotland) has developed standards for breast cancer, breast screening, colorectal and ovarian cancers and for specialist palliative care. Similarly, programmes of audit at national level are now evolving. This does not diminish the need for audit of local practices. In Scotland NHS QIS has audited implementation of the standards for specialist palliative care (Clinical Standards Board for Scotland 2002) in primary and secondary care providers.

For providers of specialist palliative care these set the standards for service provision and ensuring that they are met is a crucial aspect of clinical governance and effectiveness. These standards are linked to clinical guidelines where available (www.sign.ac.uk) and relate to access to specialist palliative care services, key elements of specialist palliative care, managing people and resources, professional education, interprofessional communication, communication with patients and carers, therapeutic interventions and patient activity.

INTEGRATED CARE PATHWAYS

The most recent developments in quality have been the development of integrated care pathways (ICPs). There has been some resistance towards implementing guidelines and ICPs from practitioners who fear that they may detract from individualised care (Fowell et al 2002). However emerging research is highlighting the positive impact of ICPs on patient care (Jack et al 2003). While guidelines and pathways can inform and guide practice, they cannot provide a blueprint. Fowell et al (2002) assert that it is important to recognise that variances from pathways are to be expected. Auditing such variances from the ICP is important to inform future practice and further development of the pathway.

One way of ensuring clinical guidelines and standards are incorporated into patient care is through the development and implementation of integrated care pathways (ICP). Integrated care pathways are structured multidisciplinary care plans which detail essential steps in the care of patients with a specific clinical problem. They have been proposed as a way of encouraging the translation of national guidelines into local protocols and their subsequent application to clinical practice. They are also a means of improving systematic collection and abstraction of clinical data for audit and of promoting change in practice.

Campbell et al 1998

Care pathways are therefore plans that describe the process of care at different stages of the illness journey, detail the expected processes and standards of care for particular conditions and provide data for audit and research (Box 12.11).

Care pathways are being used and developed in palliative care and their use is a way of ensuring quality improvement and clinical effectiveness. For example, Cringles (2002) reports a project established between primary, secondary and tertiary care settings to establish an integrated care pathway for the management of chronic cancer pain. This project improved communication across care settings and resulted in systematic approaches to the assessment and management of chronic cancer pain through the integration of ICP documentation in a patient-held record.

In palliative care, one of the challenges facing health professionals is that of providing appropriate care for the dying patient in the last hours or days of life – the so called process of 'diagnosing dying'. At this stage of the illness journey, care aims should be refocused and the ICP for the dying patient developed by the Royal Liverpool University Hospitals Trust and the Marie Curie Centre Liverpool (Fig. 12.2) provides a model for care. The ICP has three sections: initial assessment and care, ongoing care and care after death, so it integrates care for the patient and family.

Implementation of this ICP has resulted in measurable outcomes of care and allowed the standards of care within the hospital setting and specialist palliative care unit to be compatible (Ellershaw & Ward 2003). A recent research study

Box 12.11

Advantages of care pathways

- Incorporate guidelines into records, so prompt and remind staff

- Highlight explicit standards to be met – thus facilitating the audit process

- Are multiprofessional, so can improve communication and avoid duplication of documentation

- Can reduce variation in clinical practice

- Can improve standards of documentation

AN EXAMPLE OF PART OF THE LIVERPOOL CARE PATHWAY FOR THE DYING PATIENT USED FOR 4-HOURLY ASSESSMENT IN THE HOSPITAL SETTING (ADAPTED FROM THE LIVERPOOL CARE PATHWAY FOR THE DYING PATIENT — ONGOING CARE Ellershaw et al 2003)

Integrated care pathway for the dying patient

Name: _____

Unit No:_____   Date:_____

Codes (Please enter in columns) A = Achieved V = Variance

Section 2 Patient problem or focus	08:00	12:00	16:00	20:00	24:00	04:00
Assessment pain/comfort measures						
Pain *Goal : Patient is pain free* • Verbalised by patient if conscious • Pain-free on movement • Appears peaceful • Move only for comfort						
Agitation *Goal : Patient is not agitated* • Patient does not display signs of delirium, terminal anguish or restlessness (thrashing, plucking twitching) • Exclude retention of urine as a cause						
Respiratory tract secretions *Goal : Patient's breathing is not made difficult by respiratory tract secretions* • Patient will be breathing comfortably						
Nausea and vomiting *Goal : Patient does not feel nauseous or vomit* • Patient verbalises if conscious						
Other symptoms (e.g. dyspnoea) a) _____						

Figure 12.2 An example of part of the Liverpool Care Pathway for the dying patient used for 4-hourly assessment in the hospital setting (adapted from Ellershaw & Ward 2003).

conducted to assess nurses' perceptions of the Liverpool ICP in the acute hospital setting reported that nurses perceived it to have made a positive impact on the care of dying patients (Jack et al 2003). The participants in the study reported improvements in symptom control, an improvement in anticipatory prescribing, and improvements in communications with relatives. The impact of the ICP on nurses was also found to be positive as nurses felt empowered by their increased confidence and knowledge in caring for dying patients.

The process for developing ICPs reflects that involved in producing clinical guidelines. Time, energy and leadership are essential to the process and ensuring the degree of flexibility required to account for individualised care is challenging. However, rendering the invisible visible is important if practice is to be evidence-based and outcomes of care for patients and families requiring palliative care are to be improved.

CONCLUSIONS

The aim of this chapter has been to provide a framework for practising nurses to explore the basis of their own day-to-day practice and to identify strategies to help render the often 'invisible work' of nurses visible and transparent. The complexities involved in uncovering the knowledge on which practice is, and should be, based are many. However, better educational opportunities and increasing numbers of nurses undertaking graduate and postgraduate study should result in increased competence in appraising and applying evidence to practice. Furthermore, sustained and continued growth in nursing and healthcare research will strengthen the evidence base for practice. Nurses caring for patients and families who require palliative care have a professional responsibility to ensure that they are delivering excellent, effective and appropriate care. Such care can only be achieved if nurses:

- Accept their role in the generation and use of knowledge for palliative care nursing
- Plan and implement changes to palliative care practice on the basis of sound evidence
- Research questions relevant to nursing
- Evaluate the effectiveness of care through research and audit
- Contribute to the research and audit agenda at local, national and international levels.

REFERENCES

Aaronson N K, Ahmedzai S, Bergman B et al 1993 The European organisation for research and treatment of cancer. QLQ-30: a quality of life instrument for use in international clinical trials in oncology. Journal of the National Cancer Institute 85:35–75
Atkinson P 1995 Some perils of paradigms. Qualitative Health Research 5:117–124

Bailey C, Froggatt K, Field D, Krishnasamy M 2002 The nursing contribution to qualitative research in palliative care 1990–1999: a critical evaluation. Journal of Advanced Nursing 40:48–60

Benton D C, Cormack D F S 2000 Gaining access to the research site. In: Cormack D (ed.) The research process in nursing, 4th edn. Blackwell Science, Oxford

Bruera E, Kuehn N, Millar M et al 1991 The Edmonton symptom assessment chart (ESES): a simple method for the assessment of palliative care patients. Journal of Palliative Care 7:6–9

Bryman A 2001 Social research methods. Oxford University Press, New York

Burns R B 2000 Introduction to research, 4th edn. Sage, London

Campbell H, Hotchkiss R, Bradshaw N, Porteous M 1998 Integrated care pathways. British Medical Journal 316:133–137

Carper B 1978 Fundamental patterns of knowing in nursing. Advances in Nursing Science 1:13–23

Carr L T 1994 The strengths and weaknesses of quantitative and qualitative research: what method for nursing? Journal of Advanced Nursing 20:716–721

Cerinus M 2001 The ethics of research. Nurse Researcher 8:72–89

Clark D 1997 What is qualitative research and what can it contribute to palliative care? Palliative Medicine 11:159–166

Clinical Standards Board for Scotland 2002 Clinical standards: specialist palliative care. NHS Quality Improvement Scotland, Edinburgh

Cohen M 1987 A historical overview of the phenomenological movement. Journal of Nurse Scholarship 19:31–34

Copp G, Richardson A, McDaid P, Marshall-Searson D A 1998 A telephone survey of the provision of palliative day care services. Palliative Medicine 12:161–170

Cringles M 2002 Developing an integrated care pathway to manage cancer pain across primary, secondary and tertiary care. International Journal of Palliative Nursing 8:247–255

Daut R L, Cleeland C S, Flanery R C 1983 Development of the Wisconsin brief pain questionnaire to assess pain and other diseases. Pain 17:197–210

Davies B, Oberle K 1990 Dimensions of the supportive role of the nurse in palliative care. Oncology Nursing Forum 17:87–94

De Haes J M, van Knippenberry F C E, Neijt J P 1990 Measuring psychological and physical distress in cancer patients: structure and application of the Rotterdam symptom checklist. British Journal of Cancer 62:1034–1038

Deighan M, Boyd K 1996 Defining evidence-based health care: a health-care learning strategy. NT Research 1:332–339

Denzin N, Lincoln Y (eds) 1994 Handbook of qualitative research. Sage, Newbury Park, CA

Department of Health 1993 Report of the taskforce on the strategy for research in nursing, midwifery and health visiting. Department of Health, London

Department of Health 1994 Clinical audit in nursing and therapy professions. HMSO, London

Department of Health 1996 Promoting clinical effectiveness: a framework for action in and through the NHS. HMSO, London

Department of Health 1998 A first class service: quality in the new NHS. Health Service Circular: HSC(98) 113. DH, London

Department of Health 1999a Clinical governance: quality in the new NHS. NHS Executive, Leeds

Department of Health 1999b Making a difference: strengthening the nursing, midwifery and health visiting contribution to health and healthcare. DH, London

Department of Health and Social Security 1972 Report of the committee on nursing. HMSO, London

Dey I 1993 Qualitative data analysis. Routledge, London

Donabedian A 1980 Explorations in quality assessment and monitoring. Health Administration Press, Ann Arbor, MI

Donnelly S, Walsh D 1996 Quality of life assessment in advanced cancer. Palliative Medicine 10:275–283

Ellershaw J, Ward C 2003 Care of the dying patient: the last hours or days of life. British Medical Journal 326:30–34

Ellershaw J E, Peat S J, Boys L C 1995 Assessing the effectiveness of a hospital palliative care team. Palliative Medicine 9:145–152

Elstein A, Bordage G 1979 Psychology of clinical reasoning. In: Stone G, Cohen F, Alder N (eds) Health psychology. Jossey-Bass, San Francisco, CA

Fowell A, Finlay I, Johnstone R, Minto L 2002 An integrated care pathway for the last two days of life: Wales-wide benchmarking in palliative care. International Journal of Palliative Nursing 8:566–573

Froggatt K A, Poole K, Hoult L 2002 The provision of palliative care in nursing homes and residential care homes: a survey of clinical nurse specialist work. Palliative Medicine 16:481–487

Glaser B, Strauss A 1967 The discovery of grounded theory. Aldine Press, Chicago, IL

Gold R 1958 Roles in sociological field observation. Social Forces 36:217–223

Hammersley M, Atkinson P 1995 Ethnography: principles in practice. Routledge, London

Hearn J, Higginson I J 1999 Development and validation of a core outcome measure for palliative care: the palliative care outcome scale. Quality in Health Care 8:219–227

Hearn J, Feuer D, Higginson I J, Sheldon T 1999 Systematic reviews. Palliative Medicine 13:75–80

Herth K 1990 Fostering hope in terminally ill people. Journal of Advanced Nursing 15:1250–1259

Higginson I 1993 Clinical audit in palliative care. Radcliffe Medical, Oxford

Higginson I J, Finlay I, Goodwin D M et al 2002 Do hospital-based palliative care teams improve care for patients or families at the end of life? Journal of Pain and Symptom Management 23:96–106

Hodgson H 2000 Does reflexology impact on cancer patients' quality of life? Nursing Standard 14(31):33–38

Holloway I, Wheeler S 1996 Qualitative research for nurses. Blackwell Science, Oxford

Holmes S 1989 Use of a modified symptom distress scale in assessment of the cancer patient. International Journal of Nursing Studies 26:69–78

Jack B, Gambles M, Murphy D, Ellershaw J 2003 Nurses' perceptions of the Liverpool Care Pathway for the dying patient in the acute hospital setting. International Journal of Palliative Nursing 9:375–381

Jacobs-Kramer M, Chinn P 1988 Perspectives on knowing: a model of nursing knowledge. Scholarly Inquiry in Nursing Practice 2:129–139

Kennedy C 1998 Ways of knowing in palliative nursing. International Journal of Palliative Nursing 4:240–245

Kennedy C 1999 Participant observation as a research tool in a practice based profession. Nurse Researcher 7:56–65

Kennedy C 2002 The work of district nurses: first assessment visits. Journal of Advanced Nursing 40:710–720

Kubler-Ross E 1970 On death and dying. Tavistock, London

Kvale S 1983 The qualitative research interview: a phenomenological and a hermeneutical mode of understanding. Journal of Phenomenological Psychology 14:171–198

Lawton J 1998 Contemporary hospice care: the sequestration of the unbounded body and 'dirty dying'. Sociology of Health and Illness 20:121–143

Le Fevre P, Devereaux J, Smith S et al 1999 Screening for psychiatric illness in the palliative care inpatient setting: a comparison between the Hospital Anxiety and Depression Scale and the General Health Questionnaire 12. Palliative Medicine 13:399–407

Leininger M M 1985 Qualitative research methods in nursing. Grune & Stratton, New York

Lincoln Y, Guba E 1985 Naturalistic enquiry. Sage, Newbury Park, CA

Linklater G T, Leng M E F, Tiernan E J J et al 2002 Pain management services in palliative care: a national survey. Palliative Medicine 16:435–439

Luker K, Kenrick M 1992 An exploratory study of the sources of influence on the clinical decisions of community nurses. Journal of Advanced Nursing 17:457–466

MacKenzie A 1994 Evaluating ethnography: considerations for analysis. Journal of Advanced Nursing 19:774–781

Macleod M 1996 Practising nursing – becoming experienced. Churchill Livingstone, Edinburgh

McCaffery M, Ferrell B 1997 Nurses' knowledge of pain assessment and management: how much progress have we made? Journal of Pain and Symptom Management 14:175–188

McCorkle R, Young K 1978 Development of a symptom distress scale. Cancer Nursing 1:373–378

McIntyre R 1996 Nursing support for relatives of dying cancer patients in hospital: improving standards by research. Department of Nursing and Community Health, Glasgow Caledonian University, Glasgow

Meerabeau L (ed.) 1995 The nature of practitioner knowledge. Practitioner research in health care. Chapman & Hall, London

Morse J, Field P 1996 Nursing research. The application of qualitative approaches. Chapman & Hall, London

NHS Executive 1996 Achieving effective practice: a clinical effectiveness and research information pack for nurses, midwives and health visitors. NHSE, Leeds

NHS Management Executive 1994 Research and the development in the new NHS: functions and responsibilities. DH, London

North Glasgow University Hospitals NHS Trust 2005 World Medical Association – Declaration of Helsinki. Available on line at: www.ngt.org.uk/research/forms/helsinki.htm

Nursing and Midwifery Council 2002 Code of professional conduct. NMC, London

Omery A 1983 Phenomenology: a method for nursing research. Advances in Nursing Science 5:49–63

Parahoo K 1997 Nursing research: principles, process and issues. Macmillan, Basingstoke

Patton M 1980 Qualitative evaluation and research methods. Sage, Newbury Park, CA

Polit D, Hungler B 1995 Nursing research: principles and methods. J B Lippincott, Philadelphia, PA

Porter S, Carter D E 2000 Common terms and concepts in research. In: Cormack D (ed.) The research process in nursing, 4th edn. Blackwell Science, Oxford

Randall F, Downie R S 1999 Palliative care ethics: a companion for all specialities, 2nd edn. Oxford University Press, Oxford

Rathbone G V, Horsley S, Goacher J 1994 A self evaluated assessment suitable for seriously ill hospice patients. Palliative Medicine 8:29–34

Rolfe G 1998 Expanding nursing knowledge. Butterworth-Heinemann, Oxford

Royal College of Nursing 1996 The RCN clinical effectiveness initiative: a strategic initiative. RCN, London

Royal College of Nursing 2003 Clinical governance: an RCN resource guide. RCN, London. Available on line at: www.rcn.org.uk

Schipper H, Clinch J, McMurray A, Levitt M 1984 Measuring the quality of life of cancer patients: the functional living index – cancer: development and validation. Journal of Clinical Oncology 2:472–483

Scott P A, Valimaki M, Leino-Kilpi H et al 2003 Autonomy, privacy and informed consent 1: concepts and definitions. British Journal of Nursing 12:43–47

Sibbald B, Roland M 1998 Understanding controlled trials: why are randomised controlled trials so important? British Medical Journal 316:201

SIGN/Scottish Cancer Therapy Network 2000 Control of pain in patients with cancer: a national clinical guideline. SIGN Publication Number 44, SIGN/SCTN, Edinburgh

Spitzer W O, Dobson A L, Hall J et al 1981 Measuring the quality of life of cancer patients: a concise Q1 index for use by physicians. Journal of Chronic Disability 34:585–596

Strauss A 1987 Qualitative analysis for social scientists. Cambridge University Press, New York

Strauss A, Corbin J 1990 Basics of qualitative research. Sage, Newbury Park, CA

Swinscow T D V, Campbell M J 2002 Statistics at square one, 10th edn. BMJ Publishing, London

Tesch R 1990 Qualitative analysis: analysis types and software tools. Falmer Press, London

Walsche M, Ford P 1995 Nursing rituals – research and rationale actions. Butterworth-Heinemann, Oxford

Watt E, Whyte M 2003 The experience of dysphagia and its effect on the quality of life of patients with oesophageal cancer. European Journal of Cancer Care 12:183–193

White J 1995 Patterns of knowing: review, critique, and update. Advances in Nursing Science 17:73–86

Wiffen P 1998 Editorial. Evidence-based care at the end of life. Palliative Medicine 12:1–3

Wilkinson S M, Gambles M, Roberts A 2002 The essence of cancer care: the impact of training on nurses' ability to communicate effectively. Journal of Advanced Nursing 40:731–738

Wilson-Barnett J 1998 Evidence for nursing practice – an overview. NT Research 3:12–18

Wright J, Hill P 2003 Clinical governance. Churchill Livingstone, Edinburgh

Zigmund A, Snaith R P 1983 The hospital anxiety and depression scale. Acta Psychiatrica Scandinavica 67:361–370

Journals subscribed to by the Marie Curie Cancer Care Library Service

British Journal of Nursing
British Medical Journal
Cancer Nursing
Cancer Nursing Practice
European Journal of Cancer Care
European Journal of Oncology Nursing
European Journal of Pain
European Journal of Palliative Care
Evidence Based Nursing
Health Service Journal
Hospice Bulletin, *renamed* Hospice Information Bulletin
Hospice Journal
International Journal of Palliative Nursing
Journal of Advanced Nursing
Journal of Pain and Symptom Management
Journal of Palliative Care
Nurse Education Today
Nurse Researcher
Nursing Ethics
Nursing Standard
Nursing Times
Oncology Nurses Today
Oncology Nursing Forum
Pain
Palliative Care Index
Palliative Care Today
Palliative Medicine
Professional Nurse
Progress in Palliative Care

INDEX

Page numbers in *italics* denote figures, tables and boxes; *a* indicates appendix; *passim* refers to numerous scattered mentions within page range.